Biologic Therapies of Immunologic Diseases

Editors

BRADLEY E. CHIPPS
STEPHEN P. PETERS

IMMUNOLOGY AND ALLERGY CLINICS OF NORTH AMERICA

www.immunology.theclinics.com

Consulting Editor
STEPHEN A. TILLES

May 2017 • Volume 37 • Number 2

ELSEVIER

1600 John F. Kennedy Boulevard • Suite 1800 • Philadelphia, Pennsylvania, 19103-2899
http://www.theclinics.com

IMMUNOLOGY AND ALLERGY CLINICS OF NORTH AMERICA Volume 37, Number 2
May 2017 ISSN 0889-8561, ISBN-13: 978-0-323-52842-9

Editor: Jessica McCool
Developmental Editor: Kristen Helm

Immunology and Allergy Clinics of North America (ISSN 0889–8561) is published quarterly by Elsevier Inc., 360 Park Avenue South, New York, NY 10010-1710. Months of issue are February, May, August, and November. Periodicals postage paid at New York, NY and additional mailing offices. Subscription prices are $320.00 per year for US individuals, $528.00 per year for US institutions, $100.00 per year for US students and residents, $395.00 per year for Canadian individuals, $220.00 per year for Canadian students, $670.00 per year for Canadian institutions, $445.00 per year for international individuals, $670.00 per year for international institutions, $220.00 per year for international students. To receive student/resident rate, orders must be accompanied by name of affiliated institution, date of term, and the *signature* of program/residency coordinator on institution letterhead. Orders will be billed at individual rate until proof of status is received. Foreign air speed delivery is included in all *Clinics* subscription prices. All prices are subject to change without notice. **POSTMASTER**: Send address changes to *Immunology and Allergy Clinics of North America,* Elsevier Health Sciences Division, Subscription Customer Service, 3251 Riverport Lane, Maryland Heights, MO 63043. **Customer Service: 1-800-654-2452 (U.S. and Canada); 314-447-8871 (outside U.S. and Canada). Fax: 314-447-8029. E-mail: journalscustomerservice-usa@elsevier.com (for print support); journalsonlinesupport-usa@elsevier.com (for online support).**

Reprints. For copies of 100 or more, of articles in this publication, please contact the Commercial Reprints Department, Elsevier Inc., 360 Park Avenue South, New York, New York 10010-1710. Tel. 212-633-3874, Fax: 212-633-3820, E-mail: reprints@elsevier.com.

Immunology and Allergy Clinics of North America is covered in MEDLINE/PubMed (Index Medicus), Current Contents/Life Sciences, Science Citation Index, ISI/BIOMED, Chemical Abstracts, and EMBASE/Excerpta Medica.

Contributors

CONSULTING EDITOR

STEPHEN A. TILLES, MD
Executive Director, ASTHMA Inc. Clinical Research Center; Partner, Northwest Asthma and Allergy Center; Clinical Professor of Medicine, University of Washington, Seattle, Washington

EDITORS

BRADLEY E. CHIPPS, MD, FAAP, FACAAI, FAAAAI, FCCP
President-Elect, American College of Allergy, Asthma & Immunology, Medical Director, Capital Allergy & Respiratory Disease Center, Sacramento, California

STEPHEN P. PETERS, MD, PHD, FACP, FAAAAI, FCCP, FCPP
Thomas H Davis Chair in Pulmonary Medicine, Chief, Section on Pulmonary, Critical Care, Allergy & Immunologic Diseases, Professor of Internal Medicine, Pediatrics and Translational Science, Associate Director, Center for Genomics and Personalized Medicine Research, Executive Director, Respiratory Service Line, Wake Forest Baptist Health, Wake Forest School of Medicine, Winston-Salem, North Carolina

AUTHORS

DENNIS C. ANG, MD
Associate Professor, Section on Rheumatology and Immunology, Wake Forest Baptist Health, Medical Center, Winston-Salem, North Carolina

DON A. BUKSTEIN, MD
Allergy, Asthma & Sinus Center, Madison, Wisconsin; Allergy, Asthma & Sinus Center, Milwaukee, Wisconsin

WILLIAM J. CALHOUN, MD
Professor and Vice Chair for Research, Division of Allergy and Clinical Immunology, University of Texas Medical Branch, Galveston, Texas

THOMAS B. CASALE, MD
Professor of Medicine and Pediatrics, Division of Allergy and Immunology, Department of Internal Medicine, Morsani College of Medicine, University of South Florida, Tampa, Florida

JONATHAN CORREN, MD
Associate Clinical Professor of Medicine, Department of Medicine, Section of Clinical Immunology and Allergy, David Geffen School of Medicine at UCLA, Los Angeles, California

STEVEN DRAIKIWICZ, MD
Fellow, Division of Allergy and Immunology, New Jersey Medical School, Newark, New Jersey

ANTHONY P. FERNANDEZ, MD, PhD
Staff, Departments of Dermatology and Pathology, Cleveland Clinic Foundation, Cleveland, Ohio

JAMES M. FERNANDEZ, MD, PhD
Associate Staff, Department of Allergy and Clinical Immunology, Respiratory Institute, Cleveland Clinic Foundation, Cleveland, Ohio

ANNE-MARIE IRANI, MD
Professor of Pediatrics, Division of Allergy and Immunology, Children's Hospital of Richmond, Virginia Commonwealth University, Richmond, Virginia

DAVID A. KHAN, MD
Professor, Division of Allergy and Immunology, University of Texas Southwestern Medical Center, Dallas, Texas

SANTHOSH KUMAR, MD
Assistant Professor of Pediatrics, Division of Allergy and Immunology, Children's Hospital of Richmond, Virginia Commonwealth University, Richmond, Virginia

DAVID M. LANG, MD
Professor of Medicine and Chairman, Department of Allergy and Clinical Immunology, Respiratory Institute, Cleveland Clinic Foundation, Cleveland, Ohio

DENNIS K. LEDFORD, MD, FAAAI
Professor of Medicine and Pediatrics, Division of Allergy and Immunology, Department of Internal Medicine, Morsani College of Medicine, James A. Haley VA Hospital, University of South Florida, Tampa, Florida

STELLA E. LEE, MD
Department of Otolaryngology, Head & Neck Surgery, University of Pittsburgh Medical Center, Pittsburgh, Pennsylvania

ALLAN T. LUSKIN, MD
Healthy Airways, Madison, Wisconsin

JENNIFER L. McCRACKEN, MD
Assistant Professor of Medicine, Division of Allergy and Clinical Immunology, University of Texas Medical Branch, Galveston, Texas

ROBERT M. NACLERIO, MD
Section of Otolaryngology, Head & Neck Surgery, The University of Chicago Medical Center, Chicago, Illinois

KARI C. NADEAU, MD, PhD
Department of Medicine, Sean N. Parker Center for Allergy and Asthma Research, Stanford University, Palo Alto, California

JOHN OPPENHEIMER, MD
Clinical Professor of Medicine, Division of Allergy and Immunology, New Jersey Medical School, Newark, New Jersey

IRIS M. OTANI, MD
Department of Medicine, Sean N. Parker Center for Allergy and Asthma Research, Stanford University, Palo Alto, California

SHEENAL V. PATEL, MD
Division of Allergy and Immunology, University of Texas Southwestern Medical Center, Dallas, Texas

BROOKE I. POLK, MD
Division of Allergy, Asthma and Immunology, Children's Mercy Hospital, Kansas City, Missouri

LANNY J. ROSENWASSER, MD
Department of Medicine, University of Missouri Kansas City School of Medicine, Kansas City, Missouri

FARNAZ TABATABAIAN, MD
Assistant Professor of Medicine, Division of Allergy and Immunology, Department of Internal Medicine, Morsani College of Medicine, University of South Florida, Tampa, Florida

JULIA W. TRIPPLE, MD
Assistant Professor of Medicine, Division of Allergy and Clinical Immunology, University of Texas Medical Branch, Galveston, Texas

SWAMY VENUTURUPALLI, MD, FACR
Associate Clinical Professor of Medicine, UCLA, Division of Rheumatology, Cedars Sinai Medical Center, Beverly Hills, Los Angeles, California

BRANT R. WARD, MD, PhD
Assistant Professor of Medicine, Division of Rheumatology, Allergy, and Immunology; Affiliate Assistant Professor of Microbiology and Immunology; Affiliate Assistant Professor of Pediatrics, Division of Allergy and Immunology, Children's Hospital of Richmond, Virginia Commonwealth University, Richmond, Virginia

THOMAS J. WILLSON, MD
Department of Otolaryngology, Head & Neck Surgery, University of Pittsburgh Medical Center, Pittsburgh, Pennsylvania

RACHEL M. WOLFE, MD
Assistant Professor, Section on Rheumatology and Immunology, Wake Forest Baptist Health, Medical Center, Winston-Salem, North Carolina

Contents

Jonathan Corren

> A number of chronic inflammatory diseases are associated with IgE-mediated immunologic hypersensitivity, including atopic dermatitis, chronic rhinosinusitis, and asthma. Pathogenetic studies of well-characterized patient groups has allowed investigators to more precisely define the molecular pathways involved in these diseases. Specific cytokines and chemokines, as well as other unique proteins, have now been identified in each of these common disorders and a number of medications are currently in development for inhibiting their actions. Continual refinement of our understanding of the pathogenesis of these diseases will undoubtedly yield increasingly precise, and potentially more effective, treatments.

Brooke I. Polk and Lanny J. Rosenwasser

> The immune system possesses a vast number of potential targets for therapeutic intervention. Although therapies for many pathways have been pursued, only few have yielded significant success. Hindrances in altering biologic pathways include the potential for unwanted downstream effects, ineffectiveness owing to biological redundancy, recognition of a therapeutic molecule as foreign by the body's innate immune system, and the risks of subsequent malignancy and/or autoimmunity. This article covers currently available biotherapeutic agent classes as well as potential direction for future therapy.

Steven Draikiwicz and John Oppenheimer

> Progress in the understanding of disease processes has provided additional therapeutic targets, best exemplified by the increasing role of biologics in the clinical armamentarium. This article provides a focused review of current treatment paradigms and pathophysiology for asthma, atopic dermatitis, urticaria, as well as C1 inhibitor deficiency. It elucidates the populations in which biologics were studied for the aforementioned

disease states, emphasizing characteristics to consider when selecting therapy. It is important to correctly estimate patient outcome before starting therapy based on cost analysis. Treatment decisions need to be guided by appropriate patient stratification based on each individual's underlying phenotype.

fit this phenotype of disease and have fewer effective therapeutic options. In the clinical setting, total IgE, FeNO and peripheral blood eosinophils are important tools in defining Th2 high patients with asthma. However, precise biomarkers to predict better response to one specific Th2 high asthma therapy versus another is lacking. It is important to recognize that none of the current medications targeting the Th2 pathway induces persistent immunomodulation or remission.

IMMUNOLOGY AND ALLERGY CLINICS OF NORTH AMERICA

THE CLINICS ARE AVAILABLE ONLINE!
Access your subscription at:
www.theclinics.com

Erratum

In the February 2017 issue of *Immunology and Allergy Clinics of North America* (Volume 37, Issue 1), in the article "Infectious Complications in Atopic Dermatitis," the Key Points listed are incorrect. The Key Points have been corrected in the online version and are stated below:

- Infections are a major complication of atopic dermatitis.
- These complications include S. aureus infections, eczema herpeticum, eczema coxsackium and eczema vaccinatum.
- An understanding of the mechanisms of these infections is important for prevention and treatment.
- The article includes clinical pearls for clinicians in the recognition and management of these complications.

Immunol Allergy Clin N Am 37 (2017) xiii
http://dx.doi.org/10.1016/j.iac.2017.02.003
immunology.theclinics.com

Foreword

Biopharmaceuticals in Allergic Disease: Finding the Right Patients at the Right Time

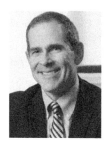

Stephen A. Tilles, MD
Consulting Editor

Since awarding the Nobel Prize to César Milstein and Niels Jerne in 1984 in recognition of their development of the hybridoma technique to produce monoclonal antibodies, the scientific community has buzzed about the idea of applying "designer" techniques to produce magic bullets to cure human diseases. By 2005, there were more than 10 FDA-approved monoclonal antibodies in use for selected diseases, including omalizumab for allergic asthma. In recent years, more diversified targets and techniques have enriched the biologic armamentarium at an astounding rate. For example, in 2015 alone, the FDA approved 13 biological products for various applications. This is innovation at its finest.

Although malignancy and autoimmunity dominated the biological drug development focus early on, we now have multiple biologic therapeutic options for patients with allergic and immunologic diseases, and while is it unclear if any deserve the "magic bullet" label, there is no doubt that thousands of our patients have benefited from these therapies, and many thousands more stand to benefit in the future. In parallel with these amazing advances, there have been both an evolution in patient care toward a "precision medicine" model and an increasingly problematic pharmacoeconomic system when attempting to implement therapeutic choices.

In this issue of *Immunology and Allergy Clinics of North America*, coeditors Bradley E. Chipps and Stephen P. Peters have assembled an impressive array of authors to address important and timely topics, including discussions of the use of biologics for asthma, chronic pulmonary obstructive disease, nasal polyps, atopic dermatitis, eosinophilic esophagitis, and food allergy. There are additional articles focusing on autoimmune disease applications, adverse reactions, individualization of biologic therapy, and pharmacoeconomics. Given the complexities involved with understanding how and when to use these therapies, this *Immunology and Allergy Clinics of North*

Immunol Allergy Clin N Am 37 (2017) xv–xvi
http://dx.doi.org/10.1016/j.iac.2017.02.002
0889-8561/17/© 2017 Published by Elsevier Inc.
immunology.theclinics.com

America issue should serve as an essential reference for all allergy/immunology specialists in practice.

Stephen A. Tilles, MD
ASTHMA Inc. Clinical Research Center
Northwest Asthma and Allergy Center
University of Washington
9725 Third Avenue NE, Suite 500
Seattle, WA 98115, USA

E-mail address:
stilles@nwasthma.com

Preface

Biologic Therapies of Immunologic Diseases

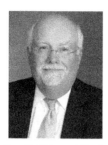 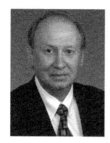

Bradley E. Chipps, MD, FAAP,   Stephen P. Peters, MD, PHD, FACP,
FACAAI, FAAAAI, FCCP   FAAAAI, FCCP, FCPP
Editors

Biologic therapies are revolutionizing our understanding of and the approach to treating diseases across the spectrum of medicine. This issue of *Immunology and Allergy Clinics of North America* focuses on their use in immunologic diseases. We begin with a discussion of the basic science aspects of these intervention strategies and then focus on the disease states that may be appropriately treated with them. We also provide insights in how precision medicine–based therapy may be applied to these patients.

The issue's initial two articles deal with the immunopathogenesis and the implications for treatment of immunologic diseases (Corren) and the biologic therapies for immunologic diseases that set the stage for the strategies for immunologic interventions (Polk and Rosenwasser). We are then able to understand the characteristics of patients who may be treated with these agents and how to provide precision medicine to determine which biologic would be important for each patient (Draikiwicz and Oppenheimer). The biologic therapies for autoimmune connective tissue diseases are discussed in detail (Wolfe and Ang), and special attention is given to the new mechanism of rheumatoid arthritis (Venuturupalli). Other important chronic skin disorders that may be modulated with biologic therapies are discussed (J. Fernandez, A. Fernandez, and Lang). The new biologic therapies for asthma (Tabatabaian, Ledford, and Casale) are very important as this is a rapidly expanding area where new treatment interventions are becoming available each year. This may also be extended to chronic obstructive lung disease, described by Tripple, McCracken, and Calhoun. The upper airway is addressed with the use of monoclonal antibodies for treatment of nasal polyps (Willson, Naclerio, and Lee) and biologic therapies for IgE-mediated food allergy and eosinophilic esophagitis (Otani and Nadeau). All these biologic products may exhibit adverse reactions, and this is discussed in detail by Patel and Kahn. A very important topic concerns the pharmacoeconomics of biologic therapy. All these therapies are quite costly,

Immunol Allergy Clin N Am 37 (2017) xvii–xviii
http://dx.doi.org/10.1016/j.iac.2017.02.001
0889-8561/17/© 2017 Published by Elsevier Inc.

immunology.theclinics.com

and a provocative and insightful discussion is provided by Bukstein and Luskin in this regard. The issue ends with a look to the future for new therapies that will be emerging for the treatment of immunologic disease (Kumar, Ward, and Irani).

This is an exciting time as novel biologic therapies emerge as effective treatment options for many patients with immunologic diseases. But we are only at the beginning of understanding key pathophysiologic mechanisms they highlight as well as specific disease phenotypes for which they will provide effective treatment.

Bradley E. Chipps, MD, FAAP, FACAAI, FAAAAI, FCCP
American College of Allergy
Asthma & Immunology
Capital Allergy & Respiratory Disease Center
5609 J Street, Suite C
Sacramento, CA 95819, USA

Stephen P. Peters, MD, PHD, FACP, FAAAAI, FCCP, FCPP
Section on Pulmonary, Critical Care
Allergy & Immunologic Diseases
Internal Medicine, Pediatrics
and Translational Science
Center for Genomics and
Personalized Medicine Research
Respiratory Service Line
Wake Forest Baptist Health
Wake Forest School of Medicine
Medical Center Boulevard
Winston-Salem, NC 27157, USA

E-mail addresses:
bchipps@capitalallergy.com (B.E. Chipps)
sppeters@wakehealth.edu (S.P. Peters)

Inflammatory Disorders Associated with Allergy

Overview of Immunopathogenesis and Implications for Treatment

Jonathan Corren, MD

KEYWORDS

- Cytokine • Eosinophil • Atopic dermatitis • Chronic rhinosinusitis • Nasal polyp
- Asthma • Monoclonal antibody

KEY POINTS

- Over the past 2 decades, the pathogenesis of chronic inflammatory conditions associated with allergy has been increasingly characterized.
- A large number of T-cell subsets have been identified that appear to play active roles in coordinating the pathologic responses in atopic dermatitis, chronic rhinosinusitis, and asthma.
- With the improved understanding of potential molecular targets in these diseases, it is now possible to provide specific therapies that block relevant cytokines.

INTRODUCTION

Over the past 2 decades, we have witnessed consistent increases in the prevalence of chronic inflammatory diseases that are associated with immunoglobulin (Ig)E-mediated immunologic hypersensitivity. During this same period, there have been major advances in our understanding of the natural history and pathogenesis of these diseases. Innovative use of mouse experiments has helped uncover the presence of new T-cell subtypes and cytokines and the development of relevant knockout models has been essential in characterizing the functionality of these cells and proteins. Subsequent studies in humans have sought to determine the relevance of these cells to specific forms of allergic disease. In addition to these developments, a great deal has been learned about the clinical and pathogenetic heterogeneity of atopic diseases. Large-scale epidemiologic studies have revealed that there are distinct phenotypes that are characterized by differences in both clinical (eg, age of onset, severity

Department of Medicine, Section of Clinical Immunology and Allergy, David Geffen School of Medicine at UCLA, 10780 Santa Monica Boulevard, Suite 280, Los Angeles, CA 90025, USA
E-mail address: jcorren@ucla.edu

Immunol Allergy Clin N Am 37 (2017) 233–246
http://dx.doi.org/10.1016/j.iac.2017.01.001
0889-8561/17/© 2017 Elsevier Inc. All rights reserved.

immunology.theclinics.com

level, medication responsiveness, specific IgE, and eosinophils in body fluids) and molecular (eg, cytokines, chemokines, and protein products) profiles. In this review, the pathogenesis of atopic dermatitis, chronic rhinosinusitis with nasal polyposis, and asthma is considered, with a special emphasis on relevant inflammatory cells and molecules that might ultimately serve as therapeutic targets.

ATOPIC DERMATITIS

Atopic dermatitis (AD) is a chronic inflammatory skin disorder characterized by skin dryness, pruritis, erythema, papule formation, and lichenification. It most often begins in early childhood but occasionally starts during the adult years. It is usually the first of the chronic allergy-associated inflammatory diseases to be expressed. It is associated with elevated serum IgE and often occurs with other atopic diseases, including asthma, rhinitis, and food allergy. There are a number of important factors that contribute to the symptoms of AD, including alterations of the skin barrier, abnormalities in innate immune function, alterations of microbial colonization of skin, and increases in Th2 adaptive immune responses. However, despite the tremendous progress made in the characterization of the pathology and molecular biology of AD, many aspects of its pathogenesis remain poorly understood (**Fig. 1**).

Skin Barrier Function

The main function of the skin is to form a physical barrier against external insults. In patients with AD, there is a significant degree of barrier dysfunction that is central to the disease. Among the causes of altered barrier function, many patients have been

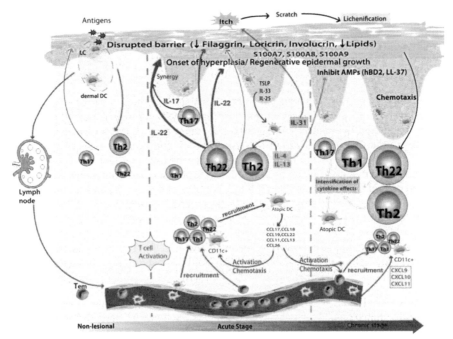

Fig. 1. Immunologic pathways involved in different phases of AD. (*From* Gittler J, Shemer A, Suárez-Farinas M, et al. Progressive activation of T(H)2/T(H) 22 cytokines and selective epidermal proteins characterizes acute and chronic atopic dermatitis. J Allergy Clin Immunol 2012;130:1344–54; with permission.)

identified with a defect in the expression of the filaggrin (FLG) gene.[1] FLG is responsible for cross-linkage of keratin filaments into tight bundles and moisturization of the stratum corneum, both of which are key elements in skin integrity.[1] Studies have demonstrated a strong link between the incidence of AD and loss-of-function variants in the FLG gene[2]; up to 50% of patients with AD carry FLG mutations. In addition, patients with AD have a significant reduction in skin ceramides, which are lipids that contribute to the regulation of water retention in the stratum corneum.[3] Patients with AD have a marked reduction of ceramides in both lesional and nonlesional skin compared with healthy individuals. Finally, there appears to be an overactivation of epidermal proteases in the skin of patients with AD. These defects are induced both by genetic variants as well as direct effects of inflammation on those proteases. This disruption of the skin barrier allows for an enhanced penetration of biologic and chemical agents through the epidermis and dermis and elicitation of immunologic activation which may cause skin inflammation.

Inflammation

Dendritic cells
Dendritic cells (DCs) play an important role in the early events of AD. Once foreign antigens have penetrated through the epidermis, they are taken up by cutaneous DCs (Langerhans cells and infiltrating inflammatory dendritic epidermal cells) and processed for presentation. Following contact with these antigens, the DCs migrate to draining lymph nodes, where they present antigens to naive T cells and then direct T-cell differentiation. During this process, thymic stromal lymphopoietin (TSLP) is released by keratinocytes, which promotes T-helper 2 (Th2) inflammation.

T cells
In the acute lesions of AD, Th2 and Th22 cells have been shown to be the predominant cell types, whereas there are lesser number of Th17 cells.[4] Cytokines produced by Th2 cells (interleukin [IL]-4, IL-13, and IL-31) and Th22 cells (IL-22) have been shown to suppress FLG and loricrin, which are critical to skin integrity[5,6]; however, this effect is observed in acute lesional skin as well as noninvolved skin of patients with AD, implying that these changes are not responsible for disease activity. IL-4 and IL-13 also regulate the class-switching of B-cell production of IgM to IgE, which is a hallmark of AD. In addition, IL-4 alone plays an important role in the maturation of naive T cells to Th2 cells. Th2-derived IL-31 has been shown to induce several chemokine genes that are associated with atopic skin inflammation, such as CCL1, CCL17 (TARC), and CCL22, which promotes ongoing skin inflammation. In addition, IL-31 appears to play a critical role in the induction of pruritus, potentially by directly stimulating nerve receptors in the skin.[7] IL-22 is produced by a unique T-cell subset, and its release is associated with marked activation of an epidermal differentiation complex (EDC) gene cluster, leading to large increases in the expression of EDC S100 proteins and subsequent increases in chemotaxis of T cells, monocytes, and neutrophils.[8] IL-17, secreted from Th17 cells, has been shown to enhance the production of IL-6 and IL-8 from keratinocytes,[9] which induce neutrophil infiltration of skin and modulates fibroblast function.[10] IL-17 also has been shown to positively affect host resistance to cutaneous infections, including cutaneous antimicrobial proteins. Given both the beneficial and deleterious effects of IL-17 in AD, it is unclear what net effect IL-17 has on AD lesions.

As AD lesions enter the chronic phase, IL-13, IL-31, and IL-22 release is intensified, whereas the release of IL-4 is diminished.[4] IL-17 release is present but to a lesser extent than in acute lesions. In addition, there appears to be activation of Th1 cells and their cytokines (eg, interferon gamma), which may be either primarily involved in pathogenesis or might be acting as a counterregulatory mechanism of the Th2 pathway. Overall, these observations suggest that maintenance of chronic AD lesions are associated with a mixed cellular response, most prominently Th2 and Th22 and to a much lesser extent Th1 and Th17.

Innate lymphoid cells

Innate lymphoid cells (ILCs) have recently been shown to play an important role in skin lesions of AD, and this effect may be most important early in the course of the disease before the arrival of antigen-specific Th2 cells. Key features of ILC2 cells include development from a common lymphoid progenitor in response to IL-7 and IL-33; lack of antigen-specific receptors; and dependence on the transcription factors GATA-3 and ROR-alpha. Like Th2 cells, ILC2 cells are a rich source of IL-5 and IL-13, but usually not IL-4. In the lesional skin of patients with AD, ILC2s are highly enriched.[11] Their function is thought to be largely regulated by keratinocyte-derived cytokines, such as IL-25 (IL-17E), IL-33, and TSLP in response to epithelial injury.

Regulatory T cells

Regulatory T cells (Tregs) are another potentially important modulator of skin immune responses. Tregs have been shown to be increased in the peripheral blood[12] but not in the skin lesions of patients with AD.[13] One interesting notion is that Tregs in patients with AD appear to decrease their immunosuppressive activity when they are activated by superantigens from *Staphylococcus aureus*.[14] This observation may contribute to *S aureus*–mediated augmentation of skin inflammation in patients with AD.

Mast cells

Mast cells express the high-affinity IgE receptor (FcεRI) and release a wide variety of proinflammatory mediators on activation. Increased mast cell numbers and activation were reported in the chronic skin lesion of AD.[15] Although they are generally considered effector cells of skin inflammation, immunosuppressive roles of mast cells also have been demonstrated in mouse AD models.

Eosinophils

Although blood and tissue eosinophilia is often observed in patients with AD, the role of eosinophils in the pathogenesis of AD has not been clearly established. During periods of increased symptoms, patients with AD demonstrate increased serum concentrations of IL-5 and eosinophil chemoattractants, such as eotaxin.[16] However, it is not clear that eosinophils are responsible for either the skin lesions or itching characteristic of AD.

Potential Immunologic Treatments

The foregoing discussion indicates that there are a number of molecular targets that are relevant to atopic dermatitis, and the inhibition of which may reduce the symptoms of AD. Clinical trials have demonstrated that antagonism of IL-4 and IL-13 by blocking the alpha subunit of the IL-4 receptor (dupilumab) results in significant reductions in disease activity.[17] It remains to be seen whether isolated inhibition of IL-13 using an anti–IL-13 antibody will have the same degree of benefit. IL-5 blockade, with attendant reductions in blood and tissue eosinophilia, did not consistently affect the signs or symptoms of AD.[18] Other molecules that will be prime candidates for drug intervention include IL-17, IL-22, IL-31, TSLP, IL-25, and IL-33.

CHRONIC RHINOSINUSITIS WITH NASAL POLYPOSIS

Chronic rhinosinusitis (CRS) is a disease with persistent or recurrent symptoms that involves the mucosa of the nose and paranasal sinuses. The presence of nasal polyps (NPs), which represent hyperplastic evaginations of sinus mucosa into the nasal passages and are present in up to one-third of patients with CRS, increases the burden of disease and the likelihood of symptom persistence after therapy. The etiology of CRS is complex and related to an interplay of genetics and environmental exposures, including allergens and microbial species (**Fig. 2**).

Mucociliary Clearance

In healthy nasal and sinus tissue, the epithelium is the body's first line of defense against inhaled noxious substances and is responsible for protecting the upper airway from infiltration by pathogens, such as viruses, bacteria, and fungi, toxic or irritating substances, and potential allergens. Respiratory epithelial cells are interconnected by tight junctions to form a protective physical barrier against these substances. Once in contact with the epithelium, particulate matter is trapped by airway mucus and then removed by movement of the mucociliary blanket. A large list of pathogens has been shown to produce compounds that impair ciliary motion, including

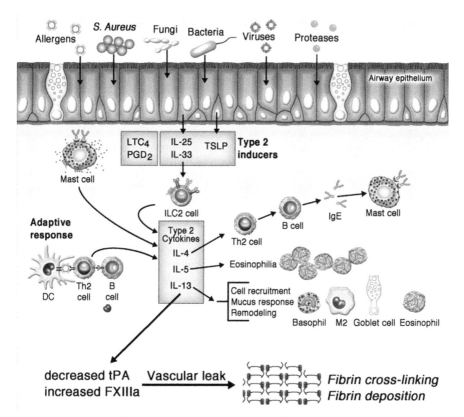

Fig. 2. Role of the host immune response in patients with CRSwNP. (*From* Stevens WW, Lee RJ, Schleimer RP, et al. Chronic rhinosinusitis pathogenesis. J Allergy Clin Immunol 2015;136(6):1448; with permission.)

Haemophilus influenzae, Staphylococcus pneumoniae, S aureus, Aspergillus fumigatus, and *Pseudomonas aeruginosa*[19] Sinus ostial obstruction caused by mucosal swelling or secretions, with subsequent sinus cavity hypoxia, also can reduce mucociliary transport.[20]

Host Defense and Inflammation

Epithelium

In addition to the production and transportation of mucus, the nasal-sinus epithelium produces a large number of antimicrobial compounds, such as lysozyme, lactoferrin, antitrypsin, defensins, *S100 proteins*, and surfactants.[21] Regulation of these substances occurs through Toll-like receptors (TLRs) that recognize microbial pathogen-associated molecular patterns and then stimulate the secretion of defense molecules, within a few hours of contact with microbes. In addition to TLRs, epithelial cells also express taste family type 2 receptor bitter taste receptors.[22] These receptors are able to detect specific molecules secreted by bacteria, which leads to very rapid increases in ciliary movement and generation of defense molecules.[22]

In addition to barrier functions and the elicitation of innate defensive molecules, epithelial cells also can release various inflammatory mediators, most notably TSLP, which acts on dendritic cells to promote the generation of Th2 cells from naive T cells.[23] In addition, TSLP acts to augment the release of type 2 cytokines (IL-4, IL-5, and IL-13) from Th2 cells, as well as innate immune cells, such as ILC2 cells. There is also evidence of IL-25 and IL-33 activity in CRS with NP (CRSwNP) tissue, although much of the data are conflicting.[23] In nasal and sinus mucosa, IL-4 and IL-13 contribute to eosinophilic inflammation (via effects on eotaxins), whereas IL-5 is the key factor that regulates the release of eosinophil progenitors from the bone marrow, eosinophil activation, and eosinophil survival.

Innate lymphoid cells

Other mechanisms of innate immunity appear to be important in chronic sinusitis and NPs. ICS2 have been shown to be increased in NPs. ILC2 cells may be important early in CRSwNP following an initial event that induces epithelial damage. Following epithelial binding and activation, TSLP may be released, leading to activation of ILC2 cells and secretion of IL-5 and IL-13.[24] This local signal from ILC2 cells in the nasal and sinus tissue leads to eosinopoiesis and eosinophil ingress into the upper airway. Large numbers of mast cells and basophils also are present in patients with CRSwNP compared with healthy controls.[25] Eosinophils, mast cells, and basophils have typically been identified in the mucosa of Western patients with CRSwNP but not in individuals of Asian descent.[26] These cell types release a variety of basic proteins (eg, eosinophil cationic protein) and inflammatory mediators (lipid-derived mediators, cytokines, and chemokines) that lead to chronic mucosal injury and may help perpetuate ongoing inflammation. These inflammatory signals have been explored to a much greater extent in asthma, and are discussed at length in a later portion of this article.

T cells and B cells

Once inflammation has been induced, in part due to persistent exposure to an exogenous stimulus, such as a microbe or allergen, the adaptive immune response may come into play. NP tissue has consistently demonstrated increases in CD4+ T cells as compared with healthy nasal and sinus tissue.[27] B cells, including plasma cells, also have been shown to be increased in polyp tissue, along with multiple antibody isotypes, including IgG1, IgG2, IgG3, IgG4, IgA, IgM, and IgE.[28] For the most part, the targeted antigen for these antibodies is not known; however, a small subset of patients with CRSwNP who are colonized with *S aureus* have detectable specific IgE antibodies directed against *S aureus* enterotoxins.[29] Enterotoxins act as superantigens and broadly activate T lymphocytes, potentially increasing the inflammatory infiltrate into the local sinus tissue.

Tissue remodeling

In addition to the inflammation noted previously, NP tissue in CRSwNP shows the formation of pseudocysts and stromal edema but shows none of the fibrosis or basement membrane thickening that is seen in patients with CRS without NPs. The edema appears to be due to vascular leakage with extravasation of plasma proteins through the epithelial barrier. Recent studies have revealed that this phenomenon may, in part, be due to products of the clotting cascade, including fibrin and other factors.[30]

Potential Immunologic Treatments

One small trial of ant-IgE therapy (omalizumab) in patients with CRSwNP and anti–*Staphylococcus aureus* enterotoxin A IgE reported significant improvement in polyp symptoms and size.[31] Abrogation of tissue eosinophils using an anti-IL5 antibody is another plausible approach, and one small trial yielded positive results on polyp reduction in a subset of patients.[32] Most recently, an antibody to the IL-4 receptor alpha chain (dupilumab), blocking both IL-4 and IL-13, demonstrated significant improvement in CRSwNP.[33] Other targets that are currently being considered include TSLP and possibly IL-25 and IL-33.

ASTHMA

Asthma is a chronic airway disease characterized clinically by episodic chest symptoms related to airways obstruction and hyperresponsiveness. For many years, it has been recognized that asthma is a heterogeneous condition, both clinically and pathogenetically. One of the principal paradigms for dividing asthma into phenotypes has been based on the presence or absence of eosinophils. These differences between asthma subtypes will be highlighted in this brief review of asthma pathogenesis (**Fig. 3**).

Inflammation

Epithelial cells

Epithelial cells in the lower airways are largely responsible for mucociliary clearance of inhaled foreign material. As in the nose and sinuses, epithelial cells in the lungs are also capable of binding to inhaled substances via pattern recognition receptors, such as TLRs, leading to activation of the epithelium with subsequent generation of cytokines. TSLP, IL-25, and IL-33 have all been shown to be significantly increased in patients with asthma.[34] Two important functions of these epithelial-derived cytokines include polarization of dendritic cell function, leading to a shift toward Th2 cell development, along with an increase in cytokine release from Th2 cells and other effector cells. In ongoing disease, epithelial cells continue to drive airway inflammation by producing chemokines and cytokines that activate eosinophils, neutrophils, and other cells of the innate immune system.

Th2 cells

Pathologic studies have demonstrated that CD4+ T cells are present in increased numbers in most patients with asthma, along with elevations of the Th2 cytokines IL-4, IL-5, and IL-13.[35] In lung tissue, IL-4 and IL-13 have critical effects on most airway structures, leading to many of the pathologic hallmarks of asthma: eosinophilic inflammation (via effects of eotaxins), increased goblet cell maturation and mucus

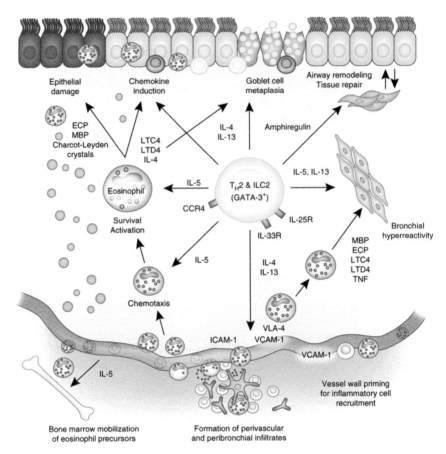

Fig. 3. Overview of functions of Th2 cells and ILC2 cells in asthma. ECP, eosinophil cationic protein; ICAM, intercellular adhesion molecule; VCAM, vascular cell adhesion molecule; VLA, very large antigen. (*From* Lambrecht BN, Hammad H. The immunology of asthma. Nat Immunol 2015;16:46; with permission.)

secretion, enhanced development of fibroblasts, increased collagen synthesis (which is incorporated into the basement membrane), and alterations in bronchial smooth muscle responsiveness to beta-adrenergic agonistis.[36] The most important immunologic effect of both IL-4 and IL-13 is the induction of switching from IgM to IgE production in B cells. IL-4, but not IL-13, also promotes the development of naive T cells into Th2 cells, a potentially important effect that leads to persistent Th2 infiltration of airway tissue.[36]

Th17 cells

Th17 cells represent a separate subset of CD4+ cells that are capable of releasing IL-17 as their principal cytokine product. Development of these cells from naive T-cell precursors is not completely understood, but appears to rely on IL-6, IL-23, and transforming growth factor (TGF)-beta.[37] IL-17 is a key member of the IL-17 family of cytokines (IL-17A, IL-17B, IL-17C, IL-17D, IL-17E [IL-25], and IL-17F). The primary identified function of IL-17A is to promote inflammation through induction of macrophage and neutrophil chemokines and growth factors including CXCL1, CXCL2 (macrophage inflammatory protein-2), CXCL5, CXCL8 (IL-8), CXCL9, CXCL10, CCL-2 (monocyte chemoattractant protein [MCP-1]), granulocyte colony-stimulating factor (CSF), and granulocyte macrophage CSF (GM-CSF).[38] There is growing evidence that Th17 cells and IL-17 are involved in human asthma. IL-17 A[+] cells along with IL-17 and other Th17 cytokines increase in the blood of individuals with asthma and appear to be correlated with the degree of severity of asthma.[39] In addition, both IL-17A and IL-8 mRNAs have been shown to be significantly increased in sputum of individuals with asthma compared with controls, and sputum IL-17A and IL-8 mRNA are more likely to be elevated in patients with more severe asthma.[40] More recently, increased numbers of IL-17A[+]CD4[+] cells have been shown to be present in the tissue of individuals with asthma.[41] Although initial hypotheses predicted that the presence of Th17 cells would be associated with increased airway neutrophils, a recent investigation demonstrated that patients with elevated numbers of Th17 cells also have elevated numbers of airway eosinophils and there were no correlations between markers of a Th17 molecular phenotype and blood, sputum, or airway tissue neutrophils.[42] It may be that the activity of airway neutrophils may be more relevant to asthma severity than their number.

Th9 cells
Th9 cells have been identified as a distinct helper T-cell subset that produces IL-9, IL-10, and IL-21.[43] IL-9 is a mast cell growth factor that promotes IL-4–driven antibody production by B cells and can also induce goblet cell metaplasia. In a knockout mouse model of allergic airway disease, IL-9 can reproduce all of the cardinal features of asthma.[44] IL-9 has high expression in the lungs of patients with allergic asthma following segmental allergen challenge,[45] however.

Innate lymphoid cell 2
Valuable information regarding the etiology of eosinophilic airway inflammation came from a recombination-activating gene recombinase knockout mouse model of asthma, in which inhalation of allergen led to bronchial eosinophilia in the complete absence of mature T and B cells.[46] These findings suggested the possibility of generating a Th2 cytokinelike profile and eosinophilia without Th2 cells. As noted previously, inhalation of an exogenous antigen, particularly those that consist of or contain a protease (eg, house dust mite) may directly induce epithelial injury, leading to epithelial IL-33 release, activation of ILC2 cells, and finally generation of IL-5 and IL-13.[46] An alternative route of ILC2 activation has been attributed to leukotriene D4 (LTD4), which has been shown to be released following a single exposure to a proteolytic allergen.[47] ILC2 cells also have been shown to express major histocompatibility complex class II and costimulatory molecules, indicating that they may act as antigen-presenting cells that activate CD4[+] T cells. In addition to their role in allergy, mouse models have demonstrated that ILC2 cells may lead to viral-induced increases in airway eosinophils and other markers of airway inflammation.[48] Although the precise signals for ILC2 recruitment are not yet fully understood, there is evidence that the receptor for prostaglandin D2 (CRTH2), for LTD4 (CysLTR1), and chemokines (CCR4 and CCR8) may be involved.[49]

Eosinophils
Approximately 50% of patients with severe asthma have evidence of airway eosinophilia. These cells, which are drawn into the systemic circulation by IL-5, make their way into the lung vasculature and then enter the airway tissue under the influence of eotaxins. Once in the tissue, eosinophils release their granule proteins, including

eosinophil cationic protein, major basic protein (MBP), eosinophil peroxidase, and eosinophil-derived neurotoxin, which are directly toxic to epithelial and other airway structures.[50] In addition, MBP has been shown to stimulate leukotriene C4 (LTC4) release from basophils, which may have clinical importance. Eosinophils also can synthesize and release a large number of proinflammatory cytokines, including IL-4, IL-5, IL-13, IL-25, GM-CSF, and IL-8, and chemokines, including RANTES (Regulated on Activation, Normal T-Cell Expressed and Secreted) and eotaxin.[51] Overall, these eosinophil-derived products augment eosinophilic inflammation in the airway and may also promote neutrophil recruitment. Important cell surface markers on eosinophils include the IL-5 receptor, CCR3 (receptor for eotaxins), CRTH2, and Siglec-8. Siglec-8 engagement on eosinophils results in apoptosis, suggesting that this receptor may play an important role in the regulation of eosinophil accumulation and survival.[52] Eosinophils have been shown to be significantly increased in patients with severe, exacerbation-prone asthma compared with individuals with mild-moderate disease, and may negatively affect lung function.[53]

Mast cells
There is strong evidence that mast cells play an important role in the early asthmatic reaction following allergen exposure with an increase in histamine, prostaglandin D_2 (PGD2) and LTC4. Mast cells also synthesize and release a vast array of proinflammatory cytokines (eg, IL-4, IL-5, IL-6, IL-13, tumor necrosis factor [TNF]-alpha) and chemokines (RANTES, MCP-1, CXCL8) that act to recruit inflammatory cells, such as eosinophils, activated macrophages, and lymphocytes.[54] However, in diseases such as asthma, mast cells within the asthmatic airways appear to be present in a chronically activated state with evidence of ongoing mediator secretion. Studies show that bronchoalveolar lavage fluid of patients with stable asthma has increased numbers of mast cells[55] and increased levels of the mast cell mediators histamine and tryptase, suggesting ongoing activation and degranulation.[55]

Airway remodeling
It has been hypothesized that chronic airway inflammation, tissue injury, and abnormal repair mechanisms lead to structural changes in the airway walls of individuals with asthma, which may lead to irreversible (or partially reversible) airflow obstruction. Pathologic characteristics of remodeling, which include goblet cell hyperplasia, subepithelial fibrosis, increased airway smooth muscle mass, and bronchial hypervascularity, have all been carefully studied in small numbers of patients and possible molecular mechanisms have been identified.[56] IL-13 may be the most instrumental of the type 2 cytokines, and plays a key role in many of these processes, particularly goblet cell hyperplasia and subepithelial fibrosis.[57] Other mediators of remodeling include vascular endothelial growth factor, which is important in neovascularization[58]; TGF-beta, which contributes to fibrosis and increased airway smooth muscle[59]; and tissue inhibitor of metalloproteinase-1, which acts as an important profibrotic factor in fibrosis.[60] A complex interplay of these and other factors makes the treatment of airway remodeling a challenge to physicians who treat asthma.

Potential Immunologic Treatments

In type-2 (eosinophilic) asthma, IL-5 and IL-4/-13 have been considered critical cytokines in both the development and persistence of asthma. Monoclonal antibodies directed against IL-5 or its receptor (mepolizumab, reslizumab, benralizumab) have demonstrated significant reductions in asthma exacerbations and variable improvements in FEV1 (forced expiratory volume in 1 second) and patient-reported outcomes.[61–63] Similarly, antibodies against IL-13 or the IL-4 receptor (lebrikizumab, tralokinumab, dupilumab) also have shown significant improvements in exacerbations,[64,65] FEV1,[64–66] and patient-reported outcomes. Efforts to inhibit IL-9 did not result in changes in any clinical parameters of asthma.[67] Epithelial-derived cytokines, including TSLP, IL-25, and IL-33, are all plausible targets in type-2 asthma, and a proof-of-concept study of anti-TSLP (AMG 157) demonstrated robust inhibition of the early and late asthmatic responses to allergen inhalation.[68] Other potential targets in type-2 asthma include the prostaglandin receptor CRTH2, which has shown variable success in a number of trials with different drugs.[69] In non–type 2 (low eosinophil) asthma, TH-17 and GM-CSF both represent possible targets, although monoclonal antibodies against these cytokines have not demonstrated efficacy to date, possibly due to patient selection issues.[70,71]

REFERENCES

1. McAleer MA, Irvine AD. 63 The multifunctional role of filaggrin in allergic skin disease. J Allergy Clin Immunol 2013;131:280–91.
2. Palmer CN, Irvine AD, Terron-Kwiatkowski A, et al. Common loss-of-function variants of the epidermal barrier protein filaggrin are a major predisposing factor for atopic dermatitis. Nat Genet 2006;38:441–6.
3. Lampe MA, Williams ML, Elias PM. Human epidermal lipids: characterization and modulations during differentiation. J Lipid Res 1983;24:131–40.
4. Gittler J, Shemer A, Suárez-Fariñas M, et al. Progressive activation of T(H)2/T(H)22 cytokines and selective epidermal proteins characterizes acute and chronic atopic dermatitis. J Allergy Clin Immunol 2012;130:1344–54.
5. Howell MD, Kim BE, Gao P, et al. Cytokine modulation of atopic dermatitis filaggrin skin expression. J Allergy Clin Immunol 2007;120:150–5.
6. Kim BE, Leung DY, Boguniewicz M, et al. Loricrin and involucrin expression is down-regulated by Th2 cytokines through STAT-6. Clin Immunol 2008;126:332–7.
7. Sonkoly E, Muller A, Lauerma AI, et al. L-31: a new link between T cells and pruritus in atopic skin inflammation. J Allergy Clin Immunol 2006;117(2):411–7.
8. Kypriotou M, Huber M, Hohl D. The human epidermal differentiation complex: cornified envelope precursors, S100 proteins and the 'fused genes' family. Exp Dermatol 2012;21:643–9.
9. Teunissen MB, Koomen CW, de Waal Malefyt R, et al. Interleukin-17 and interferon-γ synergize in the enhancement of proinflammatory cytokine production by human keratinocytes. J Invest Dermatol 1998;111:645–9.
10. Kolls JK, Lindén A. Interleukin-17 family members and inflammation. Immunity 2004;21:467–76.
11. Salimi M, Barlow JL, Saunders SP, et al. A role for IL-25 and IL-33–driven type-2 innate lymphoid cells in atopic dermatitis. J Exp Med 2013;210:2939–50.
12. Ito Y, Adachi Y, Makino T, et al. Expansion of FOXP3-positive CD4+ CD25+ T cells associated with disease activity in atopic dermatitis. Ann Allergy Asthma Immunol 2009;103:160–5.
13. Szegedi A, Baráth S, Nagy G, et al. Regulatory T cells in atopic dermatitis: epidermal dendritic cell clusters may contribute to their local expansion. Br J Dermatol 2009;160:984–93.
14. Ou LS, Goleva E, Hall C, et al. T regulatory cells in atopic dermatitis and subversion of their activity by superantigens. J Allergy Clin Immunol 2004;113:756–63.
15. Kawakami T, Ando T, Kimura M, et al. Mast cells in atopic dermatitis. Curr Opin Immunol 2009;21:666–78.

16. Hossny E, Aboul-Magd M, Bakr S. Increased plasma eotaxin in atopic dermatitis and acute urticaria in infants and children. Allergy 2001;56:996–1002.
17. Beck LA, Thaçi D, Hamilton JD, et al. Dupilumab treatment in adults with moderate-to-severe atopic dermatitis. N Engl J Med 2014;371:130–9.
18. Oldhoff JM, Darsow U, Werfel T, et al. Anti-IL-5 recombinant humanized monoclonal antibody (mepolizumab) for the treatment of atopic dermatitis. Allergy 2005;60:693–6.
19. Shen JC, Cope E, Chen B, et al. Regulation of murine sinonasal cilia function by microbial secreted factors. Int Forum Allergy Rhinol 2012;2:104–10.
20. Blount A, Zhang S, Chestnut M, et al. Transepithelial ion transport is suppressed in hypoxic sinonasal epithelium. Laryngoscope 2011;121:1929–34.
21. Seshadri S, Rosati M, Lin DC, et al. Regional differences in the expression of innate host defense molecules in sinonasal mucosa. J Allergy Clin Immunol 2013;132:1227–30.
22. Lee RJ, Xiong G, Kofonow JM, et al. T2R38 taste receptor polymorphisms underlie susceptibility to upper respiratory infection. J Clin Invest 2012;122:4145–59.
23. Lam M, Hull L, McLachlan R, et al. Clinical severity and epithelial endotypes in chronic rhinosinusitis. Int Forum Allergy Rhinol 2013;3:121–8.
24. Shaw JL, Fakhri S, Citardi MJ, et al. IL-33-responsive innate lymphoid cells are an important source of IL-13 in chronic rhinosinusitis with nasal polyps. Am J Respir Crit Care Med 2013;188:432–9.
25. Mahdavinia M, Carter RG, Ocampo CJ, et al. Basophils are elevated in nasal polyps of patients with chronic rhinosinusitis without aspirin sensitivity. J Allergy Clin Immunol 2014;133:1759–63.
26. Mahdavinia M, Suh LA, Carter RG, et al. Increased noneosinophilic nasal polyps in chronic rhinosinusitis in US second-generation Asians suggest genetic regulation of eosinophilia. J Allergy Clin Immunol 2015;135:576–9.
27. Derycke L, Eyerich S, Van Crombruggen K, et al. Mixed T helper cell signatures in chronic rhinosinusitis with and without polyps. PLoS One 2014;9(6):e97581.
28. Hulse KE, Norton JE, Suh L, et al. Chronic rhinosinusitis with nasal polyps is characterized by B-cell inflammation and EBV-induced protein 2 expression. J Allergy Clin Immunol 2013;131:1075–83.
29. Van Zele T, Gevaert P, Watelet JB, et al. *Staphylococcus aureus* colonization and IgE antibody formation to enterotoxins is increased in nasal polyposis. J Allergy Clin Immunol 2004;114:981–3.
30. Takabayashi T, Kato A, Peters AT, et al. Excessive fibrin deposition in nasal polyps caused by fibrinolytic impairment through reduction of tissue plasminogen activator expression. Am J Respir Crit Care Med 2013;187:49–57.
31. Gevaert P, Calus L, Van Zele T, et al. Omalizumab is effective in allergic and nonallergic patients with nasal polyps and asthma. J Allergy Clin Immunol 2013;131:110–6.
32. Gevaert P, Van Bruaene N, Cattaert T, et al. Mepolizumab, a humanized anti-IL-5 mAb, as a treatment option for severe nasal polyposis. J Allergy Clin Immunol 2011;128:989–95.
33. Bachert C, Mannent L, Naclerio RM, et al. Effect of subcutaneous dupilumab on nasal polyp burden in patients with chronic sinusitis and nasal polyposis: a randomized clinical trial. JAMA 2016;315:469–79.
34. Ying S, O'Connor B, Ratoff J, et al. Thymic stromal lymphopoietin expression is increased in asthmatic airways and correlates with expression of Th2-attracting chemokines and disease severity. J Immunol 2005;174:8183–90.

35. Robinson DS, Hamid Q, Ying S, et al. Predominant Th2-like bronchoalveolar T lymphocyte population in atopic asthma. N Engl J Med 1992;326:298–304.
36. Corren J. Role of interleukin-13 in asthma. Curr Allergy Asthma Rep 2013;13: 415–20.
37. Peng J, Yang XO, Chang SH, et al. IL-23 signaling enhances Th2 polarization and regulates allergic airway inflammation. Cell Res 2010;20:62–71.
38. Fossiez F, Djossou O, Chomarat P, et al. T cell interleukin-17 induces stromal cells to produce proinflammatory and hematopoietic cytokines. J Exp Med 1996;183: 2593–603.
39. Zhao Y, Yang J, Gao YD, et al. Th17 immunity in patients with allergic asthma. Int Arch Allergy Immunol 2010;151:297–307.
40. Bullens DM, Truyen E, Coteur L, et al. IL-17 mRNA in sputum of asthmatic patients: linking T cell driven inflammation and granulocytic influx? Respir Res 2006;7:135.
41. Pene J, Chevalier S, Preisser SL, et al. Chronically inflamed human tissues are infiltrated by highly differentiated Th17 lymphocytes. J Immunol 2008;80:7423–30.
42. Choy DF, Hart KM, Borthwick LA, et al. TH2 and TH17 inflammatory pathways are reciprocally regulated in asthma. Sci Transl Med 2015;301:7.
43. Chang HC, Sehra S, Goswami R, et al. The transcription factor PU. 1 is required for the development of IL-9-producing T cells and allergic inflammation. Nat Immunol 2010;11:527–34.
44. Staudt V, Bothur E, Klein M, et al. Interferon-regulatory factor 4 is essential for the developmental program of T helper 9 cells. Immunity 2010;33:192–202.
45. Erpenbeck VJ, Hohlfeld JM, Volkmann B, et al. Segmental allergen challenge in patients with atopic asthma leads to increased IL-9 expression in bronchoalveolar lavage fluid lymphocytes. J Allergy Clin Immunol 2003;111:1319–27.
46. Lambrect BN, Hammad H. The immunology of asthma. Nat Immunol 2015;15: 45–56.
47. Bartemes KR, Iijima K, Kobayashi T, et al. IL-33-responsive lineage- CD25[+] CD44[hi] lymphoid cells mediate innate type 2 immunity and allergic inflammation in the lungs. J Immunol 2012;188:1503–13.
48. Doherty TA, Khorram N, Lund S, et al. Lung type 2 innate lymphoid cells express cysteinyl leukotriene receptor 1, which regulates TH2 cytokine production. J Allergy Clin Immunol 2013;132:205–13.
49. Chang YJ, Kim HY, Albacker LA. Innate lymphoid cells mediate influenza-induced airway hyper-reactivity independently of adaptive immunity. Nat Immunol 2011;12:631–8.
50. Xue L, Salimi M, Panse I, et al. Prostaglandin D_2 activates group 2 innate lymphoid cells through chemoattractant receptor-homologous molecule expressed on T_H2 cells. J Allergy Clin Immunol 2014;133:1184–94.
51. Acharya KR, Ackerman SJ. Eosinophil granule proteins: form and function. J Biol Chem 2014;289:17406–15.
52. Davoine F, Lacy P. Eosinophil cytokines, chemokines, and growth factors: emerging roles in immunity. Front Immunol 2014;5:570.
53. Bochner B. Siglec-8 on human eosinophils and mast cells, and Siglec-F on murine eosinophils, are functionally related inhibitory receptors. Clin Exp Allergy 2009;39:317–24.
54. Kupczyk M, ten Brinke A, Sterk PJ, et al. Frequent exacerbators—a distinct phenotype of severe asthma. Clin Exp Allergy 2014;44:212–21.
55. Moiseeva EP, Bradding P. Mast cells in lung inflammation. Adv Exp Med Biol 2011;716:235–69.

56. Broide DH, Gleich GJ, Cuomo AJ, et al. Evidence of ongoing mast cell and eosinophil degranulation in symptomatic asthma airway. J Allergy Clin Immunol 1991; 88:637–48.

57. Shifren A, Witt A, Christie C, et al. Mechanisms of remodeling in asthmatic airways. J Allergy 2012;2012:316049.

58. Kuperman DA, Huang X, Koth LL, et al. Direct effects of interleukin-13 on epithelial cells cause airway hyperreactivity and mucus overproduction in asthma. Nat Med 2002;8:885–9.

59. Hoshino M, Takahashi M, Aoike N. Expression of vascular endothelial growth factor, basic fibroblast growth factor, and angiogenin immunoreactivity in asthmatic airways and its relationship to angiogenesis. J Allergy Clin Immunol 2001;107: 295–301.

60. Minshall EM, Leung DYM, Martin RJ, et al. Eosinophil-associated TGF-β1 mRNA expression and airways fibrosis in bronchial asthma. Am J Respir Cell Mol Biol 1997;17:326–33.

61. Mautino G, Henriquet C, Gougat C, et al. Increased expression of tissue inhibitor of metalloproteinase-1 and loss of correlation with matrix metalloproteinase-9 by macrophages in asthma. Lab Invest 1999;79:39–47.

62. Ortega HG, Liu MC, Pavord ID, et al. Mepolizumab treatment in patients with severe eosinophilic asthma. N Engl J Med 2014;371:1198–207.

63. Castro M, Zangrilli J, Wechsler ME, et al. Reslizumab for inadequately controlled asthma with elevated blood eosinophil counts: results from two multicentre, parallel, double-blind, randomised, placebo-controlled, phase 3 trials. Lancet Respir Med 2015;3:355–66.

64. Castro M, Wenzel SE, Bleecker ER, et al. Benralizumab, an anti-interleukin 5 receptor α monoclonal antibody, versus placebo for uncontrolled eosinophilic asthma: a phase 2b randomised dose-ranging study. Lancet Respir Med 2014; 2:879–90.

65. Hanania NA, Noonan M, Corren J, et al. Lebrikizumab in moderate-to-severe asthma: pooled data from two randomised placebo-controlled studies. Thorax 2015;70:748–56.

66. Wenzel S, Castro M, Corren J, et al. Dupilumab efficacy and safety in adults with uncontrolled persistent asthma despite use of medium-to-high-dose inhaled corticosteroids plus a long-acting β$_2$ agonist: a randomised double-blind placebo-controlled pivotal phase 2b dose-ranging trial. Lancet 2016;388:31–44.

67. Oh CK, Leigh R, McLaurin KK, et al. A randomized, controlled trial to evaluate the effect of an anti-interleukin-9 monoclonal antibody in adults with uncontrolled asthma. Respiratoratory Research 2013;14:93.

68. Gauvreau GM, O'Byrne PM, Boulet LP, et al. Effects of an anti-TSLP antibody on allergen-induced asthmatic responses. N Engl J Med 2014;370:2102–10.

69. Hall IP, Fowler AV, Gupta A, et al. Efficacy of BI 671800, an oral CRTH2 antagonist, in poorly controlled asthma as sole controller and in the presence of inhaled corticosteroid treatment. Pulm Pharmacol Ther 2015;32:37–44.

70. Busse WW, Holgate S, Kerwin E, et al. Randomized, double-blind, placebo-controlled study of brodalumab, a human anti-IL-17 receptor monoclonal antibody, in moderate to severe asthma. Am J Respir Crit Care Med 2013;1(188): 1294–302.

71. Molfino NA, Kuna P, Leff JA, et al. Phase 2, randomised placebo-controlled trial to evaluate the efficacy and safety of an anti-GM-CSF antibody (KB003) in patients with inadequately controlled asthma. BMJ Open 2016;6:e007709.

Biological Therapies of Immunologic Diseases

Strategies for Immunologic Interventions

Brooke I. Polk, MD[a],*, Lanny J. Rosenwasser, MD[b]

KEYWORDS

- Biotherapy • Biotherapeutic • Immunomodulatory • Monoclonal antibody

KEY POINTS

- To understand at a basic level the general classes of biological therapies.
- To understand the targets of biotherapeutics in asthma, allergies, and other immune-mediated disorders.
- To take note of up-to-date and future therapies for immune-mediated disorders.

INTRODUCTION

The immune system is a highly complex and ever-evolving network of signaling molecules and target cells, with several potential targets for therapeutic modification. Throughout the past few decades, numerous methods of immunomodulatory biological therapy have been proposed and extensively studied, yet only some have demonstrated success. The ability to concurrently alter a component of the immune system, account for several downstream effects, reduce adverse drug events, and minimize the risk of consequent autoimmunity and/or malignancy has proven extensively difficult. Nonetheless, several strategies for immunologic intervention have been successfully applied to the practice of medicine (**Table 1**). This article covers currently available biotherapeutic agent classes as well as potential direction for future therapy.

MONOCLONAL ANTIBODIES

Monoclonal antibodies (mAbs) have received considerable attention since their conception more than 40 years ago. By definition, mAbs are antibodies created

Disclosures: Dr L.J. Rosenwasser serves as a consultant for the NIH NHLBI, Sanofi, Regeneron, and Astra Zeneca. Dr B.I. Polk has no disclosures.
[a] Division of Allergy, Asthma and Immunology, Children's Mercy Hospital, 2401 Gillham Road, Kansas City, MO 64108, USA; [b] Department of Medicine, University of Missouri Kansas City School of Medicine, 2411 Holmes Street, Kansas City, MO 64108, USA
* Corresponding author.
E-mail address: bpolk@cmh.edu

Table 1
Description of biotherapeutic agent classes

Biotherapeutic Class	Description	Examples of FDA-Licensed Products
Monoclonal antibodies	Antibodies created from a single clonal line designed to target a specific epitope	*Chimeric*: infliximab (anti-TNF) *Humanized*: omalizumab (anti-IgE), mepolizumab (anti-IL5) *Human*: adalimumab (anti-TNF), canakinumab (anti-IL1B), ustekinumab (anti-IL23/13)
Cytokines	Small secreted proteins involved in cell–cell signaling, used either in natural form or via recombinant DNA technology to serve as competitive inhibitors	*Natural*: interferons (α, β, γ) *Recombinant*: anakinra (recombinant IL-1RA)
Fc fusion proteins	Proteins consisting of the Fc domain of IgG (generally IgG1) fused to a ligand or peptide antigen, produced by recombinant genetic engineering	*Competitive inhibition*: Etanercept, rilonacept *Direct receptor stimulation*: Alefacept, romiplostin
RNA		
siRNA	Small double-stranded RNA product designed to bind, cleave, and silence a target mRNA	None
Antisense oligonucleotides	Synthesized single-stranded antisense segments designed to directly regulate mRNA expression via binding through specific Watson-Crick hybridization	Fomiversen, mipomersen, pegaptanib
Kinase inhibitors	Specific inhibitors of kinases (phosphorylating enzymes), typically acting via occupation of an active binding site	Imatinib (anti Bcr-Abl, CD117, PDGFR), nintedanib (anti-FGFR), tofacitinib (anti-JAK)
Antichemokine drugs	Small molecule inhibitors designed to target chemokine receptors	None

Abbreviations: FDA, Food and Drug Administration; FGFR, fibroblast growth factor receptor; Ig, immunoglobulin; IL, interleukin; IL-1RA, interleukin-1 receptor antagonist; mRNA, messenger RNA; PDGFR, platelet-derived growth factor receptor; siRNA, short interfering RNA; TNF, tumor necrosis factor.

from a single B lymphocyte clone that bind a specific antigenic epitope.[1] The first mAbs were formed by Kohler and Milstein in 1975 via the hybridoma technique,[2] involving fusion (either chemically or virally) of immortalized myeloma cells with splenic B cells of an animal specifically inoculated with the target epitope. Cells are then grown in selective hypoxanthine-aminopterin-thymidine medium, whereby only hybridoma cells can survive. Because unfused myeloma cells lack the ability to produce hypoxanthine guanine phosphoribosyltransferase (HGPRT), they are rendered unable to replicate their own genetic material within the medium owing to aminopterin salvage pathway inactivation[3]; unfused B cells, conversely, cannot survive indefinitely on account of their short life span. Fused cells, however, possess both immortality and HGPRT and can thus proliferate. Individual hybridomas are subsequently screened for antibody production and multiplied in culture.

Early mAbs were limited by the immunogenicity of murine proteins, genetic instability, and suboptimal efficacy.[4] The first mAb approved for human use was muromonab-CD3 (OKT3, Janssen, Beerse, Belgium), an IgG2a murine antibody targeting the T-cell CD3 receptor to treat solid organ rejection[5]; owing to adverse effects including formation of human antimouse antibodies, its use has largely been superseded by newer biotherapuetics. By the late 1980s, techniques to humanize mAbs were developed,[6] and in the late 1990s, entirely human mAbs generated by phage display[7] and transgenic mice[8] were developed (**Fig. 1**). With phage display, mRNA is isolated from human B lymphocytes and reverse transcribed into complementary DNA (cDNA) using polymerase chain reaction amplification at heavy and light chain variable regions. The products are ligated and introduced into a phage vector and inserted into *Escherichia coli* to generate an antibody library.[9] Although this process immortalizes cDNA clones, which can be used repeatedly, it typically generates antibody fragments (Fab or scFv) that must still be incorporated into a full antibody. More than 400 mAbs have been developed to date, with usefulness in multiple immune diseases. A standardized nomenclature system exists, with murine mAbs given the suffix "-omab," chimeric mAbs (which contain only animal variable regions) designated "-ximab," humanized mAbs (mouse CDR only) "-zumab," and fully human mAbs "-umab."

In addition to the use of phage display, the efficacy of mAbs is enhanced by genetically modifying the Fc region. Termed "Fc optimization," this process is accomplished either by point mutations or by defucosylation of the N-linked oligosaccharides,[10,11] with the intent to improve mAb affinity for the FcγRIIIA receptor, thereby improving natural killer cell–mediated target destruction via antibody-dependent cellular cytotoxicity. The half-life of mAbs is prolonged by modifying interactions with the salvage pathway neonatal Fc receptor, FcRn, accomplished by point mutations in the CH2-CH3 domain in cetuximab and bevacizumab,[12] and by the addition of polyethylene glycol.

Biologic targets of mAbs are extensive; most are directed versus cell surface receptors or ligands, serving to inhibit a downstream signaling pathway. Many emerging mAbs target inflammatory cytokine families; for treatment of rheumatoid and juvenile idiopathic arthritis, for example, anti–tumor necrosis factor mAbs have been used since the late 1990s,[13] and within the past 10 years, additional mAbs directed against IL-1β (canakinumab)[14] and IL-6 (tocilizumab)[15] have proven effective. Psoriasis therapy now includes anti–IL-17a (secukinumab, ixekinumab)[16,17] and anti–IL-12/IL-23 (ustekinumab)[18] mAbs. mAbs for treatment of atopic disorders target Th2 cytokines, with 2 anti–IL-5 (mepolizumab, reslizumab) mAbs[19,20] approved for use in eosinophilic asthma and another (benralizumab) coming down the pipeline[21]; the anti–IL-4/IL-13 mAb dupilumab has also proven quite effective in phase III trials for atopic dermatitis.[22] In addition to targeting T-cell cytokines, a highly successful mAb, rituximab, targets B-cell CD20; interestingly, lymphocyte phenotyping in treated patients showed that CD4+ T cells could potentially be used as a biomarker for response to therapy.[23] Although the clinical indications for mAbs are expanding continually, commercial success overall is often and unfortunately limited by high cost[24] and adverse effects, including cytokine release syndrome and acute hypersensitivity reactions.[25]

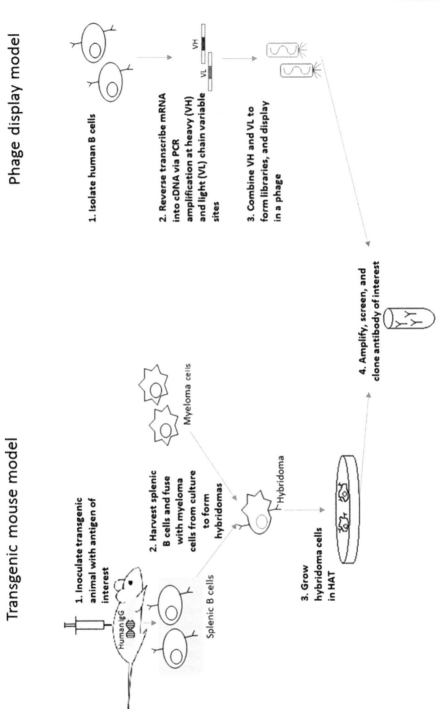

Fig. 1. Formation of monoclonal antibodies. HAT, hypoxanthine-aminopterin-thymidine; mRNA, Messenger RNA; PCR, polymerase chain reaction.

CYTOKINES

Cytokines are small secreted proteins involved in cell–cell signaling, with key roles in immune response regulation, homeostasis, and autoimmunity.[26,27] Whereas cytokine families are targeted by many emerging biotherapeutics, cytokines themselves are used as therapy in multiple immune-mediated diseases, both in unaltered form to serve natural roles and in genetically modified form to competitively inhibit in vivo cytokines. There is current clinical usefulness for multiple classes of cytokines, including interferons (IFNs) and interleukins.

A classic example of cytokine therapy is the use of IFNs. IFN-α, a type I IFN produced by leukocytes involved in innate response to viral infections, has been used as medical therapy since the 1970s, when purified topical preparations of IFN-α were deemed helpful in the prevention of viral respiratory infections[28] and in the treatment of herpesviridae skin infections.[29] A subsequent study by the same group showed success in the treatment of chronic hepatitis B infection with parenteral IFN-α.[30] Recombinant forms of IFN-α are currently used to treat hepatitis B and C, various cancers, and subsets of patients with hypereosinophilic syndromes.[31,32] IFN-β was initially used in the 1980s, when human fibroblast IFN-β administered via lumbar puncture to 10 multiple sclerosis patients resulted in improvement,[33] and this cytokine, in various forms, is still used in multiple sclerosis therapy.[31] After discovering the augmentation of macrophage oxidative metabolism by IFN-γ, its use in chronic granulomatous disease was initiated in the early 1990s[34]; it remains in use in recombinant form today.

Interleukins are also used in recombinant form as competitive endogenous inhibitors. Anakinra is a recombinant nonglycosylated interleukin-1 receptor antagonist (IL-1RA), a natural member of the IL-1 cytokine family that serves as an inhibitor of IL-1β. Prepared from cultures of genetically modified *E coli* using recombinant DNA technology, anakinra possesses an additional methionine at the amino terminus and competitively binds the IL-1 receptor.[35] Although initially marketed for rheumatoid arthritis, it has also shown recent success in cryopyrin-associated periodic syndromes (CAPS), because these patients have mutations in the cryopyrin gene leading to unregulated IL-1β production,[36] and in the treatment of systemic onset juvenile idiopathic arthritis[37] and adult-onset Still's disease.[38] Pitrakinra is a similarly modified human IL-4 that competitively binds the alpha subunit of the IL-4 receptor (IL-4Rα), acting as a competitive antagonist of both IL-4 and IL-13.[39] Pitrakinra reduced asthma exacerbations in a small subset of trial subjects, and a significant association was found between response and polymorphisms in the IL4RA gene.[40] Unfortunately, possibly owing to study design, further research on this biologic seems to have ceased. Other medical uses for interleukins include recombinant IL-11 (oprelvekin), a hematopoietic cytokine responsible for megakaryocyte maturation, for the prevention of thrombocytopenia in patient undergoing myelosuppressive chemotherapy,[41] and IL-2 has a role in treatment of cancers.

FC FUSION PROTEINS

Fusion proteins used in biological therapy are created by cDNA coding for 2 separate proteins through the use of recombinant genetic engineering. The most well-used fusion proteins are the Fc fusion proteins, which involve linking the Fc domain of human IgG (generally IgG1) to another peptide, typically a ligand or peptide antigen.[11] Fusion with the Fc domain confers the ability to interact with high affinity Fc receptors and prolongs half-life via interaction with neonatal salvage FcRn receptors, as mentioned.[42] Most Fc fusion proteins serve to competitively inhibit receptor binding (abatacept, aflibiticept, belatacept, etanercept, rilonacept), although 2 Food and Drug Administration (FDA)-approved Fc fusion proteins function as direct receptor stimulators (alefacept and romiplostin). Whereas the Fc fusion proteins are modified by Fc optimization as described for mAbs,[10] recent focus has shifted to developing new fusion platforms including the potential use of IgG3, IgG4, IgA, and IgM constructs.[11,43]

Two unique Fc fusion proteins are rilonacept and dulaglutide. Rilonacept is distinctive in that it is a dimeric fusion protein consisting of extracellular portions of both the IL-1 receptor component IL-1R1 and its accessory protein IL-1RAcP, enabling it to bind and neutralize IL-1β but also act on IL-1α and IL1-RA with reduced affinity; it was the first drug licensed for use in CAPS.[44] Dulaglutide, although used to treat type 2 diabetes, is worth noting given its distinction as the first licensed Fc fusion protein containing a non-IgG1 subclass Fc region (IgG4).[45] The 10 currently FDA-licensed Fc fusion proteins have found clinical efficacy in organ rejection, macular degeneration, CAPs, thrombocytopenia, rheumatoid arthritis, diabetes, and psoriasis. One potentially promising Fc fusion initially excited the asthma community yet failed to show efficacy in phase III trials was altrakincept, a soluble IL4R Fc fusion protein[46]; although an mAb targeting IL-4 was also ineffective in asthma treatment,[47] perhaps the ability to additionally target IL-13, as with dupilumab, could provide success.

RNA

Significant recent advances in RNA therapeutics have made it possible to target the specific nucleic acids involved in protein synthesis of particular genes of interest. Currently used RNA therapeutic techniques include double-stranded RNA-mediated interference (RNAi) and single-stranded antisense oligonucleotides (ASOs). RNAi, a posttranscriptional gene silencing mechanism, occurs naturally in human cells; in this process, a long, double-stranded RNA induces the cleavage and silencing of host mRNA, thereby preventing translation of mRNA to protein via integration with the RNA-induced silencing complex (RISC) and the endonuclease Argonaute 2.[48] This can be accomplished through the use of short interfering RNA (siRNA) or micro-RNA (miRNA), 2 types of double stranded noncoding RNA that possess subtle but important differences. The most widely examined RNAi molecules, siRNAs consist of a "passenger" sense strand that is degraded and a "guide" antisense strand that leads the RISC to the target mRNA and binds with full complementarity, inducing 5′ cleavage and silencing.[49] The antisense strand of miRNA, however, is only partially complementary to the target mRNA, and gene suppression is induced via translational repression; although this often leads to imperfect binding in therapeutic studies, a conceivable advantage of this process is the potential for miRNA to bind multiple genes.[50]

RNAi molecules face numerous challenges, including instability against extracellular and intracellular degradation (the half-life of naked siRNA is approximately 15 minutes),[50,51] weak cellular uptake, low potency, and the potential for "off-target" effects via binding to other mRNA products; improvements include the addition of viral, small molecule, and nanoparticle carriers.[52] Moreover, the human innate immune system is inherently trained to recognize double stranded RNA as foreign, thereby inducing type 1 IFNs. This process is prevented by the careful introduction of chemical modifications. Although no RNAi product is yet approved by the FDA, some siRNA-based therapies have shown promise in the treatment of "undruggable" cancer mutations,[53] although the best clinical response seems to be tumor stabilization rather than complete response. In respiratory inflammatory diseases, in vivo studies have used miRNA and siRNA to target IL-4, STAT-6, GATA3, c-kit, and other cytokines with variable success, although no drug has progressed past phase II trials.[50] Ongoing phase II trials for ALN-CC5, an siRNA targeting complement component C5, have shown promise in treatment of paroxysmal nocturnal hemoglobinuria,[54] and its creator Alnylam is pre-clinically evaluating its value in the treatment of atypical hemolytic uremic syndrome and myasthenia gravis.

Unlike siRNA and miRNA, ASOs are synthesized single-stranded antisense segments designed to directly regulate mRNA expression via binding through specific Watson-Crick hybridization.[51] ASOs are the longest studied RNA-based drugs, having been discovered more than 2 decades ago. ASOs are subject to similar limitations as siRNAs, including recognition by Toll-like receptors and other innate pattern recognition receptors, and unmodified ASOs are unable to cross plasma membranes given their negative charge[48]; to bypass these impediments, ASOs have undergone considerable modifications; reflective of sequential changes, ASOs are typically referred to as first, second, and third generation.[49] First-generation modifications include alterations to the phosphodiester backbone, primarily via phosphorothioate (PS) bonds, to increase affinity and prevent degradation.[49,54] Second-generation modifications include improving cellular uptake and target affinity via sugar moiety alterations such as 2′-O-methyl, 2′-O-methoxymethyl (2′-OMOE), and locked nucleic acid alterations,[51] and recent third-generation developments center around chimeric "gapmer" ASOs, in which a central "gap" segment that activates RNAse H is flanked by 2 to 5 chemically modified nucleotides on the 2′ ends that improve stability.[48] As of today, 3 oligonucleotide products are licensed. The first oligonucleotide to receive FDA approval in 1998, fomivirsen, is a first-generation PS-ASO used in the treatment of cytomegalovirus infection in immunocompromised individuals[49]; the other approved ASOs are mipomersen, a second-generation ASO used in familial hypercholesterolemia,[55] and pegaptanib, a pegylated antivascular endothelial growth factor aptamer used in wet macular degeneration.[56]

ASO delivery is generally accomplished via parenteral injection, although inhaled ASOs have been trialed. AIR645 was a 2′-OMOE inhaled antisense oligonucleotide targeting mRNA encoding the alpha subunit of the IL-4 receptor (IL-4Rα). Although groundbreaking in that it was the first inhaled antisense oligonucleotide of its kind, it unfortunately failed to show efficacy after phase I trials.[57] In regard to immune-mediated disease, a few novel products have recently been created. TPI ASM-8 (Pharmaxis, New South Wales, Australia) is a drug containing 2 ASOs targeting the CC chemokine receptor 3 (CCR3) and the IL-3, IL-5, and granulocyte-monocyte colony stimulating factor common beta chain, designed to block atopic inflammation. This medication showed promise and safety in the treatment of mild atopic asthma in phase I and II trials,[58] but unfortunately further progress has not been made in the past 4 years. Additionally, a fascinating antisense molecule targeting GATA3, the transcription factor essential for Th2 development, is showing potential in phase II trials for eosinophilic allergic asthma[59]; termed SB010, this DNA enzyme (DNAzyme) contains antisense base pairs targeting GATA3 mRNA on its ends and a builtin enzyme hgd40 in its center, serving as the catalytic domain to cleave and silence GATA3 mRNA.

SMALL MOLECULE KINASE INHIBITORS

Within the past 2 decades, the paradigm of chemotherapy biotherapeutics has shifted dramatically from cytotoxicity to the development of specific targeted therapies.[60] Once a potential target is identified and validated, a chemical library is screened to identify a lead compound, which is then optimized and used as a foundation for chemical modification. This modified small molecule drug is subsequently clinically validated by biomarker-led trials.[60] After discovering the involvement of protein kinases in cancer pathogenesis, significant efforts to create small molecule kinase inhibitors resulted in the identification of numerous lead compounds via these methods. Kinases activate substrates via phosphorylation by transferring phosphate from ATP to an hydroxyl group; aberrant phosphorylation has implications in numerous autoimmune and inflammatory conditions.[61] The first successfully licensed small molecule kinase inhibitor was imatinib, a modified 2-phenylaminopyrimidine designed to suppress Abelson (Abl) kinase in Bcr-Abl expressing leukemia cells via occupation of the active site of the Abl protooncogene.[62] Interestingly, imatinib also selectively inhibits tyrosine kinases c-kit (CD117) and platelet-derived growth factor receptor (PDGFR), and it is now used in a subset of systemic mastocytosis patients who are negative for the c-kit D816V gain-of-function mutation[63] and for hypereosinophilic syndrome patients possessing the FIP1L1–PDGFRA fusion kinase mutation.[64] The success of imatinib combined with the sequencing of the human kinome in 2002[65] and advances in high-throughput biochemical profiling led to influx of protein kinase inhibitors, with 33 FDA approved as of 2015.[61]

Other kinase inhibitors with nononcologic indications include nintedanib, a small molecule tyrosine kinase inhibitor specific for fibroblast growth factor receptor, vascular endothelial growth factor receptor, and PDGFR, approved in 2014 for treatment of idiopathic pulmonary fibrosis,[66] and agents dubbed "jakinibs" that target the cytoplasmic janus kinase (JAK) tyrosine kinase family.[67] There are 4 JAKs—JAK 1, 2, 3 and TYK2 (tyrosine kinase 2), each associated with a multitude of cytokines. Genome-wide association studies have linked JAKs to the development of autoimmune diseases, including lupus, Crohn's disease, and Behcet's,[27] and mutations in downstream signal transducer and activator of transcription (STAT) proteins cause immunodeficiencies. Tofacitinib, a JAK1, 3, and 2 inhibitor, the first jakinib developed for treatment of autoimmune disease, is used in rheumatoid arthritis[68]; although noninferior to etanercept for psoriasis and psoriatic arthritis,[69] it was not approved for this use. The first FDA-approved jakinib was ruxolitinib, which targets JAK1 and JAK2, initially approved for the treatment of myeloproliferative disease, but successful in a phase II trial for treatment of rheumatoid arthritis.[27] Another JAK1/2 inhibitor, baricitinib, has recently shown efficacy in the treatment of refractory rheumatoid arthritis as well, with phase III results published last month.[70] Jakinib immunomodulators allow the inhibition of multiple cytokine signals and show promise for future therapy, especially in patients who have failed traditional disease-modifying antirheumatic drugs. Adverse effects to consider include increased rates of infections as seen with other immunomodulatory medications, notably an increased risk of varicella zoster infections in tofacitinib,[27] and increases in total cholesterol likely owing to effects of IL-6, which promotes insulin resistance, and altered lipoprotein kinetics.[71]

ANTICHEMOKINE SMALL MOLECULE INHIBITORS

In the field of asthma and allergic disease, attention has been recently directed toward the development of small molecule antichemokine drugs.[72] Chemokines, by name, are chemoattractive cytokines that facilitate leukocyte recruitment and trafficking via G-protein–coupled receptors; unchecked chemokine stimulation can lead to unwanted immune responses and autoimmunity. Although antichemokine small molecule drugs have generally proven unsuccessful,[73] likely owing to redundancy in the chemokine system, there are some potentially positive recent developments in the field. CCR3 is the primary eosinophil chemokine (eotaxin) receptor, an enticing target for atopic disease. Although several small molecule CCR3 antagonists have been developed; unfortunately, none have yet progressed past phase II trials despite initial successes, primarily owing to failure to achieve efficacy.[74] One compound, BMS-629623, a novel CCR3 antagonist created by Bristol-Myers Squibb (BMS) via extensive structural modification of a prior urea-based Dupont-Merck that unfortunately antagonized CYP2D6, is reportedly undergoing phase I trials.[75] Another essential component of asthma pathogenesis involves Th2 lymphocyte recruitment. Potential chemokine receptor targets on the Th2 surface include CCR4, CCR8, and CXCR4. Thus far, blockade of CCR4 and CCR8 has regrettably shown no effect on Th2 recruitment in animal models,[76,77] although treatment of mice with the small molecule AMD3100, a CXCR4 antagonist, significantly reduced numerous inflammatory mediators in a mouse model of asthma.[78] Despite offering seemingly lucrative targets, chemokine receptor antagonists as a class have unfortunately produced scant success thus far.

SUMMARY AND FUTURE CONSIDERATIONS

Although the complete inventory of every available biotherapeutic approach to immune mediated disease is quite exhaustive, this review provides a thorough summary of general past and current methods under investigation. Potential immune system targets are vast, and the means by which to alter them even more so. The field of biotherapeutics is rapidly expanding with recent advances in biomolecular and genetic engineering, allowing for the creation of new molecules with targeted specificity and effective in vivo delivery. In addition to the methods described, fascinating new discoveries include the ability to create synthetic antibody mimetics derived from nonimmunoglobulin scaffold proteins,[79] the conjugation of oligonucleotides to siRNA products,[80] and the increasing knowledge of genomic and epigenomic engineering products. Notable advances in epigenomics include the use of transcription activator-like effectors, which are often fused to functional domains to create custom DNA-binding products to target specific genes for degradation by transcription activatorlike effector nucleases,[81] and prokaryotic clustered regularly interspaced short palindromic repeat proteins and associated Cas nucleases to target specific DNA sequences using programmable RNAs[82,83]; these interventions allow the possibility of correcting genetic abnormalities. As we move into the era of personalized precision medicine via discoveries in effective biomarkers, all of these methods carry the potential for worthwhile and efficacious clinical applications.

REFERENCES

1. Liu JK. The history of monoclonal antibody development - progress, remaining challenges and future innovations. Ann Med Surg 2014;3(4):113–6.
2. Kohler G, Milstein C. Continuous cultures of fused cells secreting antibody of predefined specificity. Nature 1975;256(5517):495–7.
3. Little M, Kipriyanov SM, Le Gall F, et al. Of mice and men: hybridoma and recombinant antibodies. Immunol Today 2000;21(8):364–70.
4. Weiner GJ. Building better monoclonal antibody-based therapeutics. Nat Rev Cancer 2015;15(6):361–70.
5. Smith SL. Ten years of Orthoclone OKT3 (muromonab-CD3): a review. J Transpl Coord 1996;6(3):109–19 [quiz: 20–1].
6. Riechmann L, Clark M, Waldmann H, et al. Reshaping human antibodies for therapy. Nature 1988;332(6162):323–7.

7. Hoogenboom HR, de Bruine AP, Hufton SE, et al. Antibody phage display technology and its applications. Immunotechnology 1998;4(1):1–20.

8. Lonberg N, Huszar D. Human antibodies from transgenic mice. Int Rev Immunol 1995;13(1):65–93.

9. Hammers CM, Stanley JR. Antibody phage display: technique and applications. J Invest Dermatol 2014;134(2):e17.

10. Yamane-Ohnuki N, Satoh M. Production of therapeutic antibodies with controlled fucosylation. MAbs 2009;1(3):230–6.

11. Czajkowsky DM, Hu J, Shao Z, et al. Fc-fusion proteins: new developments and future perspectives. EMBO Mol Med 2012;4(10):1015–28.

12. Zalevsky J, Chamberlain AK, Horton HM, et al. Enhanced antibody half-life improves in vivo activity. Nat Biotechnol 2010;28(2):157–9.

13. Venkatesha SH, Dudics S, Acharya B, et al. Cytokine-modulating strategies and newer cytokine targets for arthritis therapy. Int J Mol Sci 2015;16(1):887–906.

14. Ruperto N, Brunner HI, Quartier P, et al. Two randomized trials of canakinumab in systemic juvenile idiopathic arthritis. N Engl J Med 2012;367(25):2396–406.

15. Hashizume M, Tan SL, Takano J, et al. Tocilizumab, a humanized anti-IL-6R antibody, as an emerging therapeutic option for rheumatoid arthritis: molecular and cellular mechanistic insights. Int Rev Immunol 2015;34(3):265–79.

16. Shirley M, Scott LJ. Secukinumab: a review in psoriatic arthritis. Drugs 2016; 76(11):1135–45.

17. Vu HT, Gooderham M, Papp K. Ixekizumab for treatment of adults with moderate-to-severe plaque psoriasis and psoriatic arthritis. Expert Rev Clin Pharmacol 2016. [Epub ahead of print].

18. Kavanaugh A, Puig L, Gottlieb AB, et al. Efficacy and safety of ustekinumab in psoriatic arthritis patients with peripheral arthritis and physician-reported spondylitis: post-hoc analyses from two phase III, multicentre, double-blind, placebo-controlled studies (PSUMMIT-1/PSUMMIT-2). Ann Rheum Dis 2016;75(11): 1984–8.

19. Ortega HG, Liu MC, Pavord ID, et al. Mepolizumab treatment in patients with severe eosinophilic asthma. N Engl J Med 2014;371(13):1198–207.

20. Castro M, Zangrilli J, Wechsler ME, et al. Reslizumab for inadequately controlled asthma with elevated blood eosinophil counts: results from two multicentre, parallel, double-blind, randomised, placebo-controlled, phase 3 trials. Lancet Respir Med 2015;3(5):355–66.

21. FitzGerald JM, Bleecker ER, Nair P, et al. Benralizumab, an anti-interleukin-5 receptor alpha monoclonal antibody, as add-on treatment for patients with severe, uncontrolled, eosinophilic asthma (CALIMA): a randomised, double-blind, placebo-controlled phase 3 trial. Lancet 2016;388(10056):2128–41.

22. Simpson EL, Bieber T, Guttman-Yassky E, et al. Two phase 3 trials of dupilumab versus placebo in atopic dermatitis. N Engl J Med 2016;375(24):2335–48.

23. Lavielle M, Mulleman D, Goupille P, et al. Repeated decrease of CD4+ T-cell counts in patients with rheumatoid arthritis over multiple cycles of rituximab treatment. Arthritis Res Ther 2016;18(1):253.

24. Shaughnessy AF. Monoclonal antibodies: magic bullets with a hefty price tag. BMJ 2012;345:e8346.

25. Baldo BA. Adverse events to monoclonal antibodies used for cancer therapy: focus on hypersensitivity responses. Oncoimmunology 2013;2(10):e26333.

26. Dinarello CA. Historical insights into cytokines. Eur J Immunol 2007;37(Suppl 1): S34–45.

27. Schwartz DM, Bonelli M, Gadina M, et al. Type I/II cytokines, JAKs, and new strategies for treating autoimmune diseases. Nat Rev Rheumatol 2016;12(1):25–36.
28. Merigan TC, Reed SE, Hall TS, et al. Inhibition of respiratory virus infection by locally applied interferon. Lancet 1973;1(7803):563–7.
29. Sundmacher R, Neumann-Haefelin D, Cantell K. Letter: interferon treatment of dendritic keratitis. Lancet 1976;1(7974):1406–7.
30. Greenberg HB, Pollard RB, Lutwick LI, et al. Effect of human leukocyte interferon on hepatitis B virus infection in patients with chronic active hepatitis. N Engl J Med 1976;295(10):517–22.
31. Friedman RM. Clinical uses of interferons. Br J Clin Pharmacol 2008;65(2): 158–62.
32. Butterfield JH, Weiler CR. Use of pegylated interferon in hypereosinophilic syndrome. Leuk Res 2012;36(2):192–7.
33. Jacobs L, Salazar AM, Herndon R, et al. Intrathecally administered natural human fibroblast interferon reduces exacerbations of multiple sclerosis. Results of a multicenter, double-blind study. Arch Neurol 1987;44(6):589–95.
34. A controlled trial of interferon gamma to prevent infection in chronic granulomatous disease. The International Chronic Granulomatous Disease Cooperative Study Group. N Engl J Med 1991;324(8):509–16.
35. Mertens M, Singh JA. Anakinra for rheumatoid arthritis. Cochrane Database Syst Rev 2009;(1):CD005121.
36. Kullenberg T, Lofqvist M, Leinonen M, et al. Long-term safety profile of anakinra in patients with severe cryopyrin-associated periodic syndromes. Rheumatology 2016;55(8):1499–506.
37. Quartier P, Allantaz F, Cimaz R, et al. A multicentre, randomised, double-blind, placebo-controlled trial with the interleukin-1 receptor antagonist anakinra in patients with systemic-onset juvenile idiopathic arthritis (ANAJIS trial). Ann Rheum Dis 2011;70(5):747–54.
38. Nordstrom D, Knight A, Luukkainen R, et al. Beneficial effect of interleukin 1 inhibition with anakinra in adult-onset Still's disease. An open, randomized, multicenter study. J Rheumatol 2012;39(10):2008–11.
39. Wechsler ME, Fulkerson PC, Bochner BS, et al. Novel targeted therapies for eosinophilic disorders. J Allergy Clin Immunol 2012;130(3):563–71.
40. Slager RE, Otulana BA, Hawkins GA, et al. IL-4 receptor polymorphisms predict reduction in asthma exacerbations during response to an anti-IL-4 receptor alpha antagonist. J Allergy Clin Immunol 2012;130(2):516–22.e4.
41. Cantor SB, Elting LS, Hudson DV Jr, et al. Pharmacoeconomic analysis of oprelvekin (recombinant human interleukin-11) for secondary prophylaxis of thrombocytopenia in solid tumor patients receiving chemotherapy. Cancer 2003;97(12): 3099–106.
42. Roopenian DC, Akilesh S. FcRn: the neonatal Fc receptor comes of age. Nat Rev Immunol 2007;7(9):715–25.
43. Ammann JU, Jahnke M, Dyson MR, et al. Detection of weak receptor-ligand interactions using IgM and J-chain-based fusion proteins. Eur J Immunol 2012;42(5): 1354–6.
44. Kapur S, Bonk ME. Rilonacept (arcalyst), an interleukin-1 trap for the treatment of cryopyrin-associated periodic syndromes. P T 2009;34(3):138–41.
45. Jimenez-Solem E, Rasmussen MH, Christensen M, et al. Dulaglutide, a long-acting GLP-1 analog fused with an Fc antibody fragment for the potential treatment of type 2 diabetes. Curr Opin Mol Ther 2010;12(6):790–7.

46. Borish LC, Nelson HS, Lanz MJ, et al. Interleukin-4 receptor in moderate atopic asthma. A phase I/II randomized, placebo-controlled trial. Am J Respir Crit Care Med 1999;160(6):1816–23.
47. Kau AL, Korenblat PE. Anti-interleukin 4 and 13 for asthma treatment in the era of endotypes. Curr Opin Allergy Clin Immunol 2014;14(6):570–5.
48. Watts JK, Corey DR. Silencing disease genes in the laboratory and the clinic. J Pathol 2012;226(2):365–79.
49. Chery J. RNA therapeutics: RNAi and antisense mechanisms and clinical applications. Postdoc J 2016;4(7):35–50.
50. Qiu Y, Lam JK, Leung SW, et al. Delivery of RNAi therapeutics to the airways-from bench to bedside. Molecules 2016;21(9):E1249.
51. Barata P, Sood AK, Hong DS. RNA-targeted therapeutics in cancer clinical trials: current status and future directions. Cancer Treat Rev 2016;50:35–47.
52. Wu SY, Lopez-Berestein G, Calin GA, et al. RNAi therapies: drugging the undruggable. Sci Transl Med 2014;6(240):240ps7.
53. Ozcan G, Ozpolat B, Coleman RL, et al. Preclinical and clinical development of siRNA-based therapeutics. Adv Drug Deliv Rev 2015;87:108–19.
54. McClorey G, Wood MJ. An overview of the clinical application of antisense oligonucleotides for RNA-targeting therapies. Curr Opin Pharmacol 2015;24:52–8.
55. Santos RD, Duell PB, East C, et al. Long-term efficacy and safety of mipomersen in patients with familial hypercholesterolaemia: 2-year interim results of an open-label extension. Eur Heart J 2015;36(9):566–75.
56. Solomon SD, Lindsley K, Vedula SS, et al. Anti-vascular endothelial growth factor for neovascular age-related macular degeneration. Cochrane database Syst Rev 2014;(8):CD005139.
57. Rael EL, Lockey RF. Interleukin-13 signaling and its role in asthma. World Allergy Organ J 2011;4(3):54–64.
58. Gauvreau GM, Boulet LP, Cockcroft DW, et al. Antisense therapy against CCR3 and the common beta chain attenuates allergen-induced eosinophilic responses. Am J Respir Crit Care Med 2008;177(9):952–8.
59. Krug N, Hohlfeld JM, Kirsten AM, et al. Allergen-induced asthmatic responses modified by a GATA3-specific DNAzyme. N Engl J Med 2015;372(21):1987–95.
60. Hoelder S, Clarke PA, Workman P. Discovery of small molecule cancer drugs: successes, challenges and opportunities. Mol Oncol 2012;6(2):155–76.
61. Fabbro D, Cowan-Jacob SW, Moebitz H. Ten things you should know about protein kinases: IUPHAR Review 14. Br J Pharmacol 2015;172(11):2675–700.
62. Druker BJ, Lydon NB. Lessons learned from the development of an abl tyrosine kinase inhibitor for chronic myelogenous leukemia. J Clin Invest 2000;105(1):3–7.
63. Droogendijk HJ, Kluin-Nelemans HJ, van Doormaal JJ, et al. Imatinib mesylate in the treatment of systemic mastocytosis: a phase II trial. Cancer 2006;107(2):345–51.
64. Khoury P, Desmond R, Pabon A, et al. Clinical features predict responsiveness to imatinib in platelet-derived growth factor receptor-alpha-negative hypereosinophilic syndrome. Allergy 2016;71(6):803–10.
65. Manning G, Whyte DB, Martinez R, et al. The protein kinase complement of the human genome. Science 2002;298(5600):1912–34.
66. Mazzei ME, Richeldi L, Collard HR. Nintedanib in the treatment of idiopathic pulmonary fibrosis. Ther Adv Respir Dis 2015;9(3):121–9.
67. Kontzias A, Kotlyar A, Laurence A, et al. Jakinibs: a new class of kinase inhibitors in cancer and autoimmune disease. Curr Opin Pharmacol 2012;12(4):464–70.

68. van Vollenhoven RF, Fleischmann R, Cohen S, et al. Tofacitinib or adalimumab versus placebo in rheumatoid arthritis. N Engl J Med 2012;367(6):508–19.
69. Chiricozzi A, Faleri S, Saraceno R, et al. Tofacitinib for the treatment of moderate-to-severe psoriasis. Expert Rev Clin Immunol 2015;11(4):443–55.
70. Dougados M, van der Heijde D, Chen YC, et al. Baricitinib in patients with inadequate response or intolerance to conventional synthetic DMARDs: results from the RA-BUILD study. Ann Rheum Dis 2017;76(1):88–95.
71. He Y, Wong AY, Chan EW, et al. Efficacy and safety of tofacitinib in the treatment of rheumatoid arthritis: a systematic review and meta-analysis. BMC Musculoskelet Disord 2013;14:298.
72. Yamagata T, Ichinose M. Agents against cytokine synthesis or receptors. Eur J Pharmacol 2006;533(1–3):289–301.
73. Proudfoot AE, Power CA, Schwarz MK. Anti-chemokine small molecule drugs: a promising future? Expert Opin Investig Drugs 2010;19(3):345–55.
74. Pease JE, Horuk R. Recent progress in the development of antagonists to the chemokine receptors CCR3 and CCR4. Expert Opin Drug Discov 2014;9(5):467–83.
75. Pease J, Horuk R. Chemokine receptors in allergy, inflammation, and infectious disease. Chemokines and their receptors in drug discovery. Switzerland: Springer; 2015. p. 1–40.
76. Conroy DM, Jopling LA, Lloyd CM, et al. CCR4 blockade does not inhibit allergic airways inflammation. J Leukoc Biol 2003;74(4):558–63.
77. Chung CD, Kuo F, Kumer J, et al. CCR8 is not essential for the development of inflammation in a mouse model of allergic airway disease. J Immunol 2003;170(1):581–7.
78. Lukacs NW, Berlin A, Schols D, et al. AMD3100, a CxCR4 antagonist, attenuates allergic lung inflammation and airway hyperreactivity. Am J Pathol 2002;160(4):1353–60.
79. Al Deghaither D, Smaglo BG, Weiner LM. Beyond peptides and mAbs–current status and future perspectives for biotherapeutics with novel constructs. J Clin Pharmacol 2015;55(Suppl 3):S4–20.
80. Gooding M, Malhotra M, Evans JC, et al. Oligonucleotide conjugates - Candidates for gene silencing therapeutics. Eur J Pharm Biopharm 2016;107:321–40.
81. Mahfouz MM, Piatek A, Stewart CN Jr. Genome engineering via TALENs and CRISPR/Cas9 systems: challenges and perspectives. Plant Biotechnol J 2014;12(8):1006–14.
82. Hille F, Charpentier E. CRISPR-Cas: biology, mechanisms and relevance. Philos Trans R Soc Lond B Biol Sci 2016;371(1707).
83. Wei C, Liu J, Yu Z, et al. TALEN or Cas9-rapid, efficient and specific choices for genome modifications. J Genet 2013;40(6):281–9.

Patient Characteristics and Individualization of Biologic Therapy

Steven Draikiwicz, MD[1], John Oppenheimer, MD*

KEYWORDS

- Biologics • Patient characteristics • Asthma • Urticaria • Phenotypes

KEY POINTS

- An overview is provided of the current status of therapy for outlined disease states and the role for biologic therapy in treatment.
- Current literature is reviewed regarding studied patient characteristics and the effect on outcome in patients with asthma and urticaria.
- The need for appropriate patient phenotyping is identified and guidance on evidence-based biologic selection is provided.

INTRODUCTION

Progress in the understanding of disease processes has provided additional therapeutic targets. This progress is best exemplified by the increasing role of biologics in the clinical armamentarium. Biologic agents are therapeutics synthesized by living organisms and directed against a specific determinant.[1] This article provides a focused review of current treatment paradigms and pathophysiology for asthma and urticaria. A table highlighting the mechanisms of action of individual therapeutics is presented after each section in which they are introduced. The goal is to elucidate for practicing physicians the populations in which biologics were studied for the aforementioned disease states, emphasizing characteristics to consider when selecting therapy.

Disclosures: S. Draikiwicz has nothing to disclose. J. Oppenheimer has done consulting work for Glaxo, Myelin, Meda; adjudication for Quintiles; has research interests in AstraZenica, Genetec, Sanofi, Glaxo; has performed legal consultation for Malpractice Defense; and is a reviewer for Up-to-date, Annals of Allergy and Immunology, and the American Board of Allergy and Immunology.
Division of Allergy and Immunology, New Jersey Medical School, Newark, NJ, USA
[1] Present address: 57 Mounthaven Drive, Livingston, NJ 07039.
* Corresponding author. Pulmonary and Allergy Associates, 1 Springfield Avenue, Summit, NJ 07901, USA.
E-mail address: nallopp@optonline.net

ASTHMA

Asthma is an ongoing public health concern with more than 24 million individuals, approximately 7.3% of the total population, affected in the United States and an increase in prevalence between 2001 and 2010.[2,3] Total incremental cost of asthma in the United States was estimated to be $56 billion in 2007.[4] Current National Heart Blood and Lung Association and Global Initiative for Asthma guidelines recommend a stepwise approach to therapy.[5,6] Even with adherence to guideline therapy, including combination inhaled corticosteroids (ICS) and long-acting beta-agonist (LABA) therapy, as many as 50% of patients may continue to have suboptimal control.[7,8] Suboptimal control has been associated with lower physical and mental health–related quality of life, increased health care use, lower overall work productivity, and activity impairment.[9]

Studies show that a significant amount of uncontrolled asthma can be attributed to lack of adherence to prescribed therapy. Although approximately 60% to 70% of patients evaluated in an acute care setting fill initial prescriptions for asthma medication, one study suggests that only 14% to 16% of patients may maintain satisfactory ($\geq$80% medication availability) adherence over a 6-month period.[10,11] Beyond intentional nonadherence, failure of medication delivery may affect as many as 40% to 80% of adherent asthmatics because of inappropriate inhaler technique (nonintentional nonadherence).[12,13] Attaining control may also be impeded by obesity, active smoke exposure, allergies, psychiatric conditions, low socioeconomic status, as well as other underlying health conditions.[14,15] Accounting for these comorbidities still leaves approximately 10% or less of asthmatics on appropriate therapy who continue to have severe refractory asthma.[16] Severe asthma is classified as asthma that requires treatment with high-dose ICS plus a second controller and/or systemic corticosteroids to prevent it from becoming uncontrolled or that remains uncontrolled despite this therapy.[17] Patients with severe or difficult-to-treat asthma have higher health care use, with research showing as much as 3 times the direct medical costs and 10 times greater indirect medical costs compared with mild asthma.[18] Taken together, these patients may account for approximately 50% of direct expenditure on asthma care.[19]

Advances in the understanding of the pathophysiology of asthma have revealed that asthma is a heterogeneous disorder.[20] Multiple subgroups have been identified within the severe asthma population, which can further be stratified into specific phenotypes and endotypes.[21] The goal of phenotyping is to correlate cellular and clinical features with individual patient disease characteristics in an attempt to improve the choice of therapy.[22] Coinciding with the better understanding of the pathophysiology of asthma, the advent of immunomodulatory biologic therapy has emerged as a potential treatment option for individuals with severe refractory asthma. Omalizumab was the first monoclonal antibody approved for treatment in asthmatics in 2003, followed by mepolizumab in 2015, and reslizumab in March 2016. Multiple additional biologics are under study and are likely soon to be available for use in severe asthmatics. Choosing the optimal individual biologic requires a thorough understanding of the severe asthmatic's clinical characteristics and correlating with the patient's phenoendotype.

ASTHMA PHENOTYPING

The severe asthma phenotype characteristically has a reduced or refractory response to corticosteroid therapy.[23] Although there is no current biomarker to definitively delineate this group of individuals and classification depends on clinical course, to optimize the likelihood of clinical efficacy of biologic therapy additional phenotyping is required. Many different phenotypes of asthma have been described, including classifications stratified by causal or trigger factor, type of airflow obstruction, severity and response to treatments, radiological findings, or nature of airway inflammation.[23] A definitive method of classifying asthma phenotypes has not gained a consensus.[24]

Cluster analysis has been used in an attempt to classify underlying asthma phenotypes because of its ability to quantify similarity between individuals and use these metrics to create distinct populations in a less biased form.[25] In a 2008 study by Haldar and colleagues,[25] 4 clusters were identified in 187 refractory asthmatics receiving specialty care:

1. Early-onset atopic asthma with evidence of airway dysfunction and eosinophilic airway inflammation.
2. Obese subgroup with female preponderance with evidence of asthma symptoms but absence of eosinophilic airway inflammation.
3. Early-onset, symptom-predominant group with minimal eosinophilic disease.
4. Eosinophilic inflammation-predominant group with few symptoms, late-onset disease, and a greater proportion of men.

Cluster analysis was performed by Moore and colleagues[26] in the Severe Asthma Research Program (SARP) cohort, including 726 subjects diagnosed with severe refractory asthma. In this group, 5 distinct clusters were identified:

1. Early-onset atopic asthma with normal lung function treated with 2 or fewer controller medications.
2. Early-onset atopic asthma and preserved lung function but with increased use of medication and health care use.
3. Older obese women with late-onset nonatopic asthma, frequent oral corticosteroid use, and moderate reductions in forced expiratory volume in 1 second (FEV_1).
4. and 5. Severe airflow obstruction with bronchodilator responsiveness is shared between the groups.

However, cluster 4 had more frequent childhood onset and atopic disease with an equal gender distribution. Cluster 5 had the longest duration of asthma and a female predominance with the most severe airflow limitation at baseline and retained obstruction even after use of a bronchodilator.

The prognostic value of cluster analysis in the phenotyping of severe asthma is unclear. A subsequent analysis evaluating 4 of the SARP clusters showed no difference in asthma control–related outcomes, including exacerbation rate, time to first exacerbation, and treatment requirements.[27] The goal of identifying distinct groups is to correlate these with unique pathophysiologic mechanisms of disease to guide treatment decisions.[22] Cluster analysis elucidates the marked heterogeneity of phenotypes within the severe asthmatic population. When considering the use of a biologic agent, correlation of patient clinical clustering with type 2 high (Th2 high) biomarkers provides insight when determining anticipated response to therapy.

ASTHMA ENDOTYPES

Th2 allergic inflammation is present in up to 80% of children and 50% of adults with asthma.[28] Suggested biomarkers of Th2 high asthma phenotypes include periostin, fraction of exhaled nitric oxide, and sputum/blood eosinophils.[29] Periostin stimulates transforming growth factor-B, which leads to increased secretion of type 1 collagen by airway fibroblasts.[30] Periostin expression in airway epithelial cells is regulated by Th2 cytokines interleukin (IL)-4 and IL-13.[31] IL-13 has also been identified as a stimulator of dipeptidyl peptidase-4 (DPP4) in bronchial epithelial cells. DPP4 has been shown to increase proliferation of lung fibroblasts, bronchial smooth muscle cells, and the production of fibronectin.[32] Fractional excretion of nitric oxide (FeNO) is upregulated by cytokines IL-4 and IL-13, which induce nitric oxide synthase.[33] Besides its use as a marker of Th2 inflammation, FeNO has also been suggested as a marker of eosinophilic airway inflammation. Th2 cells release IL-5 and IL-13 into the airway epithelium and submucosa leading to the consequent increase in airway and serum eosinophilia. Genomic analysis of asthmatics has also associated increased immunoglobulin (Ig) E levels with an underlying systemic Th2 upregulation.[34] Noted that these markers in isolation are unable to classify a specific phenotype. The correlation between FeNO as a marker of a distinct eosinophilic phenotype and of Th2 inflammation has shown conflicting results. Studies involving mepolizumab have shown a dissociation between blood and sputum eosinophil counts and FeNO levels indicating that additional cytokines are responsible for regulating nitric oxide synthase, separate from those that control eosinophilia.[35] Furthermore, eosinophilic inflammation is found in both allergic as well as nonallergic patients with asthma, suggesting that eosinophilia is not the sole result of atopic habitus.[36] This suggestion is borne out by the cluster analysis from Haldar and colleagues.[25] These data suggest that further investigation is required to better delineate the likely multiple pathways that are associated with severe refractory asthma.

Data from SARP as well as prior cluster analysis have identified a distinct population of severe refractory patients with asthma with a neutrophilic predominance.[26] T-helper (Th)-1 and Th17 cell responses have been associated with this phenotype.[37] Th-1 cells are characterized by increased production of interferon-gamma, whereas Th-17 cells mediate neutrophil activation.[38] Mechanistically, Th-17 cells are also thought to contribute to steroid resistance in select populations based on mouse models.[39] In humans, bronchoalveolar levels of IL-17 have been found to correlate with disease severity in neutrophil-predominant asthma.[37] The identification of neutrophilic/Th-1 severe refractory asthma as a unique phenotype is reinforced by clinical evidence of reduced improvement in pulmonary function testing following beta-agonist treatment in this population, which is suggestive of airway remodeling.[40]

Although a significant amount of data suggests an overlap of Th-1 responses and neutrophilic asthma, Th-1 cells have also been shown to induce airway hyperreactivity independently of neutrophilic inflammation.[41] Similarly, independent environmental factors have a direct effect on neutrophilic asthma, with smoking, systemic inflammation, and infections increasing airway neutrophilia.[42–44] This finding argues against a direct correlation between an underlying Th-1 genoendotype and neutrophilic asthma as a resultant phenotype. Furthermore, an association between obesity and late-onset neutrophilic asthma has also been detected.[45]

Ultimately, sufficient data exist indicating that Th-1 and Th-17 pathways are possible therapeutic targets in asthma therapy. It is likely that a strata of subtypes exists within the non–Th2-driven asthmatic population. However, the precise clinical phenotype in which these agents offer maximal efficacy needs to be further identified.

THERAPEUTIC BIOLOGICS IN PATIENTS WITH ASTHMA
Anti–Immunoglobulin E

The first new biologic agent available for the treatment of asthma was omalizumab, which was approved by the US Food and Drug Administration in 2003 for use in patients 12 years of age and older with moderate to severe atopic asthma, a total serum IgE level between 30 and 700 IU/mL, and who are currently using ICS with incomplete control.[46] Omalizumab is a recombinant monoclonal antibody that reduces circulating IgE levels by binding to the constant region of the human IgE molecule.[47] Initial approval of omalizumab was based on 3 randomized, double-blind, placebo-controlled, multicenter trials.[46] In a trial by Busse and colleagues,[48] 525 subjects with severe allergic asthma requiring daily inhaled ICS were randomized to receive placebo or omalizumab. There were significantly fewer asthma exacerbations in the omalizumab group, with approximately a 10% absolute reduction in frequency, compared with placebo. However, similar study recruitment criteria and designs led to equivocal results in trials by Soler and colleagues[49] and Milgrom and colleagues.[50]

The EXTRA (Exploring the effects of omalizumab in allergic asthma) trial was a prospective, multicenter, randomized, parallel-group, double-blind, placebo-controlled study assessing omalizumab safety and efficacy in uncontrolled severe asthmatics. Enrolled patients required a diagnosis of severe persistent allergic asthma for greater than 1 year before trial screening and needed to remain inadequately controlled despite high-dose ICS and LABA. Omalizumab dosing was consistent with the drug's dosing table from its package insert (based on the patient's body weight and serum IgE level). Initial results indicated that asthma exacerbation rates were significantly lower during the trial period in the omalizumab group compared with the placebo group (incidence rate of 0.66 compared with 0.88).[51] Posthoc analysis divided the 850 enrolled subjects into Th2 high and low groups, with the Th2 high group having an FeNO greater than or equal to 24 parts per billion, blood eosinophil level greater than or equal to 260/μL, and serum periostin level greater than or equal to 50 ng/mL at baseline. Comparing high versus low subgroups, the Th2 high group showed significant reductions of exacerbations in the high versus low group (53% vs 16% FeNO, 32% vs 9% eosinophils, and 30% vs 3% periostin). The difference between the high and low groups has strong clinical implications reinforcing the importance of appropriate phenotypic discrimination in current practice.

A retrospective case-control study assessed allergic asthmatics, comparing the efficacy of omalizumab on pulmonary function testing in 81 asthmatic subjects with chronic rhinosinusitis and those without.[52] Analysis was performed on patients at a tertiary university clinic, analyzing outcomes of prescribed therapy over 7 years. An average treatment duration of 25 months with omalizumab revealed improved FEV_1, forced vital capacity, FEV_1/forced vital capacity ratio, and forced expiratory flow in 25% to 75% of subjects with chronic rhinosinusitis. Three of these parameters showed significant improvement compared with patients without chronic rhinosinusitis, who did not show a significant improvement in any of the study end points.

Current data indicate omalizumab to have anticipated clinical benefit in a Th2 high population and that IgE may not be the best prognostic indicator of effectiveness despite applicability criteria. Further data are required to delineate the effect of omalizumab on severe refractory intrinsic asthma compared with improved outcomes achieved from controlling exacerbating conditions, such as concomitant rhinosinusitis.

Anti–Interleukin-5

Mepolizumab is currently approved for use in patients with severe eosinophilic asthma.[53] Mepolizumab is a humanized monoclonal antibody against IL-5 that in turn reduces airway and systemic eosinophilia. Current prescribing parameters necessitate a blood eosinophil threshold of greater than or equal to 150 cell/μL at treatment initiation or blood eosinophil count of greater than or equal to 300 cells/μL in the 12 months before treatment initiation. Patients must also have uncontrolled asthma despite receiving maximal standard therapy with a high-dose ICS and at least

1 additional controller medication. Initial trials with mepolizumab failed to show significant changes in clinical measures of asthma (airway hyperresponsiveness, FEV$_1$, or peak flow recordings) despite reductions in blood and sputum eosinophil counts.[54,55] In the initial trial, 24 volunteers with mild atopic asthma controlled with short-acting beta-agonists (SABA) were recruited. Following this, a dose-ranging trial of 362 subjects enrolled subjects with persistent asthma symptoms despite the use of ICS therapy (400–1000 g µg of beclomethasone or equivalent). Subjects received injections of mepolizumab, either 250 mg, 750 mg, or placebo, at 4-week intervals for a total of 3 doses across 12 weeks. Although there was a trend toward improvement of exacerbation rates, SABA use, and quality of life in the 750-mg group, it did not reach statistical significant compared with other groups.

A subsequent trial by Haldar and colleagues[35] was conducted in a population of refractory asthmatics with a sputum eosinophil count of more than 3% on at least 1 occasion (within 2 years before study enrollment) despite high-dose ICS treatment. The study was a single-center, randomized, double-blind, placebo-controlled, parallel-group clinical trial in which subjects were randomized to receive either mepolizumab 750 mg or placebo. Subjects were treated monthly over the course of 1 year. The mepolizumab group showed an exacerbation relative risk of 0.57 compared with placebo, although there were no significant differences in change from baseline in symptom scores or between-group differences in changes in FEV$_1$ after bronchodilator use.

The DREAM (mepolizumab for severe eosinophilic asthma) trial with mepolizumab was a multicenter, double-blind, placebo-controlled trial evaluating subjects with a history of refractory asthma previously requiring systemic corticosteroid treatment 2 or more times in the period before screening and with 1 of the following criteria: a sputum eosinophil count of 3% or more, a FeNO of 50 ppb or more, serum eosinophil count of 0.3×10^9, or deterioration of asthma control following a 25% reduction or less of inhaled or oral corticosteroids.[56] Subjects were randomized in a 1:1:1:1 fashion to 75 mg, 250 mg, 750 mg of mepolizumab or placebo and received 13 infusions at 4-week intervals. Compared with placebo, the mepolizumab groups showed significant reductions in exacerbations per patient year, ranging from 39% to 52% risk reduction.

Reslizumab is a humanized monoclonal antibody composed of complementarity-determining regions of a murine antibody to human IL-5, which prevents binding of IL-5 to eosinophils.[57] Current prescribing guidelines for reslizumab indicate use in patients greater than or equal to 18 years of age as add-on maintenance therapy in patients with an eosinophilic phenotype. An initial clinical trial was conducted with 106 subjects who had incompletely controlled asthma despite treatment with high-dose ICS and at least 1 other agent.[57] Subjects required a minimum of 3% eosinophils on sputum analysis as part of recruitment criteria. The study was a randomized (1:1), double-blind, placebo-controlled, multinational study with treatment of reslizumab (3.0 mg/kg) or placebo every 4 weeks for 3 total doses. At study end, significant improvements in the primary end point Asthma Control Questionnaire score was found in the reslizumab group compared with placebo (59% compared with 40%). Statistical improvements were also evident in FEV$_1$ in the reslizumab group with an associated reduction in sputum and blood eosinophil levels.

Further study of reslizumab was conducted in 2 duplicate, multicenter, double-blind, parallel-group, randomized (1:1), placebo-controlled trials.[58] Subjects were aged 12 to 75 years with at least 400 eosinophils/µL in serum during the run-in period of 2 to 4 weeks. During this time, subjects were required to have inadequately controlled asthma while receiving at least medium-dose ICS (with or without another controller medication). Placebo or reslizumab, at 3 mg/kg, were administered every

4 weeks for a total of 13 doses, with 489 and 464 subjects randomly assigned in each study respectively. In these populations reslizumab significantly reduced the annual rate of exacerbations by 50% to 59% compared with placebo. Significant improvements were also seen in FEV_1, patient-reported quality of life, patient-reported symptoms score, and blood eosinophil count compared with placebo.

Benralizumab is a humanized monoclonal antibody that targets human IL-5 receptor-α on eosinophils and basophils.[59] Initial clinical study included adult asthmatics requiring medium-dose to high-dose ICS in combination with LABA therapy for at least 1 year with 2 to 6 exacerbations during that time who were stratified by eosinophilic phenotype. Eosinophilic phenotype was determined by FeNO (used as a surrogate marker of eosinophilic status) or increased eosinophil/lymphocyte and eosinophil/neutrophil index. Individuals with an eosinophilic phenotype were randomized (1:1:1:1) to receive 2 mg, 20 mg, 100 mg of benralizumab, or placebo. Noneosinophilic individuals were included in the study and randomized (1:1) to either 100 mg of benralizumab or placebo. Three-hundred and twenty-four individuals were randomized by eosinophilic stratification with 285 randomized to the noneosinophilic group. In the eosinophilic arm, significant reduction of annual exacerbations was found in the group receiving 100 mg of benralizumab compared with placebo but not the 2-mg or 20-mg groups. FEV_1 and Asthma Control Questionnaire-6 score were also improved compared with placebo in the eosinophilic group across all benralizumab doses. In the noneosinophilic arm, no significant difference in exacerbation rates was evident between benralizumab 100 mg and placebo but there was a trend toward reduced exacerbation rates. Additional subgroup analysis was performed using 300 eosinophils/μL as a cutoff, finding exacerbation rates were significantly reduced by 40% to 60% compared with placebo across benralizumab 20-mg and 100-mg groups. In contrast, no significant reduction in exacerbations was noted with 20 mg or 100 mg of benralizumab in the subgroup analysis in subjects with fewer than 300 eosinophils/μL. All doses of benralizumab decreased blood eosinophil counts compared with placebo.

Overall, anti–IL-5 therapy seems to be most clinically effective in patients with an eosinophilic phenotype. As previously mentioned, FeNO may not be a consistent marker of an eosinophilic phenotype, as exemplified by the discrepancy in efficacy seen in the benralizumab trial when comparing the eosinophilic study arm (stratified by FeNO) with the subsequent subgroup analysis in which subjects were stratified by serum eosinophil count (<300 or >300 eosinophils/μL). Furthermore, although serum eosinophilia of greater than 150 cells/μL is sufficient in certain circumstances to warrant mepolizumab administration, accounting for the data from anti–IL-5 agents as a whole best supports the use of these agents in asthmatics with greater than or equal to 300 eosinophils/μL.

Anti–Interleukin-13

Lebrikizumab is a humanized monoclonal antibody that binds to soluble IL-13.[60] IL-13 has been implicated in the Th2 pathway of asthma pathogenesis, has been shown to induce B-cell production of IgE, and has been strongly correlated with production of periostin.[61,62] Lebrikizumab was studied in 218 asthmatics using low-dose to high-dose ICS for 6 months before screening with evidence of uncontrolled asthma on day of randomization.[60] Subjects were allowed to continue LABA and other controller medications if already prescribed. Lebrikizumab 250 mg or placebo was given once per month for 6 total doses in this double-blind, placebo-controlled, parallel-group, multicenter study. Baseline FEV_1 was greater by 5.5% by week 12 in the lebrikizumab group compared with placebo, with effect maintained throughout the study duration.

Although not initially defined at study onset, subsequent subgroup analysis revealed a change in the baseline FEV_1 of the subjects of 8.2% in the periostin high group and 1.6% in the periostin low group compared with placebo. No significant effect was noted in exacerbation rate or asthma control scores in either the primary lebrikizumab group or analyzed subgroups. This finding highlights the importance of appropriate phenotypic discrimination and the effect it can have on therapeutic efficacy.

Subsequently a dose-ranging, randomized (1:1:1:1), double-blind, placebo-controlled study by Noonan and colleagues[63] evaluated efficacy and safety of lebrikizumab at varying doses (125 mg, 250 mg, 500 mg) in 212 subjects. Subjects were asthmatics not receiving ICS who received 4 total doses of lebrikizumab or placebo dosed every 4 weeks. Stratification across treatment arms was based on baseline IgE levels (> or <100 IU/mL) and peripheral blood eosinophil count (> or <0.14 × 10^9). No statistically significant change in FEV_1 was noted in subjects in any treatment group compared with placebo, including subsequent subgroup analysis stratified by periostin. Significant reduction of protocol-defined treatment failure and FeNO was identified in the lebrikizumab group but there was no differential response by periostin level. Discrepancy between these results and those reported earlier were attributed by the investigators to either insufficient power or IL-13 possibly having a greater role in steroid-insensitive subjects (subjects in this trial were mild asthmatics on no ICS).

Additional data regarding lebrikizumab efficacy are available in LUTE and VERSE (Lebrikizumab in moderate-to-severe asthma: pooled data from two randomized placebo-controlled studies) trials, which were replicate, randomized, double-blind, placebo-controlled studies evaluating 463 subjects.[64] Study populations were uncontrolled adult asthmatics receiving medium-dose to high-dose ICS and a second controller. Randomization occurred in a 1:1:1:1 ratio between doses of 37.5 mg, 125 mg, 250 mg of lebrikizumab, and placebo. Median duration of treatment was 24.1 weeks with dosing of study drug or placebo occurring every 4 weeks. Prespecified subgroup analysis was conducted based on periostin levels (periostin high [>50 ng/mL]) versus periostin low [<50 ng/mL] groups). There was a significant reduction in asthma exacerbations of 60% in the periostin high group compared with placebo and a nonsignificant (5% reduction) in exacerbation rates in the periostin low group. No clear dose-response relationship was observed. Mean relative change in baseline FEV_1 was 9.1% and 2.6% for the pooled periostin high and periostin low lebrikizumab groups respectively compared with placebo.

Anti–IL-13 agents have the greatest data supporting efficacy in patients with an increased periostin level (>50 ng/mL). Data are present to account for reduced exacerbation rates and improved FEV_1 in this population. Earlier studies with lebrikizumab highlight the importance of identifying appropriate candidates before initiating treatment.

Anti-Interleukin-4 and Interleukin-13

Dupilumab is a fully human monoclonal antibody to the IL-4 receptor-a, which inhibits both IL-4 and IL-13 signaling pathways.[65] IL-4 and IL-13 share redundancy in signaling and additional benefit may be seen from blocking both pathways. One-hundred and four adult moderate to severe asthmatic subjects were studied in a randomized (1:1), double-blind, placebo-controlled study. Eligible subjects required a blood eosinophil count of greater than or equal to 300 cells/μL or an increased sputum eosinophil level (≥3%) with poorly controlled symptoms despite the use of medium-dose to high-dose ICS and LABA therapy at study screen. Dupilumab 300 mg or placebo was administered once weekly for 12 weeks. A significant reduction in exacerbations of

87% was evident in the dupilumab group compared with placebo. Secondary end points, including lung function metrics, asthma symptoms, and beta-agonist rescue use, also were significantly improved compared with placebo. Although both FeNO and IgE levels were decreased in the dupilumab group, there was notably no decrease in peripheral blood eosinophils compared with placebo.

Similar to the other biologics described, dupilumab targets asthmatics with a Th2-driven response. The dual inhibition of both IL-4 and IL-13 pathways may account for what can initially be considered a more robust response compared with agents that target solely IL-4 or IL-13. More data are required to confirm its efficacy but preliminary data suggest a use in patients with an eosinophilic phenotype including increased serum or sputum eosinophil levels.

Anti–Interleukin-17

Brodalumab is a human anti–IL-17 receptor-A immunoglobulin monoclonal antibody that blocks activity of both IL-17 and IL-25.[66] Brodalumab was studied in 315 adult subjects with physician-diagnosed moderate to severe asthma who at screening were stable on ICS with or without additional LABA. Subjects were evaluated in a randomized, double-blind, placebo-controlled, dose-ranging study with randomization occurring 1:1:1:1 to receive brodalumab 140 mg, 210 mg, 280 mg, or placebo. Administration was performed subcutaneously at 7 visits across 10 weeks. No statistical significance was found in either the primary end point of improved Asthma Control Questionnaire score or in any secondary end points of lung function or asthma symptoms. The lack of clinical efficacy was suggested to be secondary to the heterogeneous nature of asthma and selective mechanism of action of monoclonal antibodies. A prespecified subgroup analysis showed a significant change in Asthma Control Questionnaire score in a subpopulation that best fit clusters 2 and 4 from the Moore and colleagues[26] cluster analysis (early-onset atopic asthma and preserved lung function and severe airflow obstruction with bronchodilator responsiveness). Study investigators hypothesized that additional study of brodalumab targeting a phenotype similar in characteristics to the aforementioned clusters may result in more significant clinical efficacy. This study highlights the importance of using phenotypic discriminators to carefully choose an optimal target population and without which a potential clinical utility may be missed.

Anti–Tumor Necrosis Factor

Infliximab is a recombinant human-murine monoclonal antibody that binds and neutralizes soluble tumor necrosis factor-alpha (TNF-a).[67] Infliximab was studied in a population of 38 adult subjects with moderate to severe persistent asthma in a double-blind, placebo-controlled, parallel-group study. Subjects underwent 1:1 randomization and received 3 infusions over a 6-week period with 5 mg/kg of infliximab or placebo. A significant increase was found in the primary end point of morning peak expiratory flow in the infliximab group. A significant difference was also found in the number exacerbations experienced in the infliximab and placebo groups, with 72% of patients in the placebo group experiencing exacerbations compared with 29% in the infliximab group. No significant difference was found between groups regarding SABA use, asthma symptom scores, or FEV_1.

Increased neutrophilia in sputum and airway responsiveness has also been observed in response to inhalation of TNF-a in normal individuals.[68] A subset of the SARP phenotype had neutrophilic-predominant asthma, suggesting a possible role for TNF-a inhibition and an effect on airway neutrophilia/inflammation. Evaluation of a TNF-a blocking agent was performed using golimumab in the uncontrolled severe asthma population.[69] The study population was limited to subjects who showed asthma symptoms on more than a third of days for at least 3 months before screening despite being on high-dose ICS and LABA therapy. Assessment was conducted in a phase 2, multicenter, randomized, double-blind, dose-ranging, placebo-controlled study. Dosing was every 4 weeks for a total of 52 weeks with either 50 mg, 100 mg, 200 mg of golimumab, or placebo based on 1:1:1:1 randomization. No significant difference was found between placebo and golimumab for exacerbations or FEV_1 during study protocol, although a trend was noted toward reduced exacerbations in the higher dose groups. However, unfavorable risk-benefit data led to discontinuation of the study because an increased number of severe adverse effects, primarily infections, were noted in the treatment arms. Of greatest concern is a significant safety signal concerning malignancy seen with the use of TNF-a blockade. In a study by Wenzel and colleagues,[69] 8 malignancies were seen in the active group of one study of 309 subjects compared with none in the placebo group.

Anti-TNF-a agents are best classified as targeting asthmatics with a Th-1 response, whereas previous biologic therapies focus on an underlying Th2 phenotype. However, safety data preclude use in this population at this time (**Table 1**).

URTICARIA

Chronic spontaneous urticaria (CSU) is the spontaneous appearance of wheals, angioedema, or both for greater than 6 weeks.[70] CSU is a significant public health concern with an annual population prevalence of approximately 0.5% to 1% and an annual lifetime prevalence of 20%.[71,72] Although most CSU resolves within 5 years, as many as 20% of cases can persist for longer.[72] Wheals are characterized by a perivascular nonnecrotizing infiltrate, primarily composed of mononuclear cells and neutrophils 60 minutes after wheal onset.[73,74] Disease activity is associated with reduced quality of life as well as increased health care use.[75]

The mechanism of CSU remains to be elucidated, although current evidence suggests that mast cells are important contributors.[70] It has been identified that as many as 30% to 40% of patients with CSU have autoimmune involvement with a circulating antibody directed to the alpha subunit of the high-affinity type I IgE receptor(FceR1) on mast cells.[76] The result of this antibody binding is degranulation of

Table 1	
The mechanisms of action of individual therapeutics	
Drug Name	**Mechanism of Action**
Omalizumab	Reduces circulating IgE by binding to the constant region of the human IgE molecule[47]
Mepolizumab Reslizumab	Binds free IL-5, which reduces airway and systemic eosinophilia[53,57]
Benralizumab	Binds IL-5 receptor-alpha on eosinophils and basophils[59]
Lebrikizumab	Binds to circulating IL-13, reducing airway periostin and DPP4 levels[60]
Dupilumab	Inhibits both IL-4 and IL-13 signaling pathways by binding to IL-4 receptor-alpha[65]
Brodalumab	Anti–IL-17 receptor-A, which blocks IL-17 and IL-25 pathways
Infliximab Golimumab	Binds and neutralizes soluble TNF-a, a key regulator of innate immunity and the Th-1 response[67,69]

the mast cell and histamine release.[77] Attempts to further classify patients with CSU include a study in which subjects were stratified into 5 groups:

- Immunoreactive histamine-releasing anti-FceR1 autoantibodies
- Immunoreactive anti-FceR1 autoantibodies without histamine-releasing activity
- Anti-IgE–like autoantibodies
- Serum with a mast cell–specific histamine-releasing factor
- Others that remain unidentified[78]

Classification of patients into these categories has direct clinical significance because patients with serum histamine-releasing activity typically have greater number, larger size, and more frequent wheals.[79]

Current guidelines recommend confirmation of CSU with the exclusion of other possible causes, including physical urticarias, drugs, foods, and infectious agents.[70] Initial therapy is with second-generation H1-antihistamines, which may be increased up to 4-times the recommended dose. In patients who fail H1-antihistamine therapy, guidelines recommend the use of either cyclosporine, montelukast, or the biologic omalizumab. Additional therapeutics have been studied either with the rationale of limiting histamine-releasing autoantibodies or reducing inflammation and coagulation biomarkers.[80]

THERAPEUTIC BIOLOGICS IN PATIENTS WITH CHRONIC SPONTANEOUS URTICARIA
Omalizumab

Omalizumab has been approved for use in patients with refractory chronic spontaneous urticaria despite high-dose H1 antihistamines since March 2014 in both the United States and Europe. The known mechanism of IgG binding to the high-affinity IgE receptor in a significant proportion of patients with chronic autoimmune urticaria prompted investigation of the use of omalizumab in these patients.

The initial proof-of-concept study of omalizumab was performed by Saini and colleagues[81] in 2011. The study was a prospective, double-blind, placebo-controlled, dose-ranging study evaluating the use of omalizumab in subjects 12 to 75 years of age with an Urticaria Activity Score of greater than 12 over 7 days despite antihistamine therapy. Ninety subjects were randomized 1:1:1:1 to receive either placebo, 75, 300, or 600 mg of omalizumab in addition to standard antihistamine therapy. Onset of effect was apparent within 1 to 2 weeks with a significant decrease in the Urticaria Activity Score in both the 300-mg and 600-mg groups with omalizumab.

Additional trials included several phase 3, multicenter, randomized, double-blind studies evaluating 323 subjects with moderate to severe chronic idiopathic urticaria who were symptomatic despite use of antihistamines.[82] Subjects were required to have a history of at least 6 months of chronic idiopathic urticaria and hives associated with itching for at least 8 consecutive weeks at a time despite use of antihistamines. Subjects with physical urticarias were excluded from these studies. Subjects were randomized to receive 3 injections every 4 weeks of either 75 mg, 150 mg, 300 mg, or placebo. Significant reductions in itch-severity score, the primary outcome measure, was evident in the 150-mg and 300-mg group at week 12 compared with baseline itch scores. Improvements were also seen in all prespecified secondary end points, including change from baseline Urticaria Activity Score, weekly number of hives, angioedema-free days over 8 weeks, and improvement in Dermatology Life Quality Index.

Subsequently a trial was performed assessing the effect of 300 mg of omalizumab in subjects aged 12 to 75 years who remained symptomatic despite treatment with H1-

antihistamines at up to 4 times the approved dose plus H2-antihistamines, leukotriene antagonists, or both.[83] Subjects were enrolled from multiple centers in a 3:1 ratio to either omalizumab (n = 252) or placebo (n = 84) with dosing at 4-week intervals for a total of 24 weeks. Subjects were required to have active disease with an Urticaria Activity Score of 16 or greater over the week before randomization. Omalizumab was effective irrespective of the combination of concomitant medications, including angioedema-free days over an 8-week period, and proportion of patients who were itch and hive free. In the omalizumab group, 34% of subjects were completely itch and hive free compared with 5% in the placebo group at 12 weeks. Clinical trials support the use of omalizumab in patients with chronic spontaneous urticaria who are refractory to initial treatment with antihistamines or leukotriene antagonists. Additional phenotypic descriptors are unavailable at this time and it should be noted that, unlike its use in asthma, studies did not stratify by IgE level. Note also that the efficacy of omalizumab exceeds the initial postulated 30% to 40% of CSU thought to be caused by chronic autoimmune urticaria. Also, efficacy is fairly robust but heterogeneous with 34% of subjects in one trial achieving complete disease remission but with 66% with residual symptoms. Initial dose-ranging studies do not suggest that this is a dose-dependent effect and further study is warranted to better determine the patients most likely to respond to therapy.

Intravenous Immunoglobulin

Intravenous immunoglobulin (IVIG) is a polyvalent antibody product derived from pooled plasma of healthy donors that is thought to act through blockade of the Fc portion of IgG molecules.[84] It has also been suggested that IVIG may have direct inhibitor effects on B-cell and T-cell function.[85,86] One study evaluated the efficacy of IVIG 2 g/kg over 2 days in 6 subjects (aged 16–72 years) with recurrent severe CSU with daily symptoms requiring high-dose corticosteroids. Infusions were given every 4 to 6 weeks. Five of the 6 subjects had a significantly improved Urticaria Activity Score after the first 3 cycles.

O'Donnell and colleagues[84] also studied the effect of IVIG in 10 patients (aged 24–75 years) with CSU. All subjects had severe CSU that was poorly responsive to conventional treatment with antihistamines. Subjects all had evidence of serum histamine-releasing activity, as shown by a positive autologous intradermal serum test. Subjects were treated with 0.4 g/kg of IVIG over 5 days. Although subjects had a varied response to therapy, 9 subjects had improvement of urticaria. The mean Urticaria Activity Score improved from baseline of 24.6 to 12.6 at 2 weeks and 7.8 at 6 weeks after treatment. These data suggest a possible benefit of IVIG in patients with refractory urticaria. There are insufficient data to classify which patients will best respond or to identify a unique phenotypes. Nonetheless, the varied response of patients to IVIG suggests a potential underlying phenotype of responders (**Table 2**).

Rituximab

Rituximab is a chimeric murine/human recombinant monoclonal antibody that binds to CD20. Rituximab treatment results in B-cell depletion with a resultant decrease in the

Table 2	
The mechanism of action of intravenous immunoglobulin	
Drug Name	**Mechanism of Action**
IVIG	Circulating immune globulin G binds to act the Fc portion of IgG molecules[84]

production of IgG antibodies. Application in CSU is targeted at reducing antibody binding to the FceR1. The use of rituximab in patients with CSU is limited to case reports.[87,88] In a case report by Chakravarty and colleagues,[87] the investigators evaluated the use of rituximab in a patient in whom other causes of urticaria had been excluded and who had positive IgG autoantibodies to FceR1 on skin biopsy of an urticarial lesion. The patient had been previously treated with oral antihistamines, cyclosporine, mycophenolate mofetil, and even oral steroids. Four weekly infusions of rituximab were given at 375 mg/m^2 concurrently with methotrexate administration of 15 to 25 mg/wk subcutaneously. Resolution of symptoms was seen within 6 weeks of completion of rituximab therapy. A case report by Steinweg and Gaspari[88] evaluated a 38-year-old woman with a 1-year history of CSU refractory to fexofenadine, ranitidine, hydroxyzine, and even high-dose (60-mg) prednisone therapy. During a breakthrough episode requiring hospitalization the subject was infused with 1 g of rituximab followed by 1 g of rituximab 2 weeks later with complete remission of symptoms for 10 months.

Insufficient data are available at this time for any recommendations involving rituximab therapy. It may be considered in patients who are refractory to other, more established therapies.

Tumor Necrosis Factor-Alpha

TNF-a promoter polymorphisms have been associated with susceptibility to CSU.[89] Despite the recognition of genetic polymorphisms, conflicting data exist regarding the significance of a correlation between TNF-a levels and CSU.[90,91] Excluding physical urticarias and urticarial vasculitis, a total of 21 documented cases exist in which TNF-a inhibitors were used in cases of refractory chronic autoimmune urticaria or CSU.[92,93] The course of disease in the case series by Wilson and colleagues[93] was varied but there was a generalized improvement with initial treatment, although further pulses of therapy were occasionally needed for relapse. Sand and Thomsen[92] reported the results of TNF-a inhibitor therapy using adalimumab or etanercept in patients who had failed high-dose antihistamines with the addition of an immunosuppressive agent. Improvement was noted in 15 of the 18 patients studied with a diagnosis of CSU or chronic autoimmune urticaria. Complete resolution was seen in 12 of these 15 patients. Response to therapy was frequently seen in the first month but patients generally relapsed within a few weeks following discontinuation.

This group needs much more research to aid in determining the best phenotypes for therapy. There seems to be some indication of efficacy of TNF-a in patients with autoimmune disease. When the practice parameter for urticaria was examined, investigators concluded that the best data regarding biologic agents were for omalizumab.[94–116] However, there is a paucity of data regarding the group most likely to respond to therapy.

SUMMARY

Most biologics currently approved and in phase II and III clinical trials for use in asthmatics have shown benefit in a common Th2 high phenoendotype. Studies with these biologics have suggested that response can be predicted based on surrogate biomarkers of Th2 activity, including serum periostin levels, total IgE, sputum and blood eosinophil count, as well as FeNO. Further data are required to determine the optimal biologic based on clinically individualized patterns of these markers. There remains a lack of therapeutic options for patients with neutrophilic asthma expressing a Th2 low, Th-1, or Th-17 phenotype. The mixed results of both brodalumab and the TNF-a inhibitors suggests there is a phenotype that may benefit from these options but this population is yet to be characterized. In the case of urticaria and atopic dermatitis, there are much less robust data regarding phenotypic discriminators of the patients most likely to benefit from therapy. It is anticipated that further phenoendotypes may be identified as the underlying mechanism of these diseases becomes better understood. The population that benefits from biologic therapy in hereditary angioedema is well characterized but the subpopulations that may respond best to respective treatments remain to be identified.

Determining those patients most likely to benefit from therapy is of critical importance because clinicians must consider the pharmacoeconomic and societal costs of these new therapeutics. Average wholesale prices vary from tens to more than $100,000 per year. Regardless of indication, there is a surprising paucity of data regarding the pharmacoeconomics of these therapies. Although clinicians focus on controlling their patients' disease, often their response to lack of disease control can be simply to add further medicines. It can easily be seen that, in a health care system that has limits, clinicians must begin to take into account costs and try to optimize less expensive medicines and institute biologic agents only in patients who are most likely to benefit from their use.

The cost of long-term prophylaxis with C1 inhibitor concentrate in patients with hereditary angioedema has been estimated to be as high as €182,000 per year in Denmark.[117] In contrast, the cost of treating attacks with icatibant on an as-needed basis would be approximately €93,000 euros per year assuming an average of 4 attacks per month. Furthermore, the price of long-term prophylaxis with danazol has been estimated to be as much as 370 times less than C1 inhibitor concentrate. On-demand therapy does not necessarily equate to cost-effective care in America, with icatibant carrying a cost of approximately $6800 per dose and other therapies for acute attacks priced similarly.[118] Prophylactic treatment of hereditary angioedema with C1-esterase inhibitor is estimated to cost approximately $487,000 per year in the United States. Estimating 6000 patients with this diagnosis actively seeking treatment per year in the United States prices the annual societal cost of therapy at $2.9 billion dollars.

Although hereditary angioedema therapy raises significant concerns regarding cost-effectiveness of therapy, the diagnosis affects a fairly small number globally. The current and anticipated use of biologics in asthma, atopic dermatitis, and urticaria do not benefit from a similar low prevalence of disease. Despite omalizumab being approved in the United States for use in asthma since 2003 and for use in urticaria since 2014, few data are available regarding cost-effectiveness in America. The estimated direct cost of omalizumab prescriptions is between $15,000 and $44,000 in asthmatics.[119] Most studies regarding omalizumab cost-effectiveness are model based and do not represent material cost savings.[120,121]

It has never been of greater importance to correctly estimate patient outcome before starting therapy based on cost analysis. The significant cost of therapy combined with the growing indications for biologics implies that a trial-by-error model would be unsustainable. Treatment decisions need to be guided by appropriate patient stratification based on an understanding of each individual's underlying phenotype.

REFERENCES

1. Boyman O, Kaegi C, Akdis M, et al. EAACI IG Biologicals Task Force paper on the use of biologic agents in allergic disorders. Allergy 2015; 70(7):727–54.

2. Blackwell DL, Lucas JW, Clarke TC. Summary health statistics for U.S. adults: National Health Interview Survey, 2012. National Center For Health Statistics. Vital Health Stat 10 2014;260.
3. Akinbami L, Moorman J, Bailey C, et al. Trends in asthma prevalence, health care use, and mortality in the United States, 2001-2010. NCHS Data Brief 2012;(94):1–8.
4. Barnett S, Nurmagambetov TA. Costs of asthma in the United States: 2002-2007. J Allergy Clin Immunol 2011;127(1):145–52.
5. Global strategy for asthma management and prevention. Available at: www.ginaasthma.org. Accessed January 20, 2017.
6. Expert Panel Report 3. Guidelines for the Diagnosis and Management of Asthma – summary report 2007. J Allergy Clin Immunol 2007;120:S94–138.
7. Bateman ED, Boushey HA, Bousquet J, et al. Can guideline-defined asthma control be achieved? The Gaining Optimal Asthma Control study. Am J Respir Crit Care Med 2004;170(8):836–44.
8. Meltzer EO, Blaiss MS, Nathan RA, et al. Asthma burden in the United States: results of the 2009 Asthma Insight and Management survey. Allergy Asthma Proc 2012;33(1):36–46.
9. Williams SA, Wagner S, Kannan H, et al. The association between asthma control and health care utilization, work productivity loss and health-related quality of life. J Occup Environ Med 2009;51(7):780–5.
10. Kaijoka EH, Itoman EM, Li ML, et al. Pediatric prescription pick-up rates after ED visits. Am J Emerg Med 2005;23(4):454–8.
11. Feehan M, Ranker L, Durante R, et al. Adherence to controller asthma medications: 6-month prevalence across a US community pharmacy chain. J Clin Pharm Ther 2015;40:590–3.
12. Melani A, Bonavia M, Cilenti V, et al. Inhaler mishandling remains common in real life and is associated with reduced disease control. Respir Med 2011;105(6):930–8.
13. Press VG, Arora VM, Shah LM, et al. Misuse of respiratory inhalers in hospitalized patients with asthma or COPD. J Gen Intern Med 2011;26(6):635–42.
14. Patel MR, Leo HL, Baptist AP, et al. Asthma outcomes in children and adolescents with multiple morbidities: findings from the National Health Interview Survey. J Allergy Clin Immunol 2015;135(6):1444–9.
15. Vernon MK, Wiklund I, Bell JA, et al. What do we know about asthma triggers? A review of the literature. J Asthma 2012;49(10):991–8.
16. Se Wenzel, Busse WW. Severe asthma: lessons from the Severe Asthma Research Program. J Allergy Clin Immunol 2007;119(1):14–21.
17. Chung KF, Wenzel SE, Brozek JL, et al. International ERS/ATS guidelines on definition, evaluation and treatment of severe asthma. Eur Respir J 2014;42(2):343–73.
18. Cisternas M, Blanc P, Yen I, et al. A comprehensive study of the direct and indirect costs of adult asthma. J Allergy Clin Immunol 2003;111(6):1212–8.
19. Menzies-Gow A, Fan Chung K. Omalizumab for the treatment of severe allergic asthma. Expert Rev Clin Immunol 2008;4(5):543–8.
20. Gibeon D, Chung KF. The investigation of severe asthma to define phenotypes. Clin Exp Allergy 2012;42(5):678–92.
21. Hekking PP, Bel EH. Developing and emerging clinical asthma phenotypes. J Allergy Clin Immunol Pract 2014;2(6):671–80.
22. Chung KF, Adcock IM. Clinical phenotypes of asthma should link up with disease mechanisms. Curr Opin Allergy Clin Immunol 2015;15(1):56–62.

23. Nair P, Dasgupta A, Brightling CE, et al. How to diagnose and phenotype asthma. Clin Chest Med 2012;33(3):445–57.
24. Baines KJ, Simpson JL, Wood LG, et al. Transcriptional phenotypes of asthma defined by gene expression profiling of induced sputum samples. J Allergy Clin Immunol 2011;127(1):153–60.
25. Haldar P, Pavord ID, Shaw DE, et al. Cluster analysis and clinical asthma phenotypes. Am J Respir Crit Care Med 2008;178(3):218–24.
26. Moore WC, Meyers DA, Wenzel SE, et al. Identification of asthma phenotypes using cluster analysis in the Severe Asthma Research Program. Am J Respir Crit Care Med 2010;181(4):315–23.
27. Bourdin A, Molinari N, Vachier I, et al. Prognostic value of cluster analysis of severe asthma phenotypes. J Allergy Clin Immunol 2014;134(5):1043–50.
28. Pearce N, Pekkanen J, Beasley R. How much asthma is really attributable to atopy? Thorax 1999;54:236–72.
29. Fajt ML, Wenzel SE. Asthma phenotypes and the use of biologic medications in asthma and allergic disease: the next steps toward personalized care. J Allergy Clin Immunol 2015;135(2):299–310.
30. Fingleton J, Braithwaite I, Travers J, et al. Serum periostin in obstructive airways disease. Eur Respir J 2016;47(5):1383–91.
31. Takayama G, Arima K, Kanaji T, et al. Periostin: a novel component of subepithelial fibrosis of bronchial asthma downstream of IL-4 and IL-13 signals. J Allergy Clin Immunol 2006;118(1):98–104.
32. Shiobara T, Chibana K, Watanabe T, et al. Dipeptidyl peptidase-4 is highly expressed in bronchial epithelial cells of untreated asthma and it increases cell proliferation along with fibronectin production in airway constitutive cells. Respir Res 2016;17:28.
33. Mummadi SR, Hahn PY. Topics in practice management: update on exhaled nitric oxide in clinical practice. Chest 2015;149(5):1340–4.
34. Woodruff PG, Modrek B, Choy DF, et al. T-helper type 2-driven inflammation defines major subphenotypes of asthma. Am J Respir Crit Care Med 2009;180(5):388–95.
35. Haldar P, Brightling CE, Hargadon B, et al. Mepolizumab and exacerbations of refractory eosinophilic asthma. N Engl J Med 2009;360:973–84.
36. Parulekar AD, Diamant Z, Hanania NA. Role of T2 inflammation biomarkers in severe asthma. Curr Opin Pulm Med 2016;22(1):59–68.
37. Trevor JL, Deshane JS. Refractory asthma: mechanisms, targets, and therapy. Allergy 2014;69(7):817–27.
38. Chung KF. Asthma phenotyping: a necessity for improved therapeutic precision and new targeted therapies. J Intern Med 2016;279(2):192–204.
39. McKinley L, Alcorn JF, Peterson A, et al. TH17 cells mediate steroid-resistant airway inflammation and airway hyperresponsiveness in mice. J Immunol 2008;181(8):4089–97.
40. Shaw DE, Berry MA, Hargadon B, et al. Association between neutrophilic airway inflammation and airflow limitation in adults with asthma. Chest 2007;132(6):1871–5.
41. Cui J, Pazdziorko S, Miyashiro JS, et al. TH1-mediated airway hyperresponsiveness independent of neutrophilic inflammation. J Allergy Clin Immunol 2005;115(2):309–15.
42. Fu JJ, Baines KJ, Wood LG, et al. Systemic inflammation is associated with differential gene expression and airway neutrophilia in asthma. OMICS 2013;17(4):187–99.

43. St-Laurent J, Bergeron C, Page N, et al. Influence of smoking on airway inflammation and remodeling in asthma. Clin Exp Allergy 2008;38(10):1852–9.
44. Thomson NC. Novel approaches to the management of noneosinophilic asthma. Ther Adv Respir Dis 2016;10(3):211–34.
45. Rasmussen F, Hancox RJ. Mechanisms of obesity in asthma. Curr Opin Allergy Clin Immunol 2014;14(1):35–43.
46. Omalizuman [Package Insert] Novartis AG. © 2016 Genentech USA, Inc. Available at: https://www.gene.com/download/pdf/xolair_prescribing.pdf. Accessed January 20, 2017.
47. Licari A, Marseglia A, Caimmi S, et al. Omalizumab in children. Paediatr Drugs 2014;16(6):491–502.
48. Busse W, Corren J, Lanier BQ, et al. Omalizumab, anti-IgE recombinant humanized monoclonal antibody, for the treatment of severe allergic asthma. J Allergy Clin Immunol 2001;108(2):184–90.
49. Soler M, Matz J, Townley R, et al. The anti-IgE antibody omalizumab reduces exacerbations and steroid requirement in allergic asthmatics. Eur Respir J 2001; 18(2):254–61.
50. Milgrom H, Berger W, Nayak A, et al. Treatment of childhood asthma with anti-immunoglobulin E antibody (omalizumab). Pediatrics 2001;108(2):E36.
51. Hanania NA, Wenzel S, Rosen K, et al. Exploring the effects of omalizumab in allergic asthma: an analysis of biomarkers in the EXTRA study. Am J Respir Crit Care Med 2013;187(8):804–11.
52. Clavenna MJ, Turner JH, Samuelson M, et al. Differential effect of omalizumab on pulmonary function in patients with allergic asthma with and without chronic rhinosinusitis. Allergy Asthma Proc 2016;37(1):23–6.
53. Teach SJ, Gill MA, Togias A, et al. Preseasonal treatment with either omalizumab or an inhaled corticosteroid boost to prevent fall asthma exacerbations. J Allergy Clin Immunol 2015;136(6):1476–85.
54. Flood-Page PT, Menzies-Gow AN, Kay AB, et al. Eosinophil's role remains uncertain as anti-interleukin-5 only partially depletes numbers in asthmatic airway. Am J Respir Crit Care Med 2003;167(2):199–204.
55. Flood-Page P, Swenson C, Faiferman I, et al. A study to evaluate safety and efficacy of mepolizumab in patients with moderate persistent asthma. Am J Respir Crit Care Med 2007;176(11):1062–71.
56. Pavord ID, Korn S, Howarth P, et al. Mepolizumab for severe eosinophilic asthma (DREAM): a multicenter, double-blind, placebo-controlled trial. Lancet 2012;380(9842):651–9.
57. Castro M, Mathur S, Hargreave F, et al. Reslizumab for poorly controlled, eosinophilic asthma: a randomized: placebo-controlled study. Am J Respir Crit Care Med 2011;184(1):1125–32.
58. Castro M, Zangrilli J, Wechsler ME, et al. Reslizumab for inadequately controlled asthma with elevated blood eosinophil counts: results from two multicenter, parallel, double-blind, randomized, placebo-controlled, phase 3 trials. Lancet Respir Med 2015;3(5):355–66.
59. Castro M, Wenzel SE, Bleecker ER, et al. Benralizumab, an anti-interleukin 5 receptor a monoclonal antibody, versus placebo for uncontrolled eosinophilic asthma: a phase 2b randomized dose-ranging study. Lancet Respir Med 2014;2(11):879–90.
60. Corren J, Lemanske RF, Hanania NA, et al. Lebrikizumab treatment in adults with asthma. N Engl J Med 2011;365(12):1088–98.

61. Brightling CE, Saha S, Hollins F. Interleukin-13: prospects for new treatments. Clin Exp Allergy 2010;40(1):42–9.
62. Li W, Gao P, Zhi Y, et al. Periostin: its role in asthma and its potential as a diagnostic or therapeutic target. Respir Res 2015;16:57.
63. Noonan M, Korenblat P, Mosesova S, et al. Dose-ranging study of lebrikizumab in asthmatic patients not receiving inhaled steroids. J Allergy Clin Immunol 2013;132(3):567–74.
64. Hanania NA, Noonan M, Corren J, et al. Lebrikizumab in moderate-to-severe asthma: pooled data from two randomized placebo-controlled studies. Thorax 2015;70(8):748–56.
65. Wenzel S, Ford L, Pearlman D, et al. Dupilumab in persistent asthma with elevated eosinophil levels. N Engl J Med 2013;368(26):2455–66.
66. Busse WW, Holgate S, Kerwin E, et al. Randomized, double-blind, placebo-controlled study of brodalumab, a human anti-IL-17 receptor monoclonal antibody, in moderate to severe asthma. Am J Respir Crit Care Med 2013; 188(11):1294–302.
67. Eric EM, Leaker BR, Nicholson GC, et al. The effects of a monoclonal antibody directed against tumor necrosis factor-alpha in asthma. Am J Respir Crit Care Med 2006;174(7):753–62.
68. Thomas PS, Yates DH, Barnes PJ. Tumor necrosis factor-alpha increases airway responsiveness and sputum neutrophilia in normal human subjects. Am J Respir Crit Care Med 1995;152(1):76–80.
69. Wenzel SE, Barnes PJ, Bleecker ER, et al. A randomized, double-blind, placebo-controlled study of tumor necrosis factor-alpha blockage in severe persistent asthma. Am J Respir Crit Care Med 2009;179(7):549–58.
70. Zuberbier T, Aberer W, Asero R, et al, European Academy of Allergy and Clinical Immunology, Global Allergy and Asthma European Network, European Dermatology Forum, World Allergy Organization. The EAACI LEN/EDF/WAO guideline for the definition, classification, diagnosis, and management of urticaria: the 2013 revision and update. Allergy 2014;69(7):868–87.
71. Cooke A, Bulkhi A, Casale TB. Role of biologics in intractable urticarial. Biologics 2015;9:25–33.
72. Saini SS. Chronic spontaneous urticarial: etiology and pathogenesis. Immunol Allergy Clin North Am 2014;34(1):33–52.
73. Mekori YA, Giorno RC, Anderson P, et al. Lymphocyte subpopulations in the skin of patients with chronic urticarial. J Allergy Clin Immunol 1983;72(6):681–4.
74. Caproni M, Giomi B, Volpi W, et al. Chronic idiopathic urticarial: infiltrating cells and related cytokines in autologous serum-induced wheals. Clin Immunol 2005; 114(3):284–92.
75. Vietri J, Turner SJ, Tian H, et al. Effect of chronic urticarial on US patients: analysis of the National Health and Wellness Survey. Ann Allergy Asthma Immunol 2015;115(4):306–11.
76. Kikuchi Y, Kaplan AP. Mechanisms of autoimmune activation of basophils in chronic urticarial. J Allergy Clin Immunol 2001;104(6):1056–62.
77. Hide M, Francis DM, Grattan CEH, et al. Autoantibodies against the high-affinity IgE receptor as a cause of histamine release in chronic urticarial. N Engl J Med 1998;328:1599–604.
78. Sabroe RA, Fiebiger E, Francis DM, et al. Classification of anti-FcepsiolonRI and anti-IgE autoantibodies in chronic idiopathic urticarial and correlation with disease severity. J Allergy Clin Immunol 2002;110(3):492–9.

79. Alyasin S, Hamidi M, Karimi AA, et al. Correlation between clinical findings and results of autologous serum skin test in patients with chronic idiopathic urticarial. South Med J 2011;104(2):111–5.

80. Cugno M, Marazano AV, Asero R, et al. Activation of blood coagulation in chronic urticaria: pathophysiological and clinical implications. Intern Emerg Med 2010;5:97–101.

81. Saini S, Rosen KE, Hseigh HJ, et al. A randomized, placebo-controlled, dose-ranging study of single-dose omalizumab in patients with H1-antihistamine-refractory chronic idiopathic urticaria. J Allergy Clin Immunol 2011;128(3): 537–73.e1.

82. Maurer M, Rosen K, Hsieh H, et al. Omalizumab for the treatment of chronic idiopathic or spontaneous urticarial. N Engl J Med 2013;368:924–35.

83. Kaplan A, Ledford D, Asthby M, et al. Omalizumab in patients with symptomatic chronic idiopathic/spontaneous urticarial despite standard combination therapy. J Allergy Clin Immunol 2013;132(1):101–9.

84. O'Donnell BF, Barr RM, Black AK, et al. Intravenous immunoglobulin in autoimmune chronic urticarial. Br J Dermatol 1998;138(1):101–6.

85. Dwyer JM. Manipulating the immune system with immune globulin. N Engl J Med 1992;326:107–16.

86. Schwab I, Nimmerjahn F. Intravenous immunoglobulin therapy: how does IgG modulate the immune system? Nat Rev Immunol 2013;13(3):176–89.

87. Chakravarty SD, Yee AF, Paget SA. Rituximab successfully treats refractory chronic autoimmune urticarial caused by IgE receptor autoantibodies. J Allergy Clin Immunol 2011;128(6):1354–5.

88. Steinweg SA, Gaspari AA. Rituximab for the treatment of recalcitrant chronic autoimmune urticarial. J Drugs Dermatol 2015;14(12):1387.

89. Tavakol M, Amirzargar AA, Movahedi M, et al. Interleukin-6 and tumor necrosis factor-alpha gene polymorphisms in chronic idiopathic urticarial. Allergol Immunopathol (Madr) 2014;42(6):533–8.

90. Piconi S, Trabattoni D, Iemoli E, et al. Immune profiles of patients with chronic idiopathic urticarial. Int Arch Allergy Immunol 2002;128(1):59–66.

91. Tedeschi A, Lorini M, Suli C, et al. No evidence of tumor necrosis factor-alpha release in blood of patients with chronic urticarial. Allergy 2006;61(4):510–1.

92. Sand FL, Thomsen SF. TNF-alpha inhibitors for chronic urticaria: experience in 20 patients. J Allergy (Cairo) 2013;2013:130905.

93. Wilson LH, Eliason MJ, Leiferman KM, et al. Treatment of refractory chronic urticarial with tumor necrosis alfa inhibitors. J Am Acad Dermatol 2011;64(6): 1221–2.

94. Bernstein J, Lang D, Khan D, et al. The diagnosis and management of acute and chronic urticarial: 2014 update. J Allergy Clin Immunol 2014;133(5): 1270–7.e66.

95. Donaldson VH, Evans RR. A biochemical abnormality in hereditary angioneurotic edema: absence of serum inhibitor of C1-esterase. Am J Sci 1963;31: 37–44.

96. Cicardi M, Aberer W, Banerji A, et al. Classification, diagnosis, and approach to treatment for angioedema: consensus report from the Hereditary Angioedema International Working Group. Allergy 2014;69(5):602–16.

97. Zuraw BL, Bernstein JA, Lang DM, et al. A focused parameter update: hereditary angioedema, acquired C1 inhibitor deficiency, and angiotensin-converting enzyme inhibitor-associated angioedema. J Allergy Clin Immunol 2013;131(6): 1491–3.

98. Pappalardo E, Cicardi M, Duponchet C, et al. Frequent de novo mutations and exon deletions in the *C1inhibitor* gene of patients with angioedema. J Allergy Clin Immunol 2000;106(6):1147–54.

99. Dewald G, Bork K. Missense mutations in the coagulation factor XII (Hageman factor) gene in hereditary angioedema with normal C1 inhibitor. Biochem Biophys Res Commun 2006;343(4):1286–9.

100. Bygum A. Hereditary angioedema in Denmark: a nationwide survey. Br J Dermatol 2009;161(5):1153–8.

101. Bork K, Frank J, Grundt B, et al. Treatment of acute attacks in hereditary angioedema with a bradykinin receptor-2 antagonist (Icatibant). J Allergy Clin Immunol 2007;119(6):1497–503.

102. Craig T, Aygoren-Pursun E, Bork K, et al. WAO guideline for the management of hereditary angioedema. World Allergy Organ J 2012;5(12):182–99.

103. Zanichelli A, Vacchini R, Badini M, et al. Standard care impact on angioedema because of hereditary C1 inhibitor deficiency: a 21-month prospective study in a cohort of 103 patients. Allergy 2011;66(2):192–6.

104. Prematta M, Gibbs JG, Pratt EL, et al. Fresh frozen plasma for the treatment of hereditary angioedema. Ann Allergy Asthma Immunol 2007;98:383–8.

105. Gelfand JA, Sherins RJ, Alling DW, et al. Treatment of hereditary angioedema with danazol. Reversal of clinical and biochemical abnormalities. N Engl J Med 1976;295(26):1444–8.

106. Du-Thanh A, Raison-Peyron N, Drouet C, et al. Efficacy of tranexamic acid in sporadic idiopathic bradykinin angioedema. Allergy 2010;65:793–5.

107. Cicardi M, Banerji A, Bracho F, et al. Icatibant, a new bradykinin-receptor antagonist, in hereditary angioedema. N Engl J Med 2010;363(6):532–41.

108. Lumry WR, Li HH, Levy RJ, et al. Randomized placebo-controlled trial of the bradykinin B2 receptor antagonist icatibant for the treatment of acute attacks of hereditary angioedema: the FAST-3 trial. Ann Allergy Asthma Immunol 2011;107(6):529–37.

109. Sheffer AL, Campion M, Levry RJ, et al. Ecallantide (DX-88) for acute hereditary angioedema attacks: integrated analysis of 2 double-blind, phase 3 studies. J Allergy Clin Immunol 2011;128(1):153–9.

110. Levy RJ, Lumry WR, McNeil DL, et al. EDEMA4: a phase 3, double-blind study of subcutaneous ecallantide treatment for acute attacks of hereditary angioedema. Ann Allergy Asthma Immunol 2010;104(6):523–9.

111. Lumry WR, Bernstein JA, Li HH, et al. Efficacy and safety of ecallantide in treatment of recurrent attacks of hereditary angioedema: open-label continuation study. Allergy Asthma Proc 2013;34(2):155–61.

112. Crag TJ, Levy RJ, Wasserman RL, et al. Efficacy of human C1 esterase inhibitor concentrate compared with placebo in acute hereditary angioedema attacks. J Allergy Clin Immunol 2009;124(4):801–8.

113. Craig TJ, Wasserman RL, Levy RJ, et al. Prospective study of rapid relief provided by C1 esterase inhibitor in emergency treatment of acute laryngeal attacks in hereditary angioedema. J Clin Immunol 2010;30(6):823–9.

114. Craig TJ, Bewtra AK, Bahna SL, et al. C1 esterase inhibitor concentrate in 1085 hereditary angioedema attacks – final results of the IMPACT2 study. Allergy 2011;66(12):1604–11.

115. Zuraw BL, Kalfus I. Safety and efficacy of prophylactic nanofiltered C1-inhibitor in hereditary angioedema. Am J Med 2012;125(9):938.

116. Lumry W, Manning ME, Hurewitz DS, et al. Nanofiltered C1-esterase inhibitor for the acute management and prevention of hereditary angioedema attacks due to C1-inhibitor deficiency in children. J Pediatr 2013;162(5):1017–22.
117. Rasmussen ER, Aagaard L, Bygum A. Real-life experience with long-term prophylactic C1 inhibitor concentrate treatment of patients with hereditary angioedema: effectiveness and cost. Ann Allergy Asthma Immunol 2016;116(5):476–7.
118. Tilles SA, Borish L, Cohen JP. Management of hereditary angioedema in 2012: scientific and pharmacoeconomic perspectives. Ann Allergy Asthma Immunol 2013;110(2):70–4.
119. Belliveau PP, Lahoz MR. Evaluation of omalizumab from a health plan perspective. J Manag Care Pharm 2005;11(9):735–45.
120. Zelger RS, Schatz M, Dalal AA, et al. Utilization and costs of severe uncontrolled asthma in a managed-care setting. J Allergy Clin Immunol Pract 2016;4(1):120–9.
121. Wu AC, Paltiel AD, Kuntz KM, et al. Cost-effectiveness of omalizumab in adults with severe asthma: results from the Asthma Policy Model. J Allergy Clin Immunol 2007;120(5):1146–52.

Biologic Therapies for Autoimmune and Connective Tissue Diseases

Rachel M. Wolfe, MD, Dennis C. Ang, MD*

KEYWORDS

- Biologic therapy • Rheumatoid arthritis • Psoriatic arthritis • Ankylosing spondylitis
- Gout • Lupus

KEY POINTS

- The available clinical data supporting the use of various biologic therapies in autoimmune rheumatic disease are reviewed.
- The use of therapies that are not US Food and Drug Administration approved in the treatment of select rheumatic diseases is discussed.
- Drug properties and indications for the included biologic therapies are reviewed.

INTRODUCTION

Biologic therapy continues to revolutionize the treatment of autoimmune disease, especially in rheumatology. As the understanding of inflammation and autoimmune disease improves, new targets for therapy emerge.[1] Tumor necrosis factor (TNF)–alpha, interleukin (IL)-1, IL-6, as well as activated T cell and B cells have all been implicated in the pathophysiology of rheumatic diseases and have provided potential targets for therapy. New therapies continue to come to market at a rapid pace, with the most recent US Food and Drug Administration (FDA) approval of secukinumab in 2015, and the indications continue to expand for existing therapies. This article reviews biologic therapies, including off-label indications, for use in a subset of autoimmune connective tissue diseases.

RHEUMATOID ARTHRITIS

Medication trials in rheumatoid arthritis (RA) have used composite measures, including several functional and quality of life indices, as well as objective tests to assess therapeutic efficacy. Two of the most common measures are the American

Disclosures: Neither author has any disclosures.
Section on Rheumatology and Immunology, Wake Forest Baptist Health, Medical Center Boulevard, Winston Salem, NC 27157, USA
* Corresponding author.
E-mail address: dang@wakehealth.edu

College of Rheumatology 20 (ACR20) and the Disease Activity Score 28 (DAS28). An ACR20 is defined as a 20% improvement in the number of swollen and tender joints and in at least 3 of the following domains: patient and physician global assessments, pain, disability, and an acute phase reactant.[2] ACR50 and ACR70 reflect a 50% and 70% improvement respectively in those same categories. DAS28 (scale range from 0 and 10) is used to define disease activity and incorporates the number of swollen and tender joints (28 of each), patient global health assessment, and acute phase reactants.[3] These indices have been validated for the evaluation of both RA and psoriatic arthritis.[4] All of the therapies discussed later in this article are FDA approved for the treatment of RA.

Anti–Tumor Necrosis Factor Alpha Therapy

Anti-TNF agents have been a mainstay in the treatment of RA for many years. Infliximab was the first anti-TNF to be approved, followed by adalimumab, etanercept, and more recently, golimumab and certolizumab pegol. A meta-analysis of infliximab, adalimumab, and etanercept showed efficacy either as monotherapy or in combination with disease-modifying antirheumatic drugs (DMARDs) with respect to ACR20, ACR50, ACR70, and DAS28, and in slowing radiographic progression.[5] Combination of anti-TNF with conventional DMARDs was superior to TNF inhibitor therapy alone.[6] Compared with methotrexate (MTX) plus placebo, MTX plus any anti-TNF showed the following ACR20, ACR50, and ACR70 responses: 60% versus 25%, 40% versus 10%, and 20% versus 5%, respectively. Although trial data are limited, observational studies support the benefit of switching from one anti-TNF agent to another anti-TNF agent after failing the initial therapy.[7,8] The order of the various anti-TNF agents does not seem to matter with regard to subsequent efficacy. No direct head-to-head trials of various anti-TNF agents have been done but data from observational studies suggest equal efficacy among the different anti-TNF agents.[9–11] Anti-TNF therapy, either as monotherapy or in combination with DMARDs, is efficacious for the treatment of active RA.

Tocilizumab

Tocilizumab (TCZ), an IL-6 receptor antagonist, has been FDA approved to treat RA since 2010. In a phase II trial (CHARISMA), MTX plus TCZ (at doses of 2 mg/kg, 4 mg/kg, and 8 mg/kg) was superior to MTX alone with respect to ACR20 at week 16.[12] Only the 8-mg/kg dose of TCZ was superior to MTX alone with regard to ACR50 and ACR70.

Among patients with RA with an inadequate response to prior TNF agents (≥1), TCZ 8 mg/kg was more efficacious than 4-mg/kg dosing and placebo.[13] A meta-analysis of 8 randomized controlled trial (RCTs) found a significant improvement in clinical indices in the 8-mg/kg dose rather than the 4-mg/kg dose regardless of prior DMARD or biologic therapy.[14] In a cohort study, TCZ plus any DMARD were superior to DMARD therapy alone at 24 weeks in terms of ACR20, ACR50, ACR70, and DAS28 remission criteria.[15]

Although TCZ is clearly efficacious for the treatment of active RA, there is only 1 head-to-head trial of TCZ versus another biologic. In ADACTA, more than 300 patients with active RA intolerant to MTX were randomized to either TCZ 8 mg/kg or adalimumab 40 mg every other week.[16] Compared with the adalimumab group, the TCZ group achieved higher response rates for DAS28 remission (39.9% vs 19.8%), and for ACR20, ACR50, and ACR70 (65% vs 49%, 47% vs 27%, and 32% vs 17%).

In 3 RCTs, TCZ subcutaneous (SC) has shown noninferiority to TCZ intravenous (IV) 8 mg/kg every 4 weeks[17,18] as well as treatment benefit compared with placebo.[19] In an open-label extension of the MUSASHI trial, in which patients were either switched from TCZ 8 mg/kg IV every 4 weeks to TCZ 162 mg SC every other week or remained on TCZ 162 mg SC every other week, continued efficacy was noted regardless of prior treatment with the exception of those patients weighing more than 100 kg.[20] In another trial, weekly dosing of TCZ 162 mg SC among patients weighing more than 100 kg showed clinical efficacy.[17]

In summary, TCZ is an effective medication for the treatment of active RA, with most benefit at the 8-mg/kg dose. Subcutaneous TCZ is equally efficacious but dosing adjustments need to be made by weight.

Abatacept

Abatacept (ABA) is a fusion protein of CTLA-4 (cytotoxic T-lymphocyte-associated protein 4) that inhibits the second signal of T-cell activation. Several studies have shown efficacy of ABA IV dosing in patients with active RA who were incomplete responders (IRs) to either MTX or anti-TNF agents.[21] More recent studies have examined the efficacy of an SC route of administration for ABA. In the ACQUIRE trial, MTX-IR patients with active RA were randomized to MTX plus either ABA IV (10 mg/kg at week 0, 2, and 4, and then every 4 weeks) or ABA SC (125 mg weekly with loading IV dose of 10 mg/kg on day 1).[22] Subcutaneous ABA was noninferior to IV ABA at 6 months with respect to the ACR20. In an open-label extension of the ACQUIRE trial, all patients on ABA 125 mg SC weekly were followed for 44 months. Benefit in clinical indices and remission rates were sustained during the open-label extension.

The AMPLE trial compared ABA SC (125 mg SC weekly without a loading dose) with adalimumab (40 mg SC every other week) in patients with active RA who were MTX-IR and biologic naive.[23] ABA was not inferior to adalimumab at 1 year and benefit was sustained for a second year's extension of this trial. In a post-hoc analysis of both the ACQUIRE and AMPLE trials, there were no statistical differences in efficacy in SC ABA with or without an IV loading dose.[21] Another study showed no difference in concomitant use of MTX versus ABA SC as monotherapy.[24]

In summary, regardless of route of administration, ABA is efficacious in the treatment of active RA.

Rituximab

Several RCTs have established the efficacy of rituximab (RTX), a monoclonal antibody that inhibits CD20, for the treatment of RA. In the REFLEX trial, patients with active RA who failed at least 1 prior TNF agent were randomized to MTX plus either RTX 1 g at weeks 0 and 2 or placebo.[25] Compared with subjects in the MTX plus placebo group, significantly more subjects in the RTX plus MTX group achieved an ACR20. In the open-label extension of this trial, retreatment (up to 12 courses over 5 years) of RTX showed sustained benefits in all RA-relevant outcome measures, including less radiologic joint damage.[26]

The best dosing regimen for RTX has been harder to evaluate. In the IMAGE study, MTX-naive patients with early, active RA were randomized to MTX plus either RTX 0.5 (given 2 weeks apart), 1 g (given 2 weeks apart), or placebo.[27] Only the RTX 1-g treatment arm met the primary end point of reduced radiographic joint damage at week 52.

In contrast, the SERENE trial evaluated biologic-naive patients with active RA who were on MTX to either RTX 0.5 g or 1 g 2 weeks apart, or placebo.[28] ACR20 response rates were statistically higher in both RTX arms compared with placebo. There was no statistical difference between the two RTX treatment arms. Two other RCTs have confirmed the results of the SERENE trial.[29,30]

In an observational cohort of patients with RA, the comparison of RTX 0.5 g and 1 g (2 doses separated by 2 weeks) revealed no difference in clinical outcomes once adjusted for baseline differences.[31] RTX is an effective therapy for the treatment of RA in patients who have previously failed DMARD or anti-TNF agents. Standard dosing is effective but there is some evidence to support the use of 0.5-g dosing.

Tofacitinib

Tofacitinib is a Janus-associated kinase (JAK) inhibitor that became FDA approved for the treatment of RA in 2012. In a meta-analysis of 3 phase II trials, IRs to DMARD therapy with active RA were randomized to either tofacitinib 5 mg twice daily or 10 mg twice daily, or to placebo.[32] At 12 weeks, the ACR20 response rates were significantly higher in both active treatment arms and were sustained at week 24. In addition, significant improvements in the following domains were observed in the active treatment arms: number of tender joints, swollen joints, pain, patient and physician global assessments, functional impairment, and C-reactive protein.

Another meta-analysis of 4 phase II trials and 5 phase III trials found similar results of improvement in ACR20 and other efficacy end points for both the tofacitinib 5 mg twice daily and 10 mg twice daily groups.[33] The response rates comparing biologic-naive patients with biologic IRs showed numerically greater (but not statistically significant) clinical response in the biologic-naive patients. In summary, tofacitinib is efficacious in both biologic-naive and biologic-IR patients with active RA.

SYSTEMIC LUPUS ERYTHEMATOSUS
Food and Drug Administration–approved Therapy

Belimumab

Belimumab, monoclonal antibody that inhibits B-lymphocyte stimulator (BLyS), is the only biologic therapy approved by the FDA for the treatment of lupus. In a phase III trial of patients with lupus (without active kidney or central nervous system involvement), belimumab (dosed at 1 mg/kg and 10 mg/kg at days 0, 14, and 28, and every 28 days until week 48) was compared with placebo with improvement in the Systemic Lupus Erythematosus (SLE) Responder Index (SRI) at week 52 as the primary end point.[34] SRI is a composite measure of disease activity that evaluates symptoms, organ involvement, and physician global assessment. At 48 weeks, the primary end point was achieved in both treatment arms with associated steroid-sparing effect.

A second trial with the same study design found similar results at week 72, with the exception that only the belimumab 10-mg/kg arm achieved significant improvement in the SRI compared with placebo.[35] Although not statistically significant, the change in the SRI in the belimumab 1-mg/kg arm was numerically greater than the placebo.

Pooling data from both trials, musculoskeletal and mucosal domains seemed to be most responsive to belimumab.[36] Moreover, patients with higher disease activity scores, low complement levels, anti–double-stranded DNA positivity, and current steroid use were reported to experience greater benefits from belimumab.[37]

Belimumab is the first FDA-approved therapy for lupus in many years and may provide benefit in a select group of patients with active SLE. There have been no trials to date evaluating belimumab for lupus nephritis.

Non–Food and Drug Administration–approved Therapy

Rituximab

The literature is mixed on the effectiveness of RTX in SLE. There have been 2 RCTs to date; both failed to meet primary and secondary end points. The first study (LUNAR) enrolled patients with class III or class IV lupus nephritis on a background of mycophenolate mofetil and GC (glucocorticoid).[38] Participants were randomized to either RTX dosed at 1000 mg on days 1, 15, 168, and 182, or placebo. However, the primary renal end point (measured by specific improvements in serum creatinine level, urine protein creatinine ratio, and the lack of active urine sediment) at week 52 was not met in this study.

The second trial, EXPLORER, was also a double-blind RCT that compared RTX (dosed at 1000 mg on days 1, 15, 168, and 182) versus placebo in patients with active lupus (excluding lupus nephritis).[39] Participants were allowed to continue their base-line immunosuppression. This study failed to meet its primary end point (reduction in lupus disease activity) and there was also no steroid-sparing effect from RTX.

In contrast, data from observational studies have been more favorable for the use of RTX therapy in SLE. Based on the analyses of pooled data (n>450), RTX was associ-ated with a 60% reduction in lupus disease activity.[40] A more recent review in 2014 (n = 1231) also reported improvements in the following disease activity parameters: overall disease activity, arthritis, thrombocytopenia, and reduced steroid dose.[41] Despite the negative RCTs, RTX may be a reasonable therapy to use in choice circum-stances (such as the parameters noted earlier) in patients with active SLE.

Abatacept

Given that T-cell activation is thought to be involved in the pathogenesis of SLE, aba-tacept, which blocks the second signal of T-cell activation, has been a target for possible therapy for SLE.[42] Askanase and colleagues[43] evaluated ABA as a mainte-nance agent for patients with active lupus nephritis postinduction. The induction regimen included cyclophosphamide (CTX) plus GC followed by AZA (azathioprine). In this phase IIB study, ABA was not superior to placebo.

A similar trial of patients with lupus on a background of MMF (mycophenolate mofe-til) did not show treatment benefits from ABA.[44] However, post-hoc analysis sug-gested that benefits may not have been adequately captured by the predetermined end points. In another phase IIb RCT study, ABA did not improve the non–life-threat-ening manifestations of lupus either.[45]

At this time, there is no evidence to suggest the efficacy of ABA for lupus nephritis or non–life-threatening symptoms. It is hoped that ongoing trials that circumvent previ-ous design flaws will determine the role (if any) of ABA in the lupus treatment armamentarium.[46]

INFLAMMATORY MYOSITIS

There are no FDA-approved biologic therapies for the treatment of inflammatory myositis.

Rituximab

RTX has shown benefit in small observational studies of patients with inflammatory myositis. A recent review reported a 78.3% clinical response rate in 485 patients with inflammatory myositis.[47] There has been only 1 RCT to date in patients with re-fractory inflammatory myositis that compared early dosing of RTX versus late dosing of RTX (750 mg/m2 up to 1 g at either weeks 0 and 1 or weeks 8 and 9 with placebo infusions as appropriate for the treatment arm).[48] In terms of time to improvement of overall disease activity, which included muscle strength, there was no difference in early versus late dosing; however, 83% of all participants, regardless of treatment arm, achieved the definition of improvement. Moreover, RTX was associated with a steroid-sparing effect. Secondary data analyses found the presence of antisynthetase and anti–Mi-2 autoantibodies as predictors of treatment response to RTX therapy.[49]

Despite a negative trial, RTX may be a reasonable option in patients with refractory inflammatory myositis, especially with certain specific autoantibodies.

Anti–Tumor Necrosis Factor Therapy

There is no consensus about the use of anti-TNF therapy in inflammatory myositis. A few case reports and series have shown benefit, whereas others refute the usefulness of anti-TNF. In a small RCT of patients with dermatomyositis, etanercept was neither beneficial nor harmful, although a steroid-sparing effect was noted.[50] Of note, a recent literature review found 20 cases of patients with RA who later developed myositis while on anti-TNF therapy.[51] Although confirmation of the root cause can be difficult, symptoms of myositis resolved with cessation of the biologic therapy. At this time, there is no good evidence to support the use of anti-TNF therapy in inflammatory myositis.

Other Biologics

Case reports of TCZ and abatacept have suggested promising new avenues of therapy and several RCTs are currently underway.[52–54]

ANKYLOSING SPONDYLITIS

Much like drug trials for RA, medication efficacy trials in AS have developed and validated composite measures that assess clinical and quality-of-life indices specific to AS. The first important scale is the Bath AS Disease Activity Index (BASDAI), which assesses pain, tenderness, and morning stiffness.[55] The second measure is the Assessment in Ankylosing Spondylitis (ASAS20) response criteria. The ASAS20 requires greater than or equal to 20% improvement in at least 3 of 4 domains: patient global assessment, pain, physical function, and inflammation.[56]

Food and Drug Administration–approved Therapy

Anti–tumor necrosis factor therapy

Anti-TNF therapy has well-established efficacy data in AS. A recent meta-analysis of RCTs of anti-TNF inhibitors (adalimumab, certolizumab, etanercept, golimumab, or infliximab) found efficacy for any anti-TNF inhibitors compared with placebo in all measures of disease activity.[57] There was no difference in treatment response between AS or nonradiographic axial spondyloarthritis.[58] Maneiro and colleagues[59] reported the following predictors of treatment response to anti-TNF inhibitors: younger age, male gender, high BASDAI, human leukocyte antigen (HLA) B27 positivity, and increased C-reactive protein level.

Secukinumab

The most recently FDA-approved therapy for the treatment of AS is secukinumab, a monoclonal antibody that binds IL-17A. In the first large trial, secukinumab at both doses (75 mg and 150 mg) with IV loading doses met the primary end point of ASAS20 with 60% and 61% response rates respectively, compared with 29% in the placebo arm. In a second RCT, the investigators evaluated the same doses of secukinumab (75 mg and 150 mg) but with subcutaneous loading.[60] The primary end point was only met in the secukinumab 150 mg group with similar response rate of 61%. Secukinumab 150 mg also met the secondary end points, including improvement in disease activity, reduction in C-reactive protein level, and ASAS40. The benefits were sustained through week 52. Secukinumab was efficacious in patients who were anti-TNF naive, and in those who previously failed anti-TNF inhibitors. Results of these 2 trials led the FDA to approve secukinumab for AS.

PSORIATIC ARTHRITIS
Food and Drug Administration–approved Therapy

Anti–tumor necrosis factor therapy
A meta-analysis of anti-TNF inhibitors (including etanercept, infliximab, and adalimumab) in psoriatic arthritis (PsA) found statistically significant improvement in ACR20, ACR50, and ACR70 response criteria. Safety evaluation did not show any added risk associated with these medications.[61] A more recent observational study of clinic patients with axial PsA found no difference in clinical efficacy among the 3 agents included (ie, etanercept, adalimumab, or golimumab).[62] The predictors of treatment response included male sex, young age, short disease duration, and absence of enthesitis.

Ustekinumab
Ustekinumab is a monoclonal antibody that inhibits IL-12 and IL-23. In a phase III trial, patients were randomized to either placebo, 45-mg ustekinumab, or 90-mg ustekinumab at weeks 0 and 4, and then every 12 weeks with multiple escape and crossovers available.[63] Ustekinumab was efficacious in anti-TNF–naive patients in terms of ACR20 response rate at week 24. In a subsequent trial, both anti-TNF–naive and anti-TNF–experienced patients were included and were randomized into 3 arms: placebo, ustekinumab 45 mg, or ustekinumab 90 mg at weeks 0 and 4, and then every 12 weeks with placebo crossover to ustekinumab 45 mg at weeks 24, 28, and 40.[64] The trial met the primary end point of ACR20 in both the active treatment arms at week 24, with sustained benefit observed through week 52. Both active treatment arms achieved higher ACR50 response rates as well. Although both anti-TNF–naive and anti-TNF–experienced patients responded well, the benefit in the anti-TNF–experienced cohort was more pronounced.

Secukinumab
Two phase III trials examined the efficacy of secukinumab in PsA. In FUTURE 1, patients were treated with IV secukinumab 10 mg/kg at weeks 0, 2, and 4, followed by either SC 150 mg or 75 mg every 4 weeks or placebo. Patient-reported outcomes were improved in both active treatment groups compared with the placebo at week 24. These benefits were sustained throughout the full 52 weeks.[65] In FUTURE 2, patients were randomized 1:1:1:1 to receive either secukinumab 300 mg, 150 mg, or 75 mg SC, or placebo, once weekly for 4 weeks and then every 4 weeks.[66] Higher ACR20 response rates were observed in all active treatment groups with a notable dose-response relationship. The ACR50 and ACR70 response rates were statistically greater than those of placebo in the secukinumab 300 mg and 150 mg groups. These trials led to the approval of secukinumab for PsA.

VASCULITIS
Food and Drug Administration–approved Therapy

Rituximab
RTX has been evaluated in both the induction and maintenance treatment phases of ANCA (Anti-neutrophil cytoplasmic antibody)-associated vasculitis (AAV). In an induction therapy study (RAVE), RTX dosed at 375 mg/m^2 once weekly for 4 weeks was compared with oral daily CTX at dose of 2 mg/kg on the background of high-dose GC in patients with AAV.[67] The study met the primary end point of noninferiority at 6 months with respect to prednisone tapering and the Birmingham Vasculitis Activity Score (BVAS) of 0. The proportion of patients who reached the primary end point was higher in RTX versus oral daily CTX (64% vs 53%; $P = .09$).

In an open-label trial evaluating RTX for induction, subjects were randomized to either RTX plus CTX (at 15 mg/kg at weeks 0 and 3) without maintenance therapy, or CTX standard dosing plus AZA maintenance therapy.[68] There was no significant difference in sustained remission at 12 months as defined by BVAS of 0. In the extension phase of this same trial, there were also no differences in composite rates of death, end-stage renal disease, or relapse rates at 24 months between the two treatment arms.[69] Of note, patients in the RTX arm were not retreated or started on other immunosuppressant agents during the 12-month extension. Return of B-cell population heralded relapse in the RTX arm and those subjects without B-cell return (total number 10 patients) did not experience any relapses.

A more recent trial evaluated the use of RTX as a maintenance agent by comparing patients with AAV treated initially with a CTX-GC regimen with either RTX therapy (given at 500 mg at days 0 and 14 and then months 6, 12, and 18) or daily AZA.[70] Primary end point was a major relapse, defined by either a BVAS >0 and major organ involvement or a disease-related life-threatening event at month 28. The relapse rates were 5% in the RTX arm and 29% in the AZA arm. Significantly more subjects in the RTX group compared with the AZA group achieved sustained remission. Safety outcomes were comparable in the two groups.

RTX is noninferior to standard regimens for induction of AAV and can be considered for maintenance therapy.

Non–Food and Drug Administration–approved Therapy

Tocilizumab

Based on small observational studies, TCZ may be an effective treatment of giant cell arteritis (GCA). A systematic analysis of 25 patients treated with either TCZ or TCZ plus GC found disease remission in all but 1 patient.[71] A significant steroid reduction was observed in those patients on combination TCZ plus GC therapy. A retrospective review of 34 patients with GCA treated with GC and TCZ found marked improvement in clinical symptoms in all patients with complete resolution of symptoms in all but 6.[72] Steroid dose was successfully tapered from 26.3 ± 13.8 mg/d to 10.3 ± 8.3 mg/d ($P<.05$). Adverse events did occur, with infection and transient neutropenia being most common.

A randomized, double-blind, placebo-controlled trial (GiACTA) is currently underway to evaluate 4 treatment arms:

1. TCZ 162 mg weekly plus 6-month prednisone taper
2. TCZ 162 mg every other week plus 6-month prednisone taper
3. Placebo plus 6-month prednisone taper
4. Placebo plus 12-month prednisone taper[73]

The study will be blinded for 52 weeks followed by open-label extension for a total of 104 weeks. Enrollment was recently completed but the study is still ongoing.

GOUT

There are no FDA-approved biologic therapies for the treatment of gout or other crystalline arthropathies.

Non–Food and Drug Administration–approved Therapy

Given the role of inflammasome and IL-1 in the pathophysiology of acute gout, medications that block IL-1 are promising therapeutic options for patients with contraindications to traditional therapies (ie, nonsteroidal antiinflammatory drugs, colchicine, and prednisone). For anakinra, an IL-1 receptor antagonist, several small observational studies suggest potential treatment benefits. In an open-label pilot study of 10 patients with acute gout, anakinra (100 mg SC for 3 days) was associated with improvement in pain and swelling in all 10 patients by 48 hours; many had complete resolution of their symptoms.[74] Other studies have reported improvement in joint pain and swelling and with acceptable safety profiles.[75]

Canakinumab, a monoclonal antibody that inhibits IL-1, has also been evaluated for the treatment of acute gout. In 2 phase III trials, canakinumab 150 mg SC once was compared with triamcinolone 40 mg intramuscularly once.[76] There was significant and prompt improvement in pain with a decrease in the pain scores in the canakinumab group compared with the triamcinolone group at 72 hours (primary end point), with improvement observed as early as 24 hours. In addition, the time to the next gout flare in the canakinumab group was reduced by 62% compared with the triamcinolone group. Both canakinumab and anakinra may be appropriate for patients with acute gout with contraindications to standard gout therapy.

FUTURE DIRECTIONS

The advent of biologic therapy continues to revolutionize the treatment of autoimmune and connective tissue diseases. There are several new biologic agents being developed to target new aspects of the inflammatory cascade. For example, a second-generation JAK inhibitor (specifically JAK1/2), baricitinib (LY3009104), is currently enrolling in a phase III trial for the treatment of RA.[77] Not only are new mechanisms of inhibition of inflammation being investigated but older mechanisms are being reevaluated with the development of biosimilar agents. Continued research evaluating biosimilar agents for efficacy and safety are underway. Even with the established biologic therapy, surveillance (phase IV trials) to evaluate for unforeseen complications is of utmost importance. Comparative effectiveness studies of various biologic agents are warranted to help inform physicians' and patients' decision making. In addition, as clinical remission with biologic therapy becomes more of a reality, evaluation of if, when, and how to stop biologic therapy will be needed. Biologic agents continue to create promising opportunities in the treatment of autoimmune disease.

THE BIOLOGIC THERAPIES
Drug Properties[78]

Anti–tumor necrosis factor-alpha therapy (infliximab, adalimumab, etanercept, certolizumab, golimumab)

Mechanism of action: these agents bind TNF-alpha by various mechanisms, thereby preventing downstream activations of inflammatory cascades. Etanercept blocks both TNF-alpha and TNF-beta.
Prescreening: tuberculosis, hepatitis B and C.
FDA-approved indications: RA, PsA, AS.
Administration:
- Infliximab:
  ○ RA: 3 mg/kg IV at 0, 2, and 6 weeks and then every 8 weeks but may be titrated up to 10 mg/kg. With MTX therapy.
  ○ AS: 5 mg/kg IV at 2 and 6 weeks and then every 6 weeks.
  ○ PsA: 5 mg/kg IV at 2 and 6 weeks and then every 8 weeks.

- Adalimumab: 40 mg SC every other week. May increase to weekly dosing.
- Etanercept: 50 mg SC weekly.
- Golimumab: 50 mg SC monthly.
- Certolizumab pegol: 400 mg SC at weeks 0, 2, 4, followed by 200 mg every other week.

Side effects: infections, including fungal infections and tuberculosis reactivation, hepatitis B reactivation, cytopenias, heart failure, lupuslike syndrome, demyelinating disease (rare).

Tocilizumab

Mechanism of action: binds both soluble and membrane-bound IL-6 receptors, which inhibits downstream activation of inflammatory cytokine production.

Prescreening: tuberculosis, hepatitis B and C, lipid profile.

FDA-approved indications: RA.

Administration:
- Infusion: start at 4 mg/kg every 4 weeks with an increase to 8 mg/kg every 4 weeks as indicated by clinical response.
- Injection: patient weight less than 100 kg, 162 mg SC every other week; weight greater than 100 kg, 162 mg every week.

Side effects: infections, increased liver function tests, neutropenia, thrombocytopenia, increase of lipid levels, and gastrointestinal perforation (rare).

Abatacept

Mechanism of action: CTLA-4 immunoglobulin, which blocks the binding of CD80/CD86 (T cells) with CD28 (antigen-presenting cells), which then prevents T-cell activation.

Prescreening: tuberculosis.

FDA-approved indications: RA.

Administration:
- IV: patient weight less than 60 kg, 500 mg; weight 60 to 100 kg, 750 mg; weight greater than 100 kg, 1000 mg. Initial infusion given at 0, 2, 4 weeks, and then every 4 weeks.
- SC: 125 mg weekly.

Side effects: infections, increased frequency of chronic obstructive pulmonary disease exacerbations, injection site reactions, hypersensitivity reaction.

Rituximab

Mechanism of action: chimeric monoclonal antibody that binds CD20 antigen expressed on B cells, which induces lysis; thus, it prevents the B-cell contribution to the inflammatory state.

Prescreening: hepatitis B.

FDA-approved indications: patients with RA who have failed 1 or more TNF agents, granulomatosis polyangiitis (GPA) and microscopic polyangiitis (MPA), along with GC.

Administration: IV infusions.
- RA: 1000 mg × 2 doses, 2 weeks apart.
- GPA/MPA: 375 mg/m^2 weekly for 4 weeks.

Side effects: infection, infusion reactions, cytopenias, hepatitis B reactivation. Rare side effects include progressive multifocal leukoencephalopathy, cardiac arrhythmias, angina.

Tofacitinib

Mechanism of action: prevents phosphorylation of signal transducers and activators of transcription by blocking JAK, which prevents downstream activation of gene expression and immune cell function.

Prescreening: tuberculosis, lymphocyte count (>500 cells/mm^3) or absolute neutrophil count (>1000 cells/mm^3), hemoglobin level greater than 9 g/dL, hepatitis B and hepatitis C.

FDA-approved indications: RA.

Administration: 5 mg by mouth twice daily.

Side effects: infections, monitor laboratory tests, including lymphocytes, neutrophils, hemoglobin, liver enzymes, and lipids. Rarely gastrointestinal perforation.

Belimumab

Mechanism of action: human monoclonal antibody that inhibits BLyS, which is required for B-cell survival.

Prescreening: None.

FDA-approved indication: antibody-positive SLE on current immunosuppression.

Administration: IV infusion of 10 mg/kg at 2-week intervals for 3 doses then every 4 weeks.

Side effects: infection, hypersensitivity reactions, depression. progressive multifocal leukoencephalopathy (rare).

Ustekinumab

Mechanism of action: human immunoglobulin (Ig) G1κ monoclonal antibody, which binds to p40 protein subunit used by IL-12 and IL-23, which prevents IL-12/IL-23 cytokine and inflammatory cascades.

Prescreening: tuberculosis.

FDA-approved indication: PsA.

Administration: 45 mg at weeks 0 and 4, and then every 12 weeks.

Side effects: infections, tuberculosis and other mycobacterial conditions, anaphylaxis, reversible posterior leukoencephalopathy syndrome.

Secukinumab

Mechanism of action: human IgG1 monoclonal antibody, which binds IL-17A and prevents 1L-17 receptor interaction, which inhibits proinflammatory cytokine release.

Prescreening: tuberculosis.

FDA-approved indications: PsA, AS.

Administration:

- AS: with loading dose, 150 mg at weeks 0, 1, 2, 3, and 4, and every 4 weeks thereafter; without loading dose, 150 mg every 4 weeks.
- PsA: with loading dose, 150 mg at weeks 0, 1, 2, 3, and 4, and every 4 weeks thereafter; without loading dose, 150 mg every 4 weeks; consider increasing to 300 mg if continued active arthritis.

Side effects: infections, tuberculosis, reactivation, inflammatory bowel disease, and neutropenia.

Anakinra

Mechanism of action: binds IL-1 type 1 receptor, which inhibits activity of IL-1 alpha and beta, decreasing the inflammatory response.

Prescreening: complete blood count.
FDA-approved indications: RA.
Administration: 100 mg SC daily.
Side effects: infection, hypersensitivity reactions, neutropenia.

Canakinumab

Mechanism of action: human monoclonal IL-1β antibody, which binds to IL-1β and prevents binding of the IL-1 receptors.
Prescreening: hepatitis B and C.
FDA-approved indications: currently evaluating for crystalline arthritis.
Administration: 150 mg SC every 4 weeks.
Side effects: infection, cytopenias, including white blood cells, neutrophils, platelets, and increase in liver function tests.

REFERENCES

1. Choy EHS, Panayi GS. Cytokine pathways and joint inflammation in rheumatoid arthritis. N Engl J Med 2001;344:907–16.
2. Felson DT, Anderson JJ, Boers M, et al. American College of Rheumatology. Preliminary definition of improvement in rheumatoid arthritis. Arthritis Rheum 1995; 38(6):727–35.
3. Fransen J, Creemers MCW, Van Riel PL. Remission in rheumatoid arthritis: agreement of the Disease Active Score (DAS28) with the ARA preliminary remission criteria. Rheumatology (Oxford) 2004;43(1):1252–5.
4. Fransen J, Antoni C, Mease PJ. Performance of response criteria for assessing peripheral arthritis in patients with psoriatic arthritis: analysis of data from randomized controlled trials of two tumour necrosis factor inhibitors. Ann Rheum Dis 2006;65(10):1373–8.
5. Chen YF, Jobanputra P, Barton P. A systemic review of the effectiveness of adalimumab, etanercept and infliximab for the treatment of rheumatoid arthritis in adults and an economic evaluation of their cost-effectiveness. Health Technol Assess 2006;10(42):iii–iv, xi-xiii, 1–229.
6. Caporali R, Pallavicini RB, Filippini M, et al. Treatment of rheumatoid arthritis with anti-TNF-alpha agents: a reappraisal. Autoimmun Rev 2009;8:274–80.
7. Caporali R, Sarzi-Puttini P, Atzeni F, et al. Switching TNF-alpha antagonist in rheumatoid arthritis: the experience of the Lorhen registry. Autoimmun Rev 2010;9(6): 465–9.
8. Ma X, Xu S. TNF inhibitor therapy for rheumatoid arthritis. Biomed Rep 2013;1(2): 177–84.
9. Santos-Moreno P, Sanchez G, Gomez D, et al. Direct comparative effectiveness among 3 anti-tumor necrosis factor biologics in a real-life cohort of patients with rheumatoid arthritis. J Clin Rheumatol 2016;22(2):57–62.
10. Greenberg JD, Reed G, Decktor D, et al. A comparative effectiveness study of adalimumab, etanercept and infliximab in biologically naive and switched rheumatoid arthritis patients: results from the US CORRONA registry. Ann Rheum Dis 2012;71:1134–42.
11. Aaltonen KJ, Virkki LM, Malmivaara A, et al. Systemic review and meta-analysis of the efficacy and safety of existing TNF blocking agents in treatment of rheumatoid arthritis. PLoS One 2012;7(1):e30275.
12. Maini RN, Taylor PC, Szechinski J, et al. Double-blind randomized controlled clinical trial of the interleukin-6 receptor antagonist, tocilizumab, in European patients

with rheumatoid arthritis who had an incomplete response to methotrexate. Arthritis Rheum 2006;54(9):2817–29.

13. Emery P, Keystone E, Tony HP, et al. IL-6 receptor inhibition with tocilizumab improves treatment outcomes in patients with rheumatoid arthritis refractory to anti-tumour necrosis factor biologicals: results from a 24-week multicentre randomised placebo-controlled trial. Ann Rheum Dis 2008;67(11):1516–23.

14. Navarro G, Taroumian S, Barroso N. Tocilizumab in rheumatoid arthritis: a meta-analysis of efficacy and selected clinical conundrums. Semin Arthritis Rheum 2014;43:458–69.

15. Genovese MC, McKay JD, Nasonov EL, et al. Interleukin-6 receptor inhibition with tocilizumab reduces disease activity in rheumatoid arthritis with inadequate response to disease-modifying antirheumatic drugs: the Tocilizumab in Combination with Traditional Disease-modifying Antirheumatic Drug Therapy study. Arthritis Rheum 2008;58(10):2968–80.

16. Gabay C, Emery P, van Vollenhoven R, et al. Tocilizumab monotherapy versus adalimumab monotherapy for treatment of rheumatoid arthritis (ADACTA): a randomised, double-blind, controlled phase 4 trial. Lancet 2013;381:1541–50.

17. Burmester GR, Rubbert-Roth A, Cantagrel A, et al. A randomised, double-blind, parallel-group study of the safety and efficacy of subcutaneous tocilizumab versus intravenous tocilizumab in combination with traditional disease-modifying antirheumatic drugs in patients with moderate to severe rheumatoid arthritis (SUMMACTA study). Ann Rheum Dis 2014;73(1):69–74.

18. Ogata A, Tanimura K, Sugimoto T, et al. Phase III study of the efficacy and safety of subcutaneous versus intravenous tocilizumab monotherapy in patients with rheumatoid arthritis. Arthritis Care Res (Hoboken) 2014;66(3):344–54.

19. Kivitz A, Olech E, Borofsky M, et al. Subcutaneous tocilizumab versus placebo in combination with disease-modifying antirheumatic drugs in patients with rheumatoid arthritis. Arthritis Care Res (Hoboken) 2014;66(11):1653–61.

20. Ogata A, Atsumi TA, Fukuda T, et al. Sustainable efficacy of switching from intravenous to subcutaneous tocilizumab monotherapy in patients with rheumatoid arthritis. Arthritis Care Res 2015;67(10):1354–62.

21. Schiff M. Subcutaneous abatacept for the treatment of rheumatoid arthritis. Rheumatology 2013;52:986–97.

22. Genovese MC, Tena CP, Covarrubias A, et al. Subcutaneous abatacept for the treatment of rheumatoid arthritis: longterm data from the ACQUIRE trial. J Rheumatol 2014;44(4):629–39.

23. Schiff M, Weinblatt ME, Valente R. Head-to-head comparison of subcutaneous abatacept versus adalimumab for rheumatoid arthritis: two-year efficacy and safety findings from AMPLE trial. Ann Rheum Dis 2014;73:86–94.

24. Nash P, Nayiager S, Genovese M, et al. Immunogenicity, Safety, and Efficacy of Abatacept Administered Subcutaneously With or Without Background Methotrexate in Patients With Rheumatoid Arthritis: Results From a Phase III, International, Multicenter, Parallel-Arm, Open-Label Study. Arthritis Care Res (Hoboken) 2013;65(5):718–28.

25. Cohen SB, Emery P, Greenwald MW, et al. Rituximab for rheumatoid arthritis refractory to anti-tumor necrosis factor therapy: results of a multicenter, randomized, double-blind, placebo-controlled, phase III trial evaluating primary efficacy and safety at twenty-four weeks. Arthritis Rheum 2006;54:2793–806.

26. Keystone EC, Cohen SB, Emery P, et al. Multiple courses of rituximab produce sustained clinical and radiographic efficacy and safety in patients with

rheumatoid arthritis and an inadequate response to 1 or more tumor necrosis factor inhibitors: 5 year data from the REFLEX study. J Rheumatol 2012;39(12): 2238–46.

27. Tak PP, Rigby WF, Rubbert-Roth A, et al. Inhibition of joint damage and improved clinical outcomes with rituximab plus methotrexate in early active rheumatoid arthritis: the IMAGE trial. Ann Rheum Dis 2011;70(1):39–46.

28. Emery P, Deodhar A, Rigby WF, et al. Efficacy and safety of different doses and retreatment of rituximab: a randomised, placebo-controlled trial in patients who are biological naive with active rheumatoid arthritis and an inadequate response to methotrexate (Study Evaluating Rituximab's Efficacy in MTX iNadequate rEsponders (SERENE)). Ann Rheum Dis 2010;69(9):1629–35.

29. Emery P, Fleischmann R, Filipowicz-Sosnowska A, et al. The efficacy and safety of rituximab in patients with active rheumatoid arthritis despite methotrexate treatment: results of a phase IIB randomized, double-blind, placebo-controlled, dose-ranging trial. Arthritis Rheum 2006;54(5):1390–400.

30. Rubbert-Roth A, Tak PP, Zerbini C. Efficacy and safety of various repeat treatment dosing regimens of rituximab in patients with active rheumatoid arthritis: results of a phase III randomized study (MIRROR). Rheumatology (Oxford) 2010;49(9): 1683–93.

31. Chatzidionysiou K, Lie E, Nasonov E, et al. Effectiveness of two different doses of rituximab for the treatment of rheumatoid arthritis in an international cohort: data from the CERERRA collaboration. Arthritis Res Ther 2016;18:50.

32. Song GG, Bae SC, Lee YH. Efficacy and safety of tofacitinib for active rheumatoid arthritis with an inadequate response to methotrexate or disease-modifying antirheumatic drugs: a meta-analysis of randomized controlled trials. Korean J Intern Med 2014;29:656–63.

33. Charles-Schoeman C, Burmester G, Nash P, et al. Efficacy and safety of tofacitinib following inadequate response to conventional synthetic or biologic disease-modifying antirheumatic drugs. Ann Rheum Dis 2016;75(7):1293–301.

34. Navarra SV, Guzman RM, Gallacher AE, et al. Efficacy and safety of belimumab in patients with active systemic lupus erythematous: a randomized, placebo-controlled, phase 3 trial. Lancet 2011;377:721–31.

35. Furie R, Petri M, Zamani O. A phase III, randomized, placebo-controlled study of belimumab, a monoclonal antibody that inhibits B-lymphocyte stimulator, in patients with systemic lupus erythematosus. Arthritis Rheum 2011;63(12):3918–30.

36. Manzi S, Sánchez-Guerrero J, Merrill JT, et al. Effects of belimumab, a B lymphocyte stimulator-specific inhibitor, on disease activity across multiple organ domains in patients with systemic lupus erythematosus: combined results from two phase III trials. Ann Rheum Dis 2012;71(11):1833–88.

37. van Vollenhoven RF, Petri MA, Crevera R, et al. Belimumab in the treatment of systemic lupus erythematous: high disease activity predictors of response. Ann Rheum Dis 2012;71(8):1343–9.

38. Rovin BH, Furie R, Latinis K, et al. Efficacy and safety of rituximab in patients with active proliferative lupus nephritis: the lupus nephritis assessment with rituximab study. Arthritis Rheum 2012;64(4):1215–26.

39. Merrill JT, Neuwelt CM, Wallace DJ, et al. Efficacy and safety of rituximab in patients with moderately to severely active systemic lupus erythematosus: the randomized double-blind phase II/III Systemic Lupus Erythematosus Evaluation of Rituximab trial. Arthritis Rheum 2010;62(1):222–33.

40. Murray E, Perry M. Off-label use of rituximab in systemic lupus erythematosus: a systemic review. Clin Rheumatol 2010;29:707–16.

41. Cobo-Ibanez T, Loza-Santamaria E, Pego-Reigosa JM, et al. Efficacy and safety of rituximab in the treatment of non-renal systemic lupus erythematous: a systemic review. Semin Arthritis Rheum 2014;44:175–85.

42. Lobo Borba HH, Funke A, Wiens A. Update on biological therapy for systemic lupus erythematosus. Curr Rheumatol Rep 2016;18:44.

43. Askanase A, Byron M, Keyes-Elstein L, et al. Treatment of lupus nephritis with abatacept and cyclophosphamide efficacy and safety study. Arthritis Rheum 2014;66(11):3096–104.

44. Wofsy D, Hillson JL, Diamond B. Abatacept for lupus nephritis: alternative definitions of complete remission support conflicting conclusions. Arthritis Rheum 2012;64(11):3660–5.

45. Merrill JT, Burgos-Vargas R, Westhovens R, et al. The efficacy and safety of abatacept in patients with non-life-threatening manifestations of systemic lupus erythematous. Arthritis Rheum 2010;62(10):3077–87.

46. Efficacy and Safety Study of Abatacept to Treat Lupus Nephritis. Available at: https://clinicaltrials.gov/ct2/show/NCT01714817. Accessed June 29, 2016.

47. Fasano S, Gordon P, Hajji R, et al. Rituximab in treatment of inflammatory myopathies: a review. Rheumatology (Oxford) 2016;55(7):1318–24.

48. Oddis CV, Reed AM, Aggarawal R, et al. Rituximab in the treatment of refractory adult and juvenile dermatomyositis and polymyositis: a randomized, placebo-phase trial. Arthritis Rheum 2013;65(2):314–24.

49. Aggarwal R, Bandos A, Reed AM, et al. Predictors of clinical improvement in rituximab-treated refractory adult and juvenile dermatomyositis and adult polymyositis. Arthritis Rheum 2014;66:740–9.

50. The Muscle Study Group. A randomized, pilot trial of etanercept in dermatomyositis. Ann Neurol 2011;70(3):427–36.

51. Brunasso AMG, Aberer W, Massone C. New onset of dermatomyositis/polymyositis during anti-TNF-α therapies: a systematic literature review. ScientificWorldJournal 2014;2014:179180.

52. George Washington University. Abatacept for the treatment of refractory juvenile dermatomyositis. In: ClinicalTrials.gov [Internet]. Bethesda (MD): National Library of Medicine (US); 2000. Available at: https://clinicaltrials.gov/ct2/show/NCT02043548. Accessed Jun 28, 2016. NLM Identifier: NCT02043548.

53. Moghadam-Kia S, Oddis CV, Aggarawal R. Modern therapies for idiopathic inflammatory myopathies: role of biologics. Clin Rev Allergy Immunol 2017;52(1):81–7.

54. University of Pittsburgh. Tocilizumab in the treatment of refractory polymyositis and dermatomyositis. In: ClinicalTrials.gov [Internet]. Bethesda (MD): National Library of Medicine (US); 2000. Available at: https://clinicaltrials.gov/ct2/show/NCT02594735. Accessed Jun 28, 2016. NLM Identifier: NCT02594735.

55. Garrett S, Jenkinson T, Kennedy LG. A new approach to defining disease status in ankylosing spondylitis: the Bath Ankylosing Spondylitis Disease Activity Index. J Rheumatol 1994;21(12):2286–91.

56. Anderson JJ, Baron G, van der Heijde D. Ankylosing spondylitis assessment group preliminary definition of short-term improvement in ankylosing spondylitis. Arthritis Rheum 2001;44(8):1876–86.

57. Maxwell LJ, Zochling J, Boonen A, et al. TNF-alpha inhibitors for ankylosing spondylitis. Cochrane Database Syst Rev 2015;(4):CD005468.

58. Callhoff J, Sieper J, Weiß A, et al. Efficacy of TNFα blockers in patients with ankylosing spondylitis and non-radiographic axial spondyloarthritis: a meta-analysis. Ann Rheum Dis 2015;74:1241–8.

59. Maneiro JR, Souto A, Salgado E, et al. Predictors of response to TNF antagonists in patients with ankylosing spondylitis and psoriatic arthritis: systemic review and meta-analysis. RMD Open 2015;1(1):e000017.

60. Baeten D, Sieper J, Braun J, et al. Secukinumab, an IL-17A inhibitor in ankylosing spondylitis. N Engl J Med 2015;373(26):2534–48.

61. Saad AA, Symmons DPM, Noyce PR, et al. Risks and benefits of tumor necrosis factor-alpha inhibitors in the management of psoriatic arthritis: systemic review and metaanalysis of randomized control trials. J Rheumatol 2008;35:883–90.

62. Lubrano E, Parson WJ, Perrotta FM. Assessment of response to treatment, remission and minimal disease activity in axial psoriatic arthritis treated with tumor necrosis factor inhibitors. J Rheumatol 2016;43:918–23.

63. McInnes IB, Kavanaugh A, Gottlieb AB, et al, on behalf of the PSUMMIT 1 Study Group. Efficacy and safety of ustekinumab in patients with active psoriatic arthritis: 1 year results of the phase 3, multicenter, double-blind, placebo-controlled PSUMMIT 1 trial. Lancet 2013;382:780–9.

64. Richlin C, Rahman P, Kavanaugh A, et al, on behalf of the PSUMIIT 2 Study Group. Efficacy and safety of the anti-IL-12/23 p40 monoclonal antibody, ustekinumab, in patients with active psoriatic arthritis despite conventional non-biological anti-tumor necrosis factor therapy: 6-month and 1 year results of the phase 3, multicentre, double-blinded, placebo-controlled, randomized PSUMMIT 2 trial. Ann Rheum Dis 2014;73:990–9.

65. Strand V, Mease P, Gossec L. Secukinumab improves patient-reported outcomes in subjects with active psoriatic arthritis: results from a randomized phase III trial (FUTURE 1). Ann Rheum Dis 2017;76(1):203–7.

66. McInnes IB, Mease PJ, Kirkham B, et al. Secukinumab, a human anti-interleukin-17A monoclonal antibody, in patients with psoriatic arthritis (FUTURE 2): a randomized, double-blind, placebo-controlled, phase 3 trial. Lancet 2015;386: 1137–46.

67. Stone JH, Merkel PA, Spiera R, et al. Rituximab versus cyclophosphamide in ANCA-associated vasculitis. N Engl J Med 2010;363:221–32.

68. Jones RB, Tervaert JW, Hauser T, et al. Rituximab versus cyclophosphamide in ANCA-associated renal vasculitis. N Engl J Med 2010;363:211–20.

69. Jones RB, Furuta S, Tervaert JW, et al. Rituximab versus cyclophosphamide in ANCA-associated renal vasculitis: 2 year results of randomized trial. Ann Rheum Dis 2015;74:1178–82.

70. Guillevin L, Pagnoux C, Karra S, et al. Rituximab versus azathioprine for maintenance in ANCA-associated vasculitis. N Engl J Med 2014;371:1771–80.

71. Osman M, Pagnoux C, Dryden DM, et al. The role of biological agents in the management of large vessel vasculitis (LVV): a systemic review and meta-analysis. PLoS One 2014;9(12):e115026.

72. Regent A, Redeker S, Deroux A, et al. Tocilizumab in giant cell arteritis: a multicenter retrospective study of 34 patients. J Rheumatol 2016;43(8):1547–52.

73. Tuckwell K, Collinson N, Klearman M, et al. Baseline data on patients enrolled in a randomized, double-blind trial of tocilizumab in giant cell arteritis [abstract]. Arthritis Rheumatol 2015;67(Suppl 10). Available at: http://acrabstracts.org/abstract/baseline-data-on-patients-enrolled-in-a-randomized-double-blind-trial-of-tocilizumab-in-giant-cell-arteritis/. Accessed June 29, 2016.

74. So A, Smedt DE, Revaz S, et al. A pilot study of IL-1 inhibition by anakinra in acute gout. Arthritis Res 2007;9(2):R28.

75. Schlesinger N. Anti-interleukin-1 therapy in the management of gout. Curr Rheumatol Rep 2014;16:398.

76. Schlesinger N, De Meulemeester M, Pikhlak A, et al. Canakinumab for acute gouty arthritis in patients with limited treatment options: results from two randomised, multicentre, active-controlled, double-blind trials and their initial extensions. Ann Rheum Dis 2012;71(11):1839–48.

77. Eli Lily and Company. A randomized, double-blind, placebo-controlled, phase 3 study evaluating the efficacy and safety of baricitinib in patients with moderately to severely active rheumatoid arthritis who have had an inadequate response to methotrexate therapy. In: ClinicalTrials.gov [Internet]. Bethesda (MD): National Library of Medicine (US); 2000. Available at: https://clinicaltrials.gov/ct2/show/NCT02265705. Accessed Jun 28, 2016. Identifier: NCT02265705.

78. FDA approved drug products. US Food and Drug Administration Web site. Available at: https://www.accessdata.fda.gov/scripts/cder/drugsatfda/index.cfm?fuseaction=Search.Search_Drug_Name Last updated: daily. Accessed June 15, 2016.

Immune Mechanisms and Novel Targets in Rheumatoid Arthritis

Swamy Venuturupalli, MD

KEYWORDS

- Rheumatoid arthritis • Pathophysiology • Biologics • Novel targets

KEY POINTS

- Rheumatoid arthritis (RA) is an excellent model to evaluate the impact of biologic therapies due to the extensive understanding of the pathophysiology, relatively well-defined objective outcome measures among autoimmune diseases, and rich experience with numerous biologics including those that work and those that have failed clinical trials.
- The etiopathogenesis of RA involves a complex interplay between a genetically susceptible host and environmental factors, which results in activation of the innate as well as the acquired immune system. The disease is propagated through resident cells in the synovium of the joint, which allows for targeted biologic therapies that act at various stages in the pathogenesis of this condition.
- Although the first generation of biologics primarily focused on inactivating key cytokines and effector cells of the adaptive immune system, the current focus is on developing small molecules that could disrupt intracellular signaling pathways involved in cytokine signaling.
- Future novel approaches will try to use differences in the metabolism of activated autoreactive cells, disruption of lymphoid aggregation and angiogenesis, and also harness the effects of the microbiome in developing safe and effective therapies for this condition.

INTRODUCTION

Over the past several decades, immense progress has been made in the understanding of the immune mechanisms and cytokine networks that contribute to the development and progression of autoimmune rheumatic diseases. This is most true for rheumatoid arthritis (RA), in which the basic biology of the immune response, the cytokine milieu, and pathogenesis of synovial hyperplasia are reasonably well understood. Based on this understanding, numerous biologic agents are now available for the treatment of RA, and at the time of this writing, approximately 10 biologics are approved for the treatment of RA by the US regulatory agencies.

Division of Rheumatology- Cedars Sinai Medical Center, 8750 Wilshire Blvd, Suite 350, Beverly Hills, CA 90211, USA
E-mail address: swamy.venuturupalli@cshs.org

Immunol Allergy Clin N Am 37 (2017) 301–313
http://dx.doi.org/10.1016/j.iac.2017.01.002
0889-8561/17/© 2017 Elsevier Inc. All rights reserved.

Although tremendous success has been attained through targeting of cytokines in patients via biologics (particularly tumor necrosis factor [TNF]-α and interleukin [IL]-6), the focus of the field has shifted to the use of small molecules that block cytokine production and/or signaling. In this article, we review the mechanisms of disease development in RA, and highlight some of the methods of manipulating cytokine networks in RA. Additionally, we discuss some of the novel mechanisms of controlling RA that are in the early stages of development.

Indeed, the allergy/immunology field also has made tremendous progress in the understanding of pathophysiologic mechanisms that lead to these disorders, and biologic therapies are now being used increasingly to treat allergic and immunologic disorders. The approaches used in RA are of relevance to the allergy/immunology field, and the experiences and approaches used in RA could provide valuable insights to the allergy/immunology community, which is why they are discussed in this article. The aim of this article was not to provide a comprehensive list of all the biologics in RA, but rather highlight the approaches that are considered to hold promise in the near and not too distant future.

OVERVIEW OF PATHOGENESIS OF RHEUMATOID ARTHRITIS

The initiation of RA is thought to be due to a combination of genetic and stochastic (random) events. Susceptibility to RA is defined by a pattern of inherited genes, the most important of which are the human leukocyte antigen (HLA) major histocompatability genes. Of these, the HLA DRB1 shared epitope has been implicated in conferring an increased risk for the disease.[1] Additionally, numerous other genes that contribute to susceptibility, including cytokine signaling and T-cell signaling, have been well described. However, genes alone account for a small portion of disease causation and environmental factors contribute to the pathogenesis as well. Of the environmental factors, smoking is the best defined, and confers a susceptibility risk of 20-fold to 40-fold.[1] In recent years, the importance of epigenetic factors, such as hypomethylation of DNA, dysregulated histone marks, or expression of microRNAs, have been demonstrated to play an important role in the upregulation of the proinflammatory genes and are increasingly being studied as potential targets for disease amelioration.

To enhance the understanding of these concepts, the key points are detailed in the first Box of **Fig. 1**, which details these various steps in the pathogenesis of RA.

The most likely mechanism of disease induction involves repeated stimulation of the innate immune system at mucosal surfaces, which can lead to autoantibody formation years before an unknown event triggers the development of disease in the synovium. For example, smoking induces peptidyl arginine deiminase expression in alveolar macrophages, which convert arginine to citrulline. These citrullinated peptides are presented to the immune system resulting in anticitrullinated protein antibodies (ACPAs). ACPAs have been described in other mucosal tissues, such as the gingiva, among other organs.[2]

Following the development of ACPAs, soluble immune complexes then form in the circulation and find their way to the synovium. Here they bind to mast cells, neutrophils, and monocytes in the synovial microvasculature, increasing vascular permeability. ACPAs then bind to the citrullinated epitopes in the synovium and the cartilage and can directly activate osteoclasts, ultimately leading to direct damage to chondrocytes, collagen, and proteoglycans. Synovial inflammation progresses, and there is further creation of neoepitopes with joint-specific antigens from degraded collagen and proteoglycans.

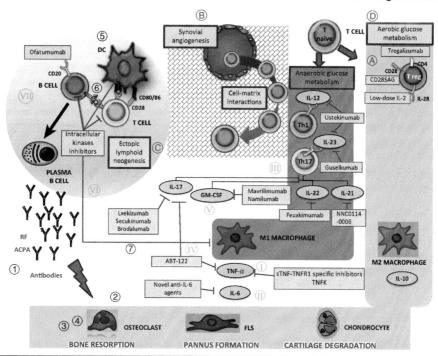

Fig. 1. Etiopathogenesis of RA and potential future targets. (*Modified from* Semerano L, Minichiello E, Bessis N, et al. Novel immunotherapeutic avenues for rheumatoid arthritis. Trends Mol Med 2016;22(3):216; with permission.)

Dendritic cells loaded with joint-specific antigens then migrate to lymph nodes, where there is activation of the acquired immune system. T-cell activation occurs in the lymph nodes, followed by epitope spreading to native antigens. This is followed by true autoimmunity; that is, B-cell and T-cell reaction to self-antigens. This cascading of events results in the activation of cytokine networks, which ultimately result in chronic and destructive synovitis. It should be noted that cytokines are not limited to the synovium and escape into the circulation causing systemic problems, such as fatigue and fever (due to IL-6 and TNF).[2]

ROLE OF CYTOKINES AND CURRENTLY AVAILABLE BIOLOGICS IN RHEUMATOID ARTHRITIS

Rheumatoid arthritis has been the most extensively studied rheumatic disease, thus allowing for the most amount of information about the cytokine networks in RA. Additionally, several therapeutic approaches to disrupt cytokine networks in RA have been performed. This has led to accumulation of a wealth of knowledge and several novel approaches to disruption of cytokines have been used and tested in RA. In this section, the major cytokines and their biological effects and feedback loops are described.

T-Cell Cytokines

Interferon (IFN) gamma was initially considered a vital cytokine in RA based on indirect observations of IFN-like activity in rheumatoid synovium. Additionally, HLA-DR expression in the rheumatoid synovium had been noted as an early observation. However, subsequently, with the use of specific IFN-gamma assays, only small amounts of INF-gamma were noted in the rheumatoid synovium, which indicated that IFN-gamma–like activity was due to other factors.[3] Most T-cell cytokines, including both TH1 and TH2 cytokines, are conspicuously absent or present at very low levels in RA synovium. On the other hand, IL-17, a Th17 cell-derived cytokine, is found in rheumatoid synovium in abundance. It acts in synergy with IL-1 and TNF-α and can independently as well as together with these cytokines induce the production of metalloproteinases, activate osteoclasts, and interact synergistically with IL-1 to amplify its effect on the rheumatoid synovium.[4]

Macrophage and Fibroblast Cytokines

In contrast to T-cell cytokines, products secreted by activated macrophages and fibroblasts are the primary cytokines involved in the pathogenesis of RA and are abundant in synovial fluid and tissue. The primary cytokines include IL-1, TNF-α, IL-6, granulocyte-macrophage colony-stimulating factor (GM-CSF), macrophage-CSF, transforming growth factor-β, and several chemokines.[5] IL-1 is one of the primary proinflammatory cytokines in RA and is secreted by synovial macrophages with multiple biological effects including the synthesis of prostaglandins, collagenase, stimulation of fibroblasts, and chemotaxis for B and T cells.[6] Although IL-1 appears to be a primary player in the RA joint, several anti–IL-1 therapies have been tried in RA with only limited success.

TNF-α is one of the most important cytokines in a variety of rheumatic diseases. It has been demonstrated in abundance in rheumatoid joints as well as circulation and stimulates collagenase and prostaglandin E2, induces bone resorption, inhibits bone formation, and stimulates resorption of proteoglycans. Both IL-1 and TNF-α enhance cytokine production, adhesion cell profile expression and production, and the production of metalloproteinases.[7]

IL-6 is highly unregulated in the rheumatoid joint and has a wide range of effects. It is the primary regulator of the acute-phase response and is responsible for the systemic features of RA, such as fatigue, cognitive dysfunction, and altered hypothalamic pituitary adrenal axis function. Interfering with the function of IL-6 through blockage of the IL-6 receptor by tocilizumab has been a successful intervention in RA[8]

Targeting of cytokines and cytokine networks using biologic agents in particular has met with significant success in RA. There are currently 5 TNF-α targeting therapies approved for use in RA, including etanercept, infliximab, adalimumab, certolizumab-pegol, and golimumab. Although these medications have revolutionized the treatment of RA, a substantial minority of patients do not respond to these medications, which has necessitated the development of other biologic agents. Biologics other than TNF blockers currently in use for RA include tocilizumab, an anti-IL6R (receptor) mAb, abatacept, a soluble fusion protein that consists of the extracellular domain of human cytotoxic T-lymphocyte–associated antigen 4 linked to the modified Fc portion of human immunoglobulin G1 (IgG1), which interferes with T-cell activation, rituximab a monoclonal antibody against the protein CD20, which is primarily found on the surface of immune system B cells, and tofacitinib. a drug of the Janus kinase inhibitor class that inhibits intracellular signaling.

THE MATURESCENCE OF CONVENTIONAL BIOLOGICS AND THE ADVENT OF NOVEL BIOLOGIC APPROACHES

Compared with other rheumatic diseases, RA has relatively well-defined outcome measures, and a thorough understanding of the pathophysiology, as described previously. As a result, biologic therapeutics in RA have been well developed. In an elegant and detailed review, Semerano and colleagues[9] described several novel immunotherapeutic avenues for RA. Although such a detailed review is beyond the scope of this article, I have summarized some of these findings in **Fig. 1** and **Table 1** and in the text below. **Table 1** summarizes selective currently available medications and novel approaches to block cytokine effects in RA. Selected important and illustrative citations also have been provided.

In general, it would be fair to say that there is increasing interest in small molecules that block cytokine production and signaling, which may have a significant competitive advantage over the monoclonal antibodies. Some of the other strategies that are in early experimental stages include interference with cell-matrix interactions and through increasing T-regulatory cell activity.

Novel strategies using anticytokine therapies, such as the development of selective inhibitors of sTNF and TNF R 1, may help by reducing infections, which is a significant limitation of current biologics.[10] Another novel strategy is the development of an anti-TNF vaccine, which involves conjugating inactivated TNF-α with a carrier protein, thus leading to the production of anti-TNF antibodies, which are polyclonal and have high avidity, thus avoiding the problems of antidrug antibodies that develop to traditional mAbs. In a phase 2 study, a TNFK showed efficacy in patients with RA who had failed traditional TNF antagonist therapy.[11]

Similarly, although a potent anti–IL-6R antibody is currently available (tocilizumab), due to significant side effects, other approaches to targeting IL-6 signaling are being actively investigated. IL-6 uses a receptor comprising 2 functional chains, namely IL-6Ra and a 130-KD non–ligand-binding but signal-transducing chain (gp130). Targeting IL-6 directly may offer a strategic advantage over targeting of the receptor itself. For example, clazakizumab, an anti–IL-6 mAb showed efficacy in patients with RA with an inadequate response to methotrexate.[12]

Table 1
Immune targets in RA including novel approaches

Target	Mechanism	Results	Comments
Cytokine targets			
Anti-TNF inhibitors			
sTNF/TNFR1 blocking agents	TNF muteins form heterodimers with sTNF-α incapable of activating TNFR1.[10]	Mouse studies showed equal efficacy to etanercept.	Selectively blocking sTNF/TNFR1 offers less risks of infection.
Anti-TNF vaccine	Inactivated TNF-α conjugated with KLH carrier protein, (TNFK) induces production of anti-TNF antibodies.	52-wk, human Phase IIa demonstrated improvement in outcomes.[11] Phase IIb study did not meet primary endpoints.	Leads to tolerance of TNF-specific B cells, but not memory T cells. Less immunogenicity due to polyclonal origin than mAbs.
Anti-IL6			
mABs against IL6-receptor (IL6R)	TCZ, an anti-IL-6R and sIL-6R humanized mAb.	Efficacy in human trials of RA is impressive.[17] Increased levels of IL-6 in circulation noted.	Elevated liver function tests, low white blood cell count, gastrointestinal perforations and infectious risks, risks thought to be due to signaling inhibition.
	Sarilumab anti- IL6R mAb. ALX-0061 nanobody.	Higher affinity for its ligand. Higher potency of trans-signaling blockade.[17]	Side effects similar to TCZ. —
mABs against IL-6	Humanized (olokizumab, clazakizumab) or fully human (sirukumab, MEDI5117).	Being tested in human trials.[12]	Side effects similar to TCZ.
Inhibitor of IL-6 trans-signaling	FE301.[18]	Shown efficacy in rat models of colitis and arthritis.	Potential to have lower side effects due to more selective effects on trans-signaling and promotes intestinal healing.

Th-17 Pathway

Targeting Th-17 differentiation	Ustekinumab and guselkumab block IL-23.	Human studies did not show benefit over placebo.[19]	IL-12 and IL-23 may not have benefit in RA, but show significant efficacy in psoriasis and PSA.
Th-17 cytokines, IL-17	Secukinumab fully human anti–IL-17A mAb	In RA-Phase II study did not show benefit over placebo,[20] being tested in Phase III.	Efficacy established in psoriasis, PSA, and AS.
	Ixekizumab humanized anti–IL-17A mAb.	Phase II trial showed efficacy in RA and confirmed in open-label extension.[21]	Now being developed only in AS and psoriasis and PSA. FDA approved for psoriasis
	Brodalumab, inhibitor of human IL-17 receptor.	Failed clinical efficacy.[22]	IL-17 inhibition may be relevant in RA, but efficacy may be lower compared with other inflammatory diseases.
Combined blockade of TNF-α and IL-17	Bispecific anti–TNF-α and anti–IL-17A mAb (ABT-122).	Synergistic benefit from combined cytokine blockade.	Demonstrated acceptable safety profile, with ongoing Phase II trials.[23]
GM-CSF	Mavrilimumab human IgG4 mAb that competitively binds to GM-CSF, blocking signal.	12-wk Phase II study, higher rates of remission and response.[24]	Safety concerns, as GM-CSF blockade promotes myeloid cell maturation. However, 74-wk exposure showed good tolerability profile and persistent clinical efficacy.
	Namilumab (neutralizing human IgG1 anti-GM-CSF mAb).	Phase 1b trial, subcutaneous injections showed rapid and persistent control.[25]	Post hoc analysis indicated rapid and persistent control of inflammation; Phase II trials ongoing.
IL-21	NNC0114-0006 (anti–IL-21 mAb).	Phase II trial, significant improvement in RA activity.	Another phase II trial, completed 2013, results have not been released
IL-22	ILV-094 (fezakinumab) human anti–IL-22 mAb.	Phase II study in patients with RA, results unknown.	

(continued on next page)

Table 1 (continued)

Target	Mechanism	Results	Comments
Cell-matrix interactions	Mediate the localization and maintenance of inflammation at the synovial membrane		
ELN	Possible involvement of LT-α in LT targeting in RA. Pacletizumab anti-LT-α mAb.	Phase II study in patients with RA, unresponsive to anti-TNF treatment, found targeting LT-α not effective.[26]	Potential alternatives are IL-27, based on mouse models showing it as a negative regulator of ELN.[27]
Regulatory cells	Restoration of immune tolerance removes reliance on immunosuppressants. Candidate approaches include activators of T-effector cell ratios in peripheral blood (T-regs).		
	Activation of DCs.	DCs adapted to 4 citrullinated peptide antigens with nuclear factor-κB inhibitor, increased T-regs.	Murine models lacking T-regs is associated with faster onset and greater severity.
Nondepleting anti-CD4	Tregalizumab (BT-061).	Activates T-regs by binding to an epitope on domain 2 of CD4.[28]	Not clinically superior to placebo in Phase II trial.
Low-dose IL-2 treatment	Activation of T-regs, independent T-effector cells.	Expansion of activated-T-reg populations.	Ongoing Phase II trials.
T-cell superagonists	TGN1412/TAB08 mAb.	Dose range critical.	Ongoing Phase I trial.
B-cell targets	B cells have multiple roles in RA. Act as antigen-presenting cells to T cells; stimulate T-cell differentiation and cytokine production; secrete proinflammatory cytokines.		
Cell-surface molecules	Rituximab (anti-CD20 chimeric mAb).	Depletes CD20-expressing B cells and CD4+ T cells and is FDA approved for RA.	Clinical development of ocrelizumab, humanized anti-CD20 mAb, was discontinued due to risk of serious infection.
	Ofatumumab (human anti-CD20 mAb).	Recognizes a distinct and proximal epitope, both in long-term and early RA.	More efficient than predecessor, rituximab. Long-term safety data have shown acceptable tolerability.[15]
	Alemtuzumab (anti-CD52 mAb).	Approved for B-cell chronic lymphocytic leukemia and multiple sclerosis.	
	MDX-1342 (anti-CD19 human mAb).	Development halted, due to safety concerns.	Toxicity issues have stopped development for RA.

Inhibition of kinase activity, centered on the following: p38 mitogen-activated protein kinase, spleen tyrosine kinase, BTK, and JAK.

Category	Agent	Mechanism	Status
Intracellular signaling			
BTK inhibitors	Ibrutinib (covalent, irreversible BTK inhibitor).	Targets B-cell CLL.	Currently being developed for CLL and B-cell non-Hodgkin lymphoma. Recruiting patients with RA for Phase II trial.
	CC-292 (covalent BTK inhibitor).	Inhibition continues well beyond plasma detection.	Currently undergoing Phase II trials in patients with RA.
JAK inhibitors	JAK inhibitors appear to be the most successful target for RA, due to their predominant role in signaling.		Deletion of JAK1 and JAK2 in mice is lethal.
	Tofacitinib.	Tofacitinib, first available JAK3 (and potentially JAK2) inhibitor. FDA approved for RA.	Linked to anemia and infection.
	Filgotinib.	30-fold selectivity in the inhibition of JAK1>>JAK2, JAK3, and Tyk2.	4-wk treatment, increased hemoglobin levels in patients with RA.
	ABT-494.	74-selective agent for JAK1>>JAK2.	Significant clinical response in Phase IIb trials.
	Decernotinib	Specific inhibitor against JAK3.	Effective in Phase II trials; currently being tested in Phase III trials.
	Baricitinib.	JAK1 and JAK2 selective inhibitor.	Successful Phase II trials, undergoing Phase III trials and expected FDA approval.[13]
Spleen tyrosine kinase inhibitors	Fostamatinib.		Successful phase II trials but Phase III trials did not achieve endpoints.[14]

Abbreviations: AS, ankylosing spondylitis; BTK, Bruton tyrosine kinase; CLL, chronic lymphocytic leukemia; DC, dendritic cell; ELN, ectopic lymphoid neogenesis; FDA, Food and Drug Administration; GM-CSF, granulocyte-macrophage colony-stimulating factor; IL-6R, interleukin-6 receptor; JAK, Janus kinase; LT, lymphotoxin; mAbs, monoclonal antibodies; PSA, Psoriatic Arthritis; RA, rheumatoid arthritis; sIL-6R, soluble IL-6 receptor; sTNF, soluble TNF; TCZ, tocilizumab; TNF, tumor necrosis factor; TNFR, TNF receptor; T-reg, regulatory T cell.

In recent years, Th-17 cells and cytokines have garnered a lot of interest, with mixed results. IL-12 and IL-23 are members of a family of cytokines that regulate the type 1 and type 17 immune responses. IL-12 has been detected in RA synovial tissues, but, when targeted in murine models of arthritis, did not show signals for improvement of arthritis. IL-12 and IL-23 share a peptide chain (p40) that can be targeted, and this forms the basis for the use of ustekinumab (anti–IL-12/23). Although Th-17 cells play an important role in RA, ustekinumab failed to show activity in RA, even though it has significant effects and is currently used in the treatment of psoriasis and Crohn disease. IL-17 molecules are associated with proinflammatory properties and are increased in synovial fluid in patients with RA. Although early clinical trials in RA suggested that IL-17 blockade using monoclonal antibodies might be effective, the results have been mixed.

Several pathways that mediate receptor signal transduction have been targeted by the use of small molecules called kinase inhibitors. The Janus kinases (JAK) are cytoplasmic protein tyrosine kinases that are critical for signal transduction to the nucleus. Some of these agents have become available for clinical use, such as tofacitinib, and others are currently in development.

Tofacitinib is a small-molecule, orally active drug that inhibits JAK-1 and JAK-3. It has shown significant efficacy in reducing the signs and symptoms of RA and can be used in combination with methotrexate or as monotherapy.

Another Jak inhibitor in development is baricitinib, which is a small-molecule, orally administered, JAK-1 and -2 inhibitor. It showed efficacy in a phase 3 randomized trial in patients with active RA refractory to TNF inhibitor therapy.[13] Another potential target is spleen tyrosine kinase (Syk), which is an intracellular cytoplasmic tyrosine kinase that mediates immune receptor signaling in macrophages, neutrophils, mast cells, and B cells. A small-molecule orally administered inhibitor of Syk, R788, or fostamatinib disodium, showed efficacy in several Phase II trials, but subsequent phase III randomized trials failed to show efficacy.[14]

Among the B-cell therapies, rituximab has shown significant efficacy in RA and is a particularly effective agent in certain subtypes of patients with high autoantibody loads. Several other B-cell–depleting therapies are in development, of which ofatumumab may be more efficient than rituximab and so far, the safety data have shown acceptable tolerability.[15]

NOVEL FUTURE APPROACHES FOR RHEUMATOID ARTHRITIS

Besides the approaches outlined previously, other opportunities exist in the treatment of RA using our understanding of the etiopathogenesis of this condition. For example, it is known that T-regulatory cells (T-regs) play an important role in suppression of the inflammatory response. Although a detailed review of the biologic effects of T-regs is beyond the scope of this article, several pieces of evidence point to an important role for T-regs in the suppression of inflammation.[9] In RA, currently, the main strategy being used is the in vivo expansion of T-regs via different means. Cell-directed treatments arming regulatory T cells (T-regs) in an antigen-independent manner have been achieved via noncytotoxic anti-CD4 mAbs (tregalizumab), T-cell superagonists (CD28SAg), or low-dose IL-2, which binds the high-affinity IL-2 receptor on T-regs. These approaches are currently in various stages of development.

Another possible approach stems from the understanding that stromal cells and cell– matrix interactions mediate the localization and maintenance of inflammation at the synovial membrane. With persistent chronic inflammation and cell influx, infiltrating lymphocytes can form tertiary lymphoid organs. Selective targeting of "ectopic lymphoid neogenesis" is appealing and has been tested in a Phase II study, of pacletizumab (MLTA3698), an anti-LT-/mAb and a Phase II study of an anti-TNF treatment, baminercept (LTBR-Ig, BG9924), a fusion product of LT-/receptor and IgG1. Neither of these showed positive results.[12] Fibroblast-like synoviocytes (FLSs) are important resident synovial cells that interact with the infiltrating immune cells (see **Fig. 1**) and are thought to orchestrate the transition from acute synovitis to chronic RA. Efforts are ongoing to identify and develop therapies that attenuate the activity of FLSs.

Synovial angiogenesis nurtures the proliferating pannus and is influenced by proinflammatory and proangiogenic factors in this acidic and hypoxic tissue microenvironment. Although the prospect of starving inflammation is intriguing, so far no anti-angiogenic treatments have been developed for RA. An interesting observation is that regulatory cells rely on aerobic glucose metabolism and effector T cells rely on anaerobic glucose metabolism. In vivo studies have demonstrated that blocking glycolysis with 2-desoxyglucose in naïve T cells hinders their differentiation into Th-17 cells.

Recently, differences in the microbiota in the intestines and oral cavity of patients with RA and controls has been reported. Interestingly, the most virulent species of bacteria in the feces predicted the response to treatment in patients. The interaction between the microbiome and the host appear to be bidirectional, and future studies will demonstrate the value of manipulation of the microbiome in controlling RA.[16]

SUMMARY

Significant progress has been made in the understanding of the pathophysiology of RA. RA is thought to occur due to activation of the innate immune system at mucosal surfaces in a genetically susceptible host. This leads to development of ACPAs that find their way to the synovium, where they activate the osteoclasts, macrophages, and the FLSs. Soluble immune complexes then migrate to lymph nodes, where the acquired immune system is activated and continues the process. Several steps in the process of development of chronic synovitis provide targets for intervention, and indeed RA has one of the most developed biologic drug profiles among rheumatic diseases. However, several questions remain regarding the ideal treatment for RA. For example, it is widely recognized that early institution of treatment is one of the best predictive factors for response to therapy. Similarly, it has been established that different cellular responses and cytokine responses are at play, not only in different patients, but also at different stages of the disease. Although several biologic drugs are currently in use in RA, there is an unmet need for additional therapies with better efficacy and fewer side effects. Several novel approaches are currently being investigated and several novel biologics are in various stages of development. In the future, with advances in the fields of proteomics, genomics, and metabolomics, specific phenotypes of the disease can be better identified and specific therapies for particular phases of the disease and specific patients will allow for improved control of this condition.

REFERENCES

1. Lundstrom E, Källberg H, Alfredsson L, et al. Gene-environment interaction between the DRB1 shared epitope and smoking in the risk of anti-citrullinated protein antibody-positive rheumatoid arthritis: all alleles are important. Arthritis Rheumatol 2009;60(6):1597–603.
2. McInnes IB, Schett G. The pathogenesis of rheumatoid arthritis. N Engl J Med 2011;365(23):2205–19.

3. Firestein GS, Zvaifler NJ. Peripheral blood and synovial fluid monocyte activation in inflammatory arthritis. II. Low levels of synovial fluid and synovial tissue interferon suggest that gamma-interferon is not the primary macrophage activating factor. Arthritis Rheumatol 1987;30(8):864–71.
4. Kotake S, Udagawa N, Takahashi N, et al. IL-17 in synovial fluids from patients with rheumatoid arthritis is a potent stimulator of osteoclastogenesis. J Clin Invest 1999;103(9):1345–52.
5. Arend WP, Dayer JM. Cytokines and cytokine inhibitors or antagonists in rheumatoid arthritis. Arthritis Rheumatol 1990;33(3):305–15.
6. Kay J, Calabrese L. The role of interleukin-1 in the pathogenesis of rheumatoid arthritis. Rheumatology (Oxford) 2004;43(Suppl 3):iii2–9.
7. Feldmann M, Maini RN. Lasker Clinical Medical Research Award. TNF defined as a therapeutic target for rheumatoid arthritis and other autoimmune diseases. Nat Med 2003;9(10):1245–50.
8. Hashizume M, Mihara M. The roles of interleukin-6 in the pathogenesis of rheumatoid arthritis. Arthritis 2011;2011:765624.
9. Semerano L, Minichiello E, Bessis N, et al. Novel immunotherapeutic avenues for rheumatoid arthritis. Trends Mol Med 2016;22(3):214–29.
10. Shibata H, Yoshioka Y, Ohkawa A, et al. The therapeutic effect of TNFR1-selective antagonistic mutant TNF-α in murine hepatitis models. Cytokine 2008;44(2):229–33.
11. Durez P, Vandepapeliere P, Miranda P, et al. Therapeutic vaccination with TNF-Kinoid in TNF antagonist-resistant rheumatoid arthritis: a phase II randomized, controlled clinical trial. PLoS One 2014;9(12):e113465.
12. Weinblatt ME, Mease P, Mysler E, et al. The efficacy and safety of subcutaneous clazakizumab in patients with moderate-to-severe rheumatoid arthritis and an inadequate response to methotrexate: results from a multinational, phase IIb, randomized, double-blind, placebo/active-controlled, dose-ranging study. Arthritis Rheumatol 2015;67(10):2591–600.
13. Genovese MC, Kremer J, Zamani O, et al. Baricitinib in patients with refractory rheumatoid arthritis. N Engl J Med 2016;374(13):1243–52.
14. Weinblatt ME, Genovese MC, Ho M, et al. Effects of fostamatinib, an oral spleen tyrosine kinase inhibitor, in rheumatoid arthritis patients with an inadequate response to methotrexate: results from a phase III, multicenter, randomized, double-blind, placebo-controlled, parallel-group study. Arthritis Rheumatol 2014; 66(12):3255–64.
15. Anand V. Ofatumumab for rheumatoid arthritis: a Cochrane systematic review and meta-analysis. Arthritis Rheumatol 2015;67 [abstract: 500].
16. Zhang X, Zhang D, Jia H, et al. The oral and gut microbiomes are perturbed in rheumatoid arthritis and partly normalized after treatment. Nat Med 2015;21(8):895–905.
17. Semerano L, Thiolat A, Minichiello E, et al. Targeting IL-6 for the treatment of rheumatoid arthritis: Phase II investigational drugs. Expert Opin Investig Drugs 2014; 23(7):979–99.
18. Nowell MA, Williams AS, Carty SA, et al. Therapeutic targeting of IL-6 trans signaling counteracts STAT3 control of experimental inflammatory arthritis. J Immunol 2009;182(1):613–22.
19. Smolen J, Agarwal SK, Ilivanova E, et al. OP0031 a phase 2 study evaluating the efficacy and safety of subcutaneously administered ustekinumab and guselkumab in patients with active rheumatoid arthritis despite treatment with methotrexate. Ann Rheum Dis 2015;74(Suppl 2):76–7.

20. Genovese MC, Durez P, Richards HB, et al. One-year efficacy and safety results of secukinumab in patients with rheumatoid arthritis: phase II, dose-finding, double-blind, randomized, placebo-controlled study. J Rheumatol 2014;41(3): 414–21.
21. Genovese MC, Braun DK, Erickson JS, et al. Safety and efficacy of open-label subcutaneous ixekizumab treatment for 48 weeks in a phase II study in biologic-naive and TNF-IR patients with rheumatoid arthritis. J Rheumatol 2016; 43(2):289–97.
22. Pavelka K, Chon Y, Newmark R, et al. A study to evlauate the safety tolerability, and efficacy of brodalumumab in subjects with rheumatoid arthritis and an inadequate response to Methotrexate. J Rheumatol 2015;42(6):912–9.
23. Ahmed G, Goss S. Pharmacokinetics of ABT-122, a dual TNF- and IL-17A-targeted DVD-IGTM, after single dosing in healthy volunteers and multiple dosing in subjects with rheumatoid arthritis. Ann Rheum Dis 2015;74(Suppl 2):479.
24. Burmester GR, Weinblatt ME, McInnes IB, et al. Efficacy and safety of mavrilimumab in subjects with rheumatoid arthritis. Ann Rheum Dis 2013;72(9):1445–52.
25. Huizinga T, et al. SAT0210 first-in-patient study of namilumab, an anti-GM-CSF monoclonal antibody, in active rheumatoid arthritis: results of the priora phase IB study. Ann Rheum Dis 2015;74(Suppl 2):733.
26. Genovese M, Greenwald MC, Maria W, et al. Efficacy and safety of baminercept in the treatment of rheumatoid arthritis (RA): results of the phase 2B study in the TNF-IR population. Arthritis Rheumatol 2009;60(Suppl 10):417.
27. Jones GW, Bombardieri M, Greenhill CJ, et al. Interleukin-27 inhibits ectopic lymphoid-like structure development in early inflammatory arthritis. J Exp Med 2015;212(11):1793–802.
28. Helling B, König M, Dälken B, et al. A specific CD4 epitope bound by tregalizumab mediates activation of regulatory T cells by a unique signaling pathway. Immunol Cell Biol 2015;93(4):396–405.

Biologic Therapy in the Treatment of Chronic Skin Disorders

James M. Fernandez, MD, PhD[a], Anthony P. Fernandez, MD, PhD[b], David M. Lang, MD[a],*

KEYWORDS

- Urticaria • Angioedema • Psoriasis • Atopic dermatitis • Biologic agents
- Omalizumab • Dupilimab

KEY POINTS

- Understanding of immune pathways involved in the pathogenesis of chronic urticaria, atopic dermatitis, and psoriasis is growing.
- Biologic therapies targeting specific immune-related targets are rapidly becoming viable options for patients with severe or refractory dermatologic diseases.
- Biologic agents allow a safe and efficacious alternative in some refractory skin diseases.

INTRODUCTION

Chronic immune-related skin diseases continue to affect patients throughout the world. In many instances the diseases are refractory to first-line therapy. As clinicians uncover immunologic pathways involved in the pathogenesis of these diseases, therapeutic agents targeting specific molecular pathways are being developed. This article reviews the use of such agents in chronic urticaria (CU), atopic dermatitis, and psoriasis.

Chronic Urticaria

Understanding of the pathogenesis of CU has improved in recent years.[1,2] Despite this, many patients affected with CU experience poor control of their disease and

Disclosure: J. Fernandez, no disclosures; A. Fernandez, speaker's bureau, research, consulting for AbbVie, consulting for Novartis; D.M. Lang (PI: ClinicalTrials.gov Identifier: NCT00555971), clinical research with, received honoraria from, and/or has served as a consultant for Adamis, AstraZeneca, Genentech (PI: ClinicalTrials.gov Identifier: NCT00555971), GlaxoSmithKline, Merck, Novartis.

[a] Department of Allergy and Clinical Immunology, Respiratory Institute, Cleveland Clinic Foundation, 9500 Euclid Avenue, Cleveland, OH 44195, USA; [b] Departments of Dermatology and Pathology, Cleveland Clinic Foundation, 9500 Euclid Avenue, Cleveland, OH 44195, USA
* Corresponding author.
E-mail address: langd@ccf.org

Immunol Allergy Clin N Am 37 (2017) 315–327
http://dx.doi.org/10.1016/j.iac.2017.01.006
0889-8561/17/© 2017 Elsevier Inc. All rights reserved.

immunology.theclinics.com

impaired quality of life.[1] An estimated 50% or more of patients with CU do not achieve satisfactory control with antihistamine treatment alone.[2]

Urticaria and pruritus are generated primarily by the action of histamine on H1 receptors located on endothelial cells (wheal) and on sensory nerves (flare). The non-necrotizing infiltrate in CU consists of CD4+ (CD, cluster of differentiation) lymphocytes, monocytes, neutrophils, eosinophils, and basophils, which may be refractory to antihistamine pharmacotherapy, even when advanced to higher than US Food and Drug Administration (FDA)–approved doses.[2] Patients with CU who do not improve with H1 and H2 antihistamine therapy, including dose advancement of a potent antihistamine (eg, doxepin or hydroxyzine) as tolerated are candidates for alternative therapies.[1] Several biologic agents have been studied in patients with antihistamine-resistant CU.

Omalizumab
Omalizumab is a chimeric human-mouse recombinant antibody, produced in a Chinese hamster ovary cell line that binds to the domain at which immunoglobulin (Ig) E binds to FCεRI (the high affinity IgE receptor) on mast cells and basophils.[3] Its mechanism of action in patients with CU has not been determined. In clinical trials of omalizumab in subjects with CU, most adverse events (AEs) were mild or moderate in severity, and did not differ remarkably compared with placebo. Severe thrombocytopenia, eosinophilic conditions, serum sickness, and hair loss have been reported.[3] The rate of anaphylaxis observed in patients with moderate-severe allergic asthma receiving omalizumab is approximately 1 in 1000.[1,3] Whether the rate of anaphylaxis will be similar in patients with CU, and whether the same precautions for omalizumab are appropriate for a population of patients with CU, is unclear. In clinical studies, malignancies were observed in clinical trials in a small number of subjects with asthma receiving omalizumab and in subjects receiving placebo.[1,3] Of 4127 subjects who received omalizumab, 20 (0.5%) developed malignancy; of 2236 who received placebo injections, 5 (0.2%) developed malignancy. A recent study,[4] with a median follow up time of approximately 5 years, compared the safety of omalizumab in 5007 asthmatics receiving omalizumab with 2829 asthmatics not receiving omalizumab. Rates of malignancy were similar: 12.3 per 1000 patient years for omalizumab, compared with 13.0 per 1000 patient years in asthmatics who did not receive omalizumab. This finding implies that omalizumab is not associated with an increased risk for malignancy. This study also found a higher rate of cardiovascular events in asthmatics receiving omalizumab (13.4 per 1000 patient years), including myocardial infarction and cerebrovascular events, compared with non–omalizumab-treated asthmatics (8.1 per 1000 patient years). Although these results suggest that omalizumab is associated with an increased risk of cardiovascular events, there were aspects of the design of this study that imply this is not the case, including baseline differences in cardiovascular risk factors. An analysis of 25 randomized controlled trials found no remarkable difference in the rate of cardiovascular events in 3342 omalizumab-treated asthmatics compared with 2895 subjects with asthma who did not receive omalizumab.[3] Efforts to further understand possible risks for malignancy and for cardiovascular disease are continuing during postmarketing surveillance.

There is evidence from case reports and case series, and high-quality evidence from randomized controlled trials, supporting the therapeutic utility of omalizumab for patients with refractory CU.[1,5–7] A recent meta-analysis[8] identified 7 randomized, double-blind, placebo-controlled studies of omalizumab, with 1312 subjects with CU. Omalizumab was administered at doses of 75 mg, 150 mg, 300 mg, or 600 mg. The 7 studies showed a low risk of bias. All used allocation concealment, and there was no evidence for publication bias detected. Omalizumab was consistently more effective than placebo. Response was dose dependent; the 300-mg dose was the most effective. Rates of complete response were statistically significantly higher in subjects randomized to omalizumab compared with placebo (RR (relative risk) = 4.55; 95% confidence interval, 3.33–6.23; $P<.00001$). Omalizumab was well tolerated; there was no remarkable difference in AEs in subjects randomized to omalizumab compared with placebo. These data imply that the effects of omalizumab in properly selected patients with CU are robust and consistent.

In one of these randomized controlled trials,[7] 336 of 480 subjects screened for participation, whose CU remained poorly controlled despite dose advancement of H1 antihistamines to 4 times the FDA-approved dose in combination with H2 antihistamines and/or an antileukotriene, received 6 injections of omalizumab 300 mg or placebo on a monthly basis. Subjects maintained their prerandomization regimens of high-dose H1 antihistamine, H2 antihistamine, and/or antileukotriene during participation; in contrast, in other randomized controlled trials,[5,6] patients were taking antihistamines at approved doses (eg, cetirizine 10 mg/d). Based on its design, this randomized controlled trial[7] enhances the strength of evidence supporting the efficacy of omalizumab for recalcitrant CU. It is also important to note that the subjects enrolled in randomized controlled studies of omalizumab for CU had a high disease burden, with a mean Urticaria Activity Score (UAS) over 7 days (UAS7) of 31, and a history of prior corticosteroid treatment in approximately 50%.[9]

Table 1 describes the proportion of subjects who were free of hives and itching (ie, achieved a UAS7 score of 0) and who had clinically significant reduction in frequency and severity of urticaria (UAS7 score <6) in 3 randomized controlled trials.[5–7] The primary outcome was the change in itch severity score compared with baseline; efficacy was assessed in each study at 12 weeks. A total of 412 subjects were randomized to 300 mg of omalizumab every 4 weeks for 12 weeks, whereas 242 received placebo. The proportions of subjects with UAS7 scores of 0 were 36% (149 out of 412) in association with 300 mg of omalizumab, and 6% (15 out of 242) in subjects randomized to placebo. The proportion of subjects with UAS7 scores less than 6 were 55% (226 out of 412) in association with 300 mg of omalizumab, and 14% (34 out of 242) in subjects randomized to placebo. This finding leads to a calculated number needed to treat of 3.3 for UAS scores of 0 and 2.4 for UAS less than 6, respectively, implying that, for every 33 patients with antihistamine-resistant CU who are treated with omalizumab at a dose of 300 mg every 4 weeks for 12 weeks, 10 will become hive and itch free; for every 24 patients treated with omalizumab, at a dose of 300 mg every 4 weeks for 12 weeks, 10 will experience clinically significant improvement. However, the potential for a salutary response to omalizumab cannot be predicted based on demographic characteristics (eg, age, gender), laboratory data (including total serum IgE level and findings reflecting autoimmunity, such as autologous serum skin test, autoantibodies to IgE or the high-affinity IgE receptor, or antithyroid antibodies), histopathology, or previous course of CU.[10] Individuals with physical urticaria syndromes were excluded from the randomized controlled trials; for this reason, the evidence describing benefit in patients with physical urticaria treated with omalizumab consists of case reports and case series, and is not high quality.[11] The optimal duration of omalizumab treatment of CU, and optimal strategies for suspending omalizumab, also merit clarification in future studies.[11]

Interleukin-1 inhibitors

Cryopyrin-associated periodic syndromes (CAPS), also referred to as cryopyrinopathies, are a group of autoinflammatory conditions, including familial cold

Table 1
Proportion of subjects in 3 randomized controlled trials evaluating the efficacy of omalizumab who became hive and itch free and who experienced clinically significant improvement

| Author, Year | Randomized Subjects | | | UAS7 = 0 | UAS7 = 0 | UAS7 <6 | UAS7 <6 |
	Study Duration (wk)	Omalizumab 300 mg	Placebo	300 mg	Placebo	300 mg	Placebo
Maurer, et al,[5] 2013	12	79	79	35 (44%)	4 (5%)	52 (66%)	15 (19%)
Kaplan, et al,[7] 2013	24[a]	252	83	85 (34%)	4 (5%)	132 (52%)	10 (12%)
Saini, et al,[6] 2015	24[a]	81	80	29 (36%)	7 (9%)	42 (52%)	9 (11%)
Totals	—	412	242	149 (36%)	15 (6%)	226 (55%)	34 (14%)

[a] Efficacy analysis at week 12; trial duration, 24 weeks.

Data from Refs.[5–7]

autoinflammatory syndrome, Muckle-Wells syndrome, and neonatal-onset multi-system inflammatory disease, characterized by abnormalities in the C1AS1 gene, which encodes for the cryopyrin protein.[1] Canakinumab is a fully human anti--IL-1β monoclonal antibody that selectively blocks IL-1β. Dramatic benefit with administration of canakinumab in CAPS has been shown in a randomized controlled trial.[12]

Schnitzler syndrome is a rare condition caused by an IgM, or less commonly IgG, monoclonal gammopathy, in which patients present with nonpruritic urticaria, bone pain, and intermittent fever.[1] Dramatic benefit has been described in several cases with administration of anakinra, a recombinant human interleukin (IL)-1 receptor antagonist (IL-1Rα), approved by the FDA for refractory rheumatoid arthritis and CAPS.[13] Because of the rarity of Schnitzler syndrome, it is unlikely that randomized controlled trials will be performed. Based on the dramatic benefit reported, anakinra may be regarded as an agent with substantial promise for successful treatment of this condition.

Efficacy of canakinumab and anakinra in cases of refractory urticarial vasculitis has also been described.[14,15]

Tumor necrosis factor-alpha inhibitors

With the understanding that tumor necrosis factor alpha (TNF-α) may play a role in the pathogenesis of some cases of CU, etanercept, adalimumab, and infliximab have been used for treatment of patients with CU or urticarial vasculitis. Sand and Thomsen[16] reported that 12 of 20 (60%) patients with refractory CU experienced resolution on therapeutic trials of either etanercept 50 mg weekly or adalimumab 40 mg twice monthly, whereas another 3 (15%) experienced partial response and 5 (25%) had no benefit. Response was observed within the first month after treatment initiation. Duration of treatment spanned 3 to 30 months. Among the 12 who experienced resolution of CU, 5 had previously suspended treatment with omalizumab either because of lack of improvement or anaphylaxis.

A case report describing dramatic improvement of refractory delayed pressure urticaria has also been reported in association with TNF-α inhibitor therapy.[17] Etanercept 25 mg twice weekly was administered for psoriasis. By the fifth day of therapy, dramatic benefit was observed. The patient was subsequently switched to infliximab for treatment of psoriasis, and remained free of urticaria or angioedema. In a case series of 6 patients with either idiopathic CU or urticarial vasculitis treated with a TNF-α inhibitor, all patients were dramatically improved.[18] TNF-α inhibitors all carry a risk of serious infections, including tuberculosis and fungal infections, and a risk for lymphomas and other malignancies. The evidence supporting use of TNF-α blockers is limited by small numbers of patients who have been reported, and lack of randomized controlled trials to establish efficacy.

Atopic Dermatitis

Atopic dermatitis (AD) is a chronic and relapsing inflammatory skin disease affecting 10% of children and 1% to 3% of adults.[19] It is highly associated with other allergic diseases such as asthma and allergic rhinitis. Typical clinical findings in AD are pruritus, facial and extensor eczema in infants and children, flexural eczema in adults, and a chronic or relapsing dermatitis. The pathophysiology of AD involves a complex interaction of multiple immunologic and inflammatory components in addition to environmental and genetic factors. The standard treatment includes skin hydration, allergen and irritant avoidance, topical corticosteroids, and topical immunosuppressant therapy. Despite these treatment measures many cases are refractory and require systemic immunomodulatory treatments.

As mentioned, AD involves many different components of the immune system. Early on there is a T-helper 2 (Th2) immune response leading to production of IL-4 and IL-13 (triggering production of IgE by B lymphocytes), IL-5 (important for recruitment and activation of eosinophils), and IL-6. The chronic effect of AD is a switch from Th2 cells to Th1 cells with the subsequent upregulation of interferon (IFN) gamma and IL-5.[20] Given this pathogenesis, biological targets within these pathways have been investigated with varying success in the treatment of refractory AD.

Omalizumab

Many patients with AD have an increased IgE level and Th2 skewing. Omalizumab is a recombinant humanized monoclonal anti-IgE antibody that blocks the interaction of IgE with high-affinity FcεRI and downregulates dendritic cell, basophil, and mast cell FcεRI expression. It reduces levels of free IgE in the serum by blocking initial antigen presentation and the additional production of IgE, and also reduces numbers of inflammatory cells.[21]

A prospective analysis was performed to assess the efficacy of 150 mg or 300 mg of omalizumab given every 2 weeks in 21 patients with moderate to severe persistent allergic asthma and AD. Patients were stratified into the following groups: very high IgE level (>700 IU/mL), high IgE level (186–700 IU/mL), and normal IgE level (0–185 IU/mL). AD severity was assessed at 0, 1, 3, 6, and 9 months via an Investigator Global Assessment (IGA) index. All 21 patients showed clinical and statistically significant improvement of their AD based on IGA scores. Some patients showed improvement as early as 1 month of therapy. When evaluating patients based on pretreatment IgE levels, improvement was noted in all 3 groups. with greater improvement in Scoring Atopic Dermatitis (SCORAD) scores being seen in those patients with normal pretreatment serum IgE levels compared with the other groups. However, it has been noted that patients with IgE levels well beyond those approved for omalizumab in the treatment of asthma (30–700 IU/mL) have shown clinical improvement of their AD with omalizumab administration.[22]

Another study investigated 150 mg of omalizumab given every 2 weeks for 10 injections in 11 patients with IgE level greater than 10,000 IU/mL. Disease severity was monitored using SCORAD and photographic documentation. Of the 11 patients, 2 responded with a very good clinical response (SCORAD reduction >50%), 4 showed satisfactory results (SCORAD reduction between 25% and 50%), 3 showed no clinically relevant changes (reduction or increase in SCORAD <25%), and 2 showed worsening of their eczema (SCORAD increase >25%).[23]

Infliximab

As previously mentioned the chronic pathogenesis of AD frequently results in a switch from a Th2 to Th1 immune response. This switch results in the production of TNF-α level and upregulation of proinflammatory cytokine levels, such as IL-1, IL-6, IL-8.[24] Patients with AD have been shown to have increased serum and tissue concentrations of TNF-α.[25] Infliximab is a chimeric monoclonal antibody that consists of a murine Fab portion specific for human TNF-α and the constant region (Fc) of human IgG1. Infliximab binds with high specificity and affinity to free and membrane-bound TNF-α. Infliximab has a dual mode of action:

1. Blocking soluble TNF-α
2. Inducing lysis of TNF receptor–bearing target cells, which requires activation of complement[25]

One study examined the efficacy of infliximab on 9 patients with moderate or severe AD refractory to conventional therapy. Infliximab 5 mg/kg was given at weeks 0, 2, 6, 14, 22, 30, and 38, and patients were followed for 46 weeks. AD was monitored by following the Eczema Area and Severity Index (EASI), Pruritus Severity Assessment (PSA), and Dermatology Life Quality Index (DLQI). Response was defined as a reduction of EASI score by 50% (excellent), by 30% to 49% (moderate), or by 29% (nonsignificant). Patients with AD who were classified as responders (reduction of EASI $\geq$30%) at week 10 entered a retreatment phase lasting up to week 46.[25] Furthermore, serologic markers including blood eosinophil count, C-reactive protein, and eosinophilic cationic protein level were monitored. At week 2, infliximab showed a significant clinical efficacy as assessed by EASI ($P = .03$) in all 9 patients with AD; mean EASI scores decreased from 22.5 (week 0) to 10.6 (week 2). Pruritus, as assessed by PSA, significantly improved in all patients with AD at week 2 (1.4; $P = .03$) and week 10 (1.6; $P = .04$) compared with week 0 (2.8). There was a significant reduction in DLQI scores from baseline among all patients at week 10 (week 0, 19; week 10, 10.9; $P = .02$). This reduction in DLQI was based primarily on a decrease in pruritus. However, the sustained response to infliximab was not seen long term on maintenance therapy in the patient responders who entered the retreatment phase. Only 2 patients maintained improvement at week 46. It is speculated that the lack of sustained response may have been caused by the development of antiinfliximab antibodies previously observed in infliximab studies for other disease states.[25]

Rituximab

Given that AD shows a heavy Th2 bias with downstream B-cell activation and resulting IgE production, it has been postulated that intervention with anti–B cell therapy may be beneficial.

Rituximab is a chimeric monoclonal anti-CD20 antibody that eliminates B cells by inducing antibody-dependent cell-mediated cytotoxicity, complement-dependent toxicity, or apoptosis.[26] Six patients with severe AD (refractory to topical corticosteroids and calcineurin inhibition) received 2 doses of 1000 mg of rituximab 2 weeks apart. EASI, pruritus, total and allergen-specific IgE levels, skin histology, and inflammatory cell and cytokine expression in skin and peripheral blood before and for 22 weeks after therapy were monitored.[27] All 6 patients showed improvement of their skin symptoms within 4 to 8 weeks and this was maintained for the full 24 weeks of the study. The EASI significantly decreased from 29.4 before the study to 8.4 by week 8 and remained at or below this level at week 24. Histologic changes such as spongiosis, acanthosis, and T-cell and B-cell numbers also improved. No significant decrease was seen in allergen-specific IgE levels and total IgE level. In contrast, recent case reports have not reproduced the success of rituximab seen in the previous study.[28]

Mepolizumab

Eosinophils and T cells play major roles in the pathogenesis of AD. IL-5 is a key cytokine in eosinophil differentiation and growth in the bone marrow.[29] Mepolizumab is humanized monoclonal antibody to IL-5 currently approved for eosinophilic asthma. A trial using mepolizumab in 2 doses of 750 mg, given 1 week apart, was performed on patients with moderate to severe AD using a randomized, placebo-controlled, parallel-group design. Eighteen patients received mepolizumab and 22 placebo treatment. Although peripheral blood eosinophil numbers were significantly decreased in the treatment group compared with placebo, there was no significant difference in IgA assessment, SCORAD, pruritus scoring, and serum thymus and activation-regulated chemokine (TARC) values in the mepolizumab-treated group compared with placebo.[29]

Dupilumab

Dupilumab is currently the most promising biologic treatment of AD. Dupilumab is a fully human monoclonal antibody that is directed against the shared alpha subunit of the IL-4 receptor resulting in signaling blockade of IL-4 and IL-13, which are key drivers of Th2-mediated inflammation. A double-blind, placebo-controlled trial involving adults with moderate to severe AD refractory to topical glucocorticoids and calcineurin inhibitors investigated dupilumab as monotherapy in two 4-week trials, one 12-week trial, and in combination with topical glucocorticoids in another 4-week study. EASI score, the IGA score, pruritus, safety assessments, serum Th2 biomarker levels (eosinophils, IgE, and TARC), and disease transcriptome were monitored.[30]

Both 4-week trials enrolled adults with moderate to severe AD that was not adequately controlled with topical medications such as glucocorticoids and calcineurin inhibitors. Patients were randomly assigned in one of the 4-week studies to placebo or dupilumab at 75-mg, 150-mg, or 300-mg weekly subcutaneous injections or placebo, 150 mg or 300 mg weekly in the other 4-week study. In the both 4-week trials, there was a rapid dose-dependent increase of EASI-50, as well as improvement in the pruritus numerical rating scale score. Eighteen patients from these two 4-week trials participated in gene-expression profiling through skin biopsies. Significant dose-dependent changes in the RNA-expression profile were observed in the patients after 4 weeks of treatment dupilumab with the gene-expression profiles of samples from lesions in dupilumab-treated patients more closely matching the profile of samples from nonlesional sites.[30] In the 12-week study, 109 patients were randomly assigned to receive weekly subcutaneous dupilumab at a dose of 300 mg or placebo. At 12 weeks, 85% of patients in the treatment group versus 35% in the placebo group had a 50% or greater reduction in the EASI. The dupilumab group also had a greater reduction in the body surface area affected (−60% vs −18% in placebo) and in the pruritus numerical rating scale score (−56% vs −15%). Serum biomarker profiling (eosinophil counts, TARC, and IgE) showed weak or no correlation with improvements in EASI or pruritus, although significant correlations were observed between reductions in the TARC level and changes in pruritus scores. In the combination study, patients were randomly assigned to receive 4 weekly doses of placebo or subcutaneous dupilumab at a dose of 300 mg with both groups receiving a standardized regimen of topical glucocorticoids. The primary end points were the incidence and severity of AEs. One-hundred percent of the patients in the dupilumab group, compared with 50% of those who received topical glucocorticoids with placebo injection, met the criteria for EASI-50 ($P = .002$). The percentages of patients with any AE were similar in the placebo and treatment groups. However, serious AEs, such as skin infection, occurred more frequently with placebo injections.[30]

Psoriasis

A wealth of research during the past several decades has led to detailed understanding of the pathogenesis of psoriasis vulgaris. Despite its well-known association with overexpression of proinflammatory cytokines such as IFN-δ and TNF-α, a recent paradigm shift has led to Th17 cells and cytokines such as IL-17, IL-23, and IL-12 replacing Th1 cells as what are thought to be the key mediators of tissue damage. This knowledge has led to development of biologic therapies that specifically block individual cytokines, including TNF-α inhibitors, IL-12/IL-23 inhibitors, and IL-17 inhibitors, which are extremely effective at treating moderate to severe psoriasis and/or psoriatic arthritis and have revolutionized the ability to manage psoriatic disease over the past 10 to 15 years. At present, there are 6 biologic medications (etanercept, infliximab, adalimumab, ustekinumab, secukinumab, and ixekizumab) that are FDA approved for treatment of moderate to severe psoriasis vulgaris. All except ixekizumab are also currently FDA approved for treating psoriatic arthritis.

Tumor necrosis factor-alpha inhibitors

Etanercept was FDA approved for psoriasis in 2004 and is a fusion protein containing two 75-kD TNF-α receptors linked to the Fc portion of an IgG1 antibody that binds and eliminates the activity of soluble TNF-α. In a double-blind phase 3 trial, there was an improvement from baseline of greater than or equal to 75% in the Psoriasis Area and Severity Index (PASI 75) in 4% of patients in the placebo group versus 49% of patients receiving 50 mg of etanercept twice weekly.[31] Clinical responses continued to improve with longer treatment and, at week 24, 59% of patients achieved greater than or equal to PASI 75. Etanercept was generally well tolerated, with AEs typically being mild. Another phase 3 randomized controlled trial examined safety and efficacy of etanercept dose reduction for maintenance therapy. After 12 weeks of etanercept 50 mg twice weekly, patients were transitioned to 25 mg twice weekly.[32] At week 24, PASI 75 was achieved by 54% of patients whose dose was reduced to 25 mg twice weekly, which increased from the percentage of patients who achieved PASI 75 at week 12 with 50 mg twice weekly.

Infliximab was FDA approved in 2006 and is a chimeric mouse/human IgG1 monoclonal antibody that binds and eliminates both soluble and membrane-bound TNF-α. In a double-blind, placebo-controlled trial, 88% of patients treated with infliximab (5 mg/kg) achieved greater than or equal to PASI 75 improvement from baseline compared with 6% in the placebo group.[33] Infliximab was generally well tolerated, but unique AEs include infusion reactions (other TNF-α inhibitors are given as subcutaneous injections). The most common infusion reactions with infliximab included chills, headache, flushing, nausea, and dyspnea, and most were mild or moderate in severity. In another phase 3, double-blind trial, patients were treated with infusions of either infliximab 5 mg/kg or placebo at weeks 0, 2, and 6, then every 8 weeks.[34] At week 50, 61% of patients receiving infliximab achieved PASI 75 and 45% achieved PASI 90, supporting this dosing schedule for long-term use. In an open-label, active-controlled randomized trial comparing infliximab with methotrexate (15–20 mg weekly), more patients achieved PASI 75 in the infliximab group (78%) compared with the methotrexate group (42%).[35] Although AE incidence was comparable between groups, incidence of serious and severe AEs was slightly higher in the infliximab group.

Adalimumab was FDA approved in 2008 and is a fully humanized IgG1 monoclonal antibody that, like infliximab, binds and eliminates soluble and membrane-bound TNF-α. In a phase 3, randomized controlled study, 71% of patients receiving adalimumab 40 mg every other week following a loading dose of 80 mg achieved PASI 75 at week 16, compared with 7% of placebo-treated patients.[36] Adalimumab treatment had an AE profile similar to other TNF-α inhibitors. In another study, patients receiving adalimumab 40 mg every other week were compared with patients receiving methotrexate 7.5 to 25 mg weekly.[37] After 16 weeks, 79.6% of adalimumab-treated patients achieved PASI 75, compared with 35.5% with methotrexate. In addition, AEs leading to discontinuation were more common in the methotrexate group compared with the adalimumab group. In a phase 3b randomized, double-blind, vehicle-controlled trial examining adalimumab plus or minus calcipotriol/betamethasone topical treatment, patients receiving both adalimumab and topical treatment had more rapid improvement and better efficacy after 4 weeks, but thereafter the trend was for better efficacy with adalimumab alone.[38]

Interleukin-12/interleukin-23 inhibitors

Ustekinumab was FDA approved in 2008 and is a fully humanized IgG1 monoclonal antibody that binds the shared p40 subunit of IL-12 and IL-23, blocking their ability to interact with their receptors. In a phase 3 randomized, double-blind study comparing ustekinumab every 12 weeks (following a loading dose) with placebo, approximately 67% of patients receiving ustekinumab achieved PASI 75 by week 12 versus 3.1% receiving placebo.[39] More than 35% achieved greater than or equal to PASI 90 by week 12, and at least 44% achieved PASI 90 by week 28. Most AEs were mild and did not require treatment adjustment. In another phase 3, double-blind, placebo-controlled study, 66.7% of patients receiving 45 mg and 75.7% of patients receiving 90 mg ustekinumab achieved PASI 75 by week 12.[40] Patients were followed to 52 weeks, and a higher percentage of partial responders (>PASI 50 but <PASI 75) at week 28 achieved PASI 75 at week 52 if ustekinumab dosing was decreased from every 12 weeks to every 8 weeks. The percentage of patients having mild or serious AEs was similar in the 45-mg, 90-mg, and placebo groups.

Interleukin-17 inhibitors

Secukinumab is fully human IgG1 monoclonal antibody that binds and eliminates IL-17A, and was FDA approved in 2015. In 2 phase 3, double-blind, 52-week trials comparing secukinumab with etanercept and placebo, secukinumab 300 mg every 4 weeks (following loading dosing) led to PASI 75 response in 77.1% to 81.6% by week 12, compared with 44.0% in the etanercept group and 4.9% in the placebo group.[41] AE incidences during the treatment period were similar in the secukinumab and etanercept groups, and responses were maintained in most patients through week 52.

Ixekizumab is a humanized IgG4 monoclonal antibody that binds and eliminates IL-17A, and was FDA approved in 2016. In 2 phase 3, double-blind prospective studies comparing ixekizumab 80 mg every 2 or 4 weeks versus etanercept or placebo, PASI 75 was achieved at week 12 in 87.3% to 89.7% of patients receiving ixekizumab every 2 weeks and 84.2% to 87.3% in the every-4-weeks group, compared with 41.6% to 53.4% in the etanercept group and 2.4% to 7.3% in the placebo group.[42] Again, AEs were similar in the ixekizumab, etanercept, and placebo groups.

Clearance of psoriasis has always been a possibility in some patients with systemic treatment, even with traditional systemic medications like methotrexate. However, the realization of psoriasis clearance (PASI 100) as a possibility was firmly established with the introduction of IL-17 inhibitors. In the phase 3 trials for secukinumab and ixekizumab, 24.1% to 40.5% of patients achieved complete clearance by week 12, as opposed to only 5.3% to 7.3% of patients receiving etanercept.[41,42]

Emerging biologics

The future of treatment of psoriatic disease continues to look extremely bright. At present, there are several different classes of biologic medications in phase 1 to 3 studies exploring efficacy and safety for treating psoriasis vulgaris. Brodalumab is an IL-17 receptor inhibitor that has completed phase 3 studies with exciting efficacy data showing superiority versus ustekinumab, but its future is uncertain because of several concerning adverse effects during the trials.[43] In addition, there are 3 IL-23 inhibitors in various stages of development, guselkumab, tildrakizumab, and BI 655066.[44-46] Importantly, some of these emerging medications have been evaluated in head-to-head studies in which efficacy and safety were directly compared with biologic medications currently available, including etanercept and ustekinumab. Results of these preliminary studies suggest that the emerging therapies assessed result in similar, if not superior, efficacy compared with the currently available medications with which they were compared. The AE profiles of these medications also continue to look promising, with common and unique adverse effects being mostly mild and tolerable.[47,48]

SUMMARY

Several biologic agents currently play an important therapeutic role for management of patients with CU, AD, and psoriasis, particularly omalizumab for antihistamine-resistant CU, IL-1 inhibitors for CAPS and Schnitzler syndrome, dupilumab for recalcitrant AD, and IL-17 inhibitors for psoriasis. It is likely that the therapeutic utility of biologic agents for patients with immune-related dermatologic disorders will expand in the future.

REFERENCES

1. Bernstein JA, Lang DM, Khan D, et al. The diagnosis and management of acute and chronic urticaria: 2014 update. J Allergy Clin Immunol 2014;133:1270–7.
2. Kaplan AP. Treatment of chronic spontaneous urticaria. Allergy Asthma Immunol Res 2012;4:326–31.
3. Omalizumab, Xolair, label. Available at: http://www.accessdata.fda.gov/drugsatfda_docs/label/2007/103976s5102lbl.pdf. Accessed June 25, 2015.
4. Long A, Rahmaoui A, Rothman K, et al. Incidence of malignancy in patients with moderate to severe asthma treated with or without omalizumab. J Allergy Clin Immunol 2014;134:560–7.
5. Maurer M, Rosen KE, Hsieh HJ, et al. Omalizumab for the treatment of chronic idiopathic or spontaneous urticaria. N Engl J Med 2013;368:924–35.
6. Saini S, Bindslev-Jensen C, Maurer M, et al. Efficacy and safety of omalizumab in patient with chronic idiopathic/spontaneous urticaria who remain symptomatic on H1 antihistamines: a randomized placebo controlled study. J Invest Dermatol 2015;135:67–75.
7. Kaplan A, Ledford D, Ashby M, et al. Omalizumab in patients with symptomatic chronic idiopathic/spontaneous urticaria despite standard combination therapy. J Allergy Clin Immunol 2013;132:101–9.
8. Zuo-Tao Z, Chun-Mei J, Wen-Jun Y, et al. Omalizumab for the treatment of chronic spontaneous urticaria: A meta-analysis of randomized trials. J Allergy Clin Immunol 2016;137:1742–50.
9. Rosen K, Bradley MS, Ashby M, et al. Baseline characteristics of patients with refractory chronic idiopathic/spontaneous urticaria enrolled in three phase III, randomized, placebo controlled trials of omalizumab. Ann Allergy Asthma Immunol 2013;111:A118.
10. Viswanathan RK, Moss MH, Mathur SK. Retrospective analysis of the efficacy of omalizumab in chronic refractory urticaria. Allergy Asthma Proc 2013;34:446–52.
11. Lang DM. A critical appraisal of omalizumab as a therapeutic option for chronic refractory urticaria/angioedema. Ann Allergy Asthma Immunol 2014;112:276–9.
12. Lachmann HJ, Kone-Paut I, Kuemmerle-Deschner JB, et al. Use of canakinumab in the cryopyrin-associated periodic syndrome. N Engl J Med 2009;360:2416–25.
13. Schuster C, Kranke B, Aberer E, et al. Schnitzler syndrome: response to anakinra in two cases and review of the literature. Int J Dermatol 2009;48:1190–4.

14. Krause K, Mahamed A, Weller K, et al. Efficacy and safety of canakinumab in urticarial vasculitis: an open label study. J Allergy Clin Immunol 2013;132:751–4.
15. Botsios C, Sfriso P, Punzi L, et al. Non-complementemic urticarial vasculitis: successful treatment with the IL-1 receptor antagonist, anakinra. Scand J Rheumatol 2007;36:236–7.
16. Sand FL, Thomsen SF. TNF-alpha inhibitors for chronic urticaria: experience in 20 patients. J Allergy (Cairo) 2013;2013:130905.
17. Magerl M, Philipp S, Manasterski M, et al. Successful treatment of delayed pressure urticaria with anti-TNF-alpha. J Allergy Clin Immunol 2007;119:752–4.
18. Wilson LH, Eliason MJ, Leiferman KM, et al. Treatment of refractory chronic urticaria with tumor necrosis factor-alfa inhibitors. J Am Acad Dermatol 2011;64: 1221–2.
19. Leung DY, Nicklas RA, Li JT, et al. Disease management of atopic dermatitis: an updated practice parameter. Joint Task Force on Practice Parameters, Work Group on Atopic Dermatitis. Ann Allergy Asthma Immunol 2004;93:1–21.
20. Leung DY, Soter NA. Cellular and immunologic mechanisms in atopic dermatitis. J Am Acad Dermatol 2001;44:S1–12.
21. Djukanovic R, Wilson SJ, Kraft M, et al. Effects of treatment with anti-immunoglobulin E antibody omalizumab on airway inflammation in allergic asthma. Am J Respir Crit Care Med 2004;170:583–93.
22. Sheinkopf LE, Rafi AW, Do LT, et al. Efficacy of omalizumab in the treatment of atopic dermatitis: a pilot study. Allergy Asthma Proc 2008;29(5):530.
23. Belloni B, Ziai M, Lim A, et al. Low-dose anti-IgE therapy in patients with atopic eczema with high serum IgE levels. J Allergy Clin Immunol 2007;120(5):1223.
24. Leung DYM, Bieber T. Atopic dermatitis. Lancet 2003;361:151–60.
25. Jacobi A, Antoni C, Manger B, et al. Infliximab in the treatment of moderate to severe atopic dermatitis. J Am Acad Dermatol 2005;52(3 Pt 1):522.
26. Jezirehi AR, Bonavida B. Cellular and molecular signal transduction pathways modulated by rituximab (Rituxan, anti-CD20 mAb) in non-Hodgkin's lymphoma: implications in chemosensitization and therapeutic intervention. Oncogene 2005;24:2121–43.
27. Simon D, Hösli S, Kostylina G, et al. Anti-CD20 (rituximab) treatment improves atopic eczema. J Allergy Clin Immunol 2008;121(1):122.
28. McDonald BS, Jones J, Rustin M. Rituximab as a treatment for severe atopic eczema: failure to improve in three consecutive patients. Clin Exp Dermatol 2016;41(1):45–7.
29. Oldhoff JM, Darsow U, Werfel T, et al. Anti-IL-5 recombinant humanized monoclonal antibody (mepolizumab) for the treatment of atopic dermatitis. Allergy 2005;60(5):693.
30. Beck LA, Thaçi D, Hamilton JD, et al. Dupilumab treatment in adults with moderate-to-severe atopic dermatitis. N Engl J Med 2014;371(2):130.
31. Leonardi CL, Powers JL, Matheson RT, et al, Etanercept Psoriasis Study Group. Etanercept as monotherapy in patients with psoriasis. N Engl J Med 2003; 349(21):2014–22.
32. Papp KA, Tyring S, Lahfa M, et al. Etanercept Psoriasis Study Group. A global phase III randomized controlled trial of etanercept in psoriasis: safety, efficacy, and effect of dose reduction. Br J Dermatol 2005;152(6):1304–12.
33. Gottlieb AB, Evans R, Li S, et al. Infliximab induction therapy for patients with severe plaque-type psoriasis: a randomized, double-blind, placebo-controlled trial. J Am Acad Dermatol 2004;51(4):534–42.

34. Reich K, Nestle FO, Papp K, et al. EXPRESS study investigators. Infliximab induction and maintenance therapy for moderate-to-severe psoriasis: a phase III, multicentre, double-blind trial. Lancet 2005;366(9494):1367–74.
35. Barker J, Hoffmann M, Wozel G, et al. Efficacy and safety of infliximab vs. methotrexate in patients with moderate-to-severe plaque psoriasis: results of an open-label, active-controlled, randomized trial (RESTORE1). Br J Dermatol 2011; 165(5):1109–17.
36. Menter A, Tyring SK, Gordon K, et al. Adalimumab therapy for moderate to severe psoriasis: a randomized, controlled phase III trial. J Am Acad Dermatol 2008; 58(1):106–15.
37. Saurat JH, Stingl G, Dubertret L, et al, CHAMPION Study Investigators. Efficacy and safety results from the randomized controlled comparative study of adalimumab vs. methotrexate vs. placebo in patients with psoriasis (CHAMPION). Br J Dermatol 2008;158(3):558–66.
38. Thaçi D, Ortonne JP, Chimenti S, et al. A phase IIIb, multicentre, randomized, double-blind, vehicle-controlled study of the efficacy and safety of adalimumab with and without calcipotriol/betamethasone topical treatment in patients with moderate to severe psoriasis: the BELIEVE study. Br J Dermatol 2010;163(2): 402–11.
39. Leonardi CL, Kimball AB, Papp KA, et al. PHOENIX 1 study investigators. Efficacy and safety of ustekinumab, a human interleukin-12/23 monoclonal antibody, in patients with psoriasis: 76-week results from a randomised, double-blind, placebo-controlled trial (PHOENIX 1). Lancet 2008;371(9625):1665–74.
40. Papp KA, Langley RG, Lebwohl M, et al. PHOENIX 2 study investigators. Efficacy and safety of ustekinumab, a human interleukin-12/23 monoclonal antibody, in patients with psoriasis: 52-week results from a randomised, double-blind, placebo-controlled trial (PHOENIX 2). Lancet 2008;371(9625):1675–84.
41. Langley RG, Elewski BE, Lebwohl M, et al, ERASURE Study Group, FIXTURE Study Group. Secukinumab in plaque psoriasis–results of two phase 3 trials. N Engl J Med 2014;371(4):326–38.
42. Griffiths CE, Reich K, Lebwohl M, et al. UNCOVER-2 and UNCOVER-3 investigators. Comparison of ixekizumab with etanercept or placebo in moderate-to-severe psoriasis (UNCOVER-2 and UNCOVER-3): results from two phase 3 randomised trials. Lancet 2015;386(9993):541–51.
43. Lebwohl M, Strober B, Menter A, et al. Phase 3 studies comparing brodalumab with ustekinumab in psoriasis. N Engl J Med 2015;373(14):1318–28.
44. Gordon KB, Duffin KC, Bissonnette R, et al. A phase 2 trial of guselkumab versus adalimumab for plaque psoriasis. N Engl J Med 2015;373(2):136–44.
45. Papp K, Thaçi D, Reich K, et al. Tildrakizumab (MK-3222), an anti-interleukin-23p19 monoclonal antibody, improves psoriasis in a phase IIb randomized placebo-controlled trial. Br J Dermatol 2015;173(4):930–9.
46. Krueger JG, Ferris LK, Menter A, et al. Anti-IL-23A mAb BI 655066 for treatment of moderate-to-severe psoriasis: Safety, efficacy, pharmacokinetics, and biomarker results of a single-rising-dose, randomized, double-blind, placebo-controlled trial. J Allergy Clin Immunol 2015;136(1):116–24.e7.
47. Beroukhim K, Danesh MJ, Nguyen C, et al. Anti-IL-23 phase II data for psoriasis: a review. J Drugs Dermatol 2015;14(10):1093–6.
48. Nwe SM, Champlain AH, Gordon KB. Rationale and early clinical data on IL-17 blockade in psoriasis. Expert Rev Clin Immunol 2013;9(7):677–82.

Biologic and New Therapies in Asthma

Farnaz Tabatabaian, MD[a], Dennis K. Ledford, MD[a,b], Thomas B. Casale, MD[a,c],*

KEYWORDS

- Biologics • Asthma • Anti-IL-5 • Anti-IL-13 • Anti-IL-4 • Th2 • CRTH2 • Anti-IgE

KEY POINTS

- T2-high asthma patients are identified by elevated sputum or blood eosinophils, fractional exhaled nitric oxide (FeNO), and antigen-specific immunoglobulin E (IgE).
- T2-low asthma patients are identified by increased neutrophils or paucigranulocytic findings in the sputum.
- T2-low asthma patients respond poorly to corticosteroids and new biologics approved for asthma.
- T2 targeted therapies discussed in this review include antagonists of interleukin-5 (IL-5), IL-13, IL-4, chemoattractant receptor homologous molecule on T2 cells, and IgE.

INTRODUCTION

Asthma is a complicated chronic disease that affects people from childhood to the elderly. In the United States, approximately 17.7 million adults and 6.3 million children have asthma. In 2011, 1.8 million emergency room (ER) visits carried a primary diagnosis of asthma. The average length of hospitalization for patients with asthma was 3.6 days. In 2013, the average number of lost school days was 13.8 million, and the average number of lost work days was 10.1 million. From 2006 to 2010, approximately 38% of children and 50% of adults with asthma had uncontrolled symptoms. An estimated cost of US$19.7 billion annually makes asthma 1 of the top 10 prevalent conditions impacting health care system costs.[1] The question remains, why with current therapeutic regimens are patients still uncontrolled? Phenotypic heterogeneity among asthma patients contributes to the variable severity and control of the disease.

Disclosure: See last page of article.
[a] Division of Allergy and Immunology, Department of Internal medicine, Morsani College of Medicine, University of South Florida, 13330 USF Laurel Dr. 5th Floor, MDC 80, Tampa, FL 33612-4799, USA; [b] Division of Allergy and Immunology, Department of Internal Medicine, Morsani College of Medicine, James A. Haley VA Hospital, University of South Florida, 13000 Bruce B, Downs Boulevard, Tampa, FL 33612, USA; [c] Division of Allergy and Immunology, Department of Internal Medicine, Morsani College of Medicine, University of South Florida, 12901 Bruce B Downs Boulevard, MDC 19, Tampa, FL 33612 USA
* Corresponding author.
E-mail address: tbcasale@health.usf.edu

Immunol Allergy Clin N Am 37 (2017) 329–343
http://dx.doi.org/10.1016/j.iac.2017.01.007
0889-8561/17/© 2017 Elsevier Inc. All rights reserved.

immunology.theclinics.com

Traditional classification of patients with asthma reflected associated triggers, including exercise, viruses, cigarette smoke, allergens, and aspirin. The National Institutes of Health–sponsored Severe Asthma Research Program (SARP) used cluster analysis to provide unbiased methods to define various asthma phenotypes. The SARP data, as well as other studies, indicated that early-onset disease is consistently associated with more atopy and allergic conditions over a range of severities, whereas adult-onset disease is often associated with obesity and was more common in women. A cluster of adult-onset patients with mild airflow obstruction has fewer exacerbations, but another cluster with moderate airflow obstruction is more exacerbation prone.

In categorizing patients by the observable clinical characteristics, researchers are attempting to link these to underlying molecular mechanisms of their disease, in other words, the endotype (**Fig. 1**). To date, primarily 2 endotypes of asthma are described, Th2-high (T2 high) and Th2-low (T2 low).[2–4] Patients with Th2-high asthma have increased eosinophils in their sputum and airways, whereas T2-low asthma patients have either an increase in neutrophils or a paucigranulocytic (minimal inflammatory cells) profile in their sputum and airways. In this review, the focus is on defining what is currently known about the pathophysiology of underlying inflammation intrinsic to these endotypes, including key pathways and cytokines, to better target therapy. Furthermore, the utility of point-of-care biomarkers to guide optimal treatments with controllers and especially biologics is discussed. This step is the first step in precision medicine where medications are targeted toward patients with the anticipation of optimal therapeutic effect.

PATHOPHYSIOLOGY
T2-Low Asthma or Non-T2 Asthma

Studies of patients with severe asthma unresponsive to typical therapeutic regimens in the 1990s illustrated that some of these individuals had neutrophilic inflammation.[5] Only about 50% of patients with severe asthma exhibit increased eosinophils along with heightened expression of transforming growth factor -β and increased synthesis of collagen beneath the bronchial subepithelial basement membrane.[5] The subset of patients with neutrophil predominance does not exhibit typical T2 cytokines. Neutrophil-predominant patients typically have an onset of disease in adulthood and are generally less corticosteroid responsive. Key cytokines involved in the pathogenesis of these patients include those produced by T helper 1 (Th1) and Th17 cells. The role of Th17 cells and IL-17 in asthma is not defined; however, in experimental asthma models, IL-17A contributes to airway remodeling by stimulating fibroblast proliferation.[6,7] IL-17 is also increased in sputum of patients with severe asthma and can induce the production of IL-8, a potent neutrophil chemoattractant. In a clinical trial targeting IL-17A, IL-17F, and IL-25 via inhibition of the IL-17 receptor α, there was little benefit in patients with mild to moderate asthma.[8] It is important to note that patients with sputum neutrophilia were not enriched for in this study, and this could have resulted in the overall lack of efficacy. Other targets evaluated for this endotype include antagonists of tumor necrosis factor (TNF)-α and IL-1. These proinflammatory cytokines are upregulated in asthmatics with neutrophilic inflammation.[9] Blocking TNF-α in severe asthma has had variable success, but a relatively high risk of adverse effects has resulted in a lack of further clinical development for asthma.[10]

Interleukin-8 (IL-8) is a potent mediator of neutrophil chemotaxis through the chemokine receptor CXCR2. A CXCR2 antagonist has been studied for potentially treating neutrophilic airway inflammation. In preliminary study of 12 patients with increased

T2 Low Asthma

T2 High Asthma

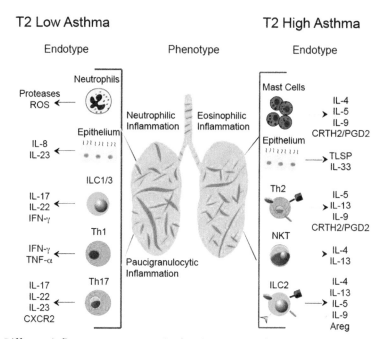

Fig. 1. Different inflammatory patterns in the airways contribute to the underlying inflammation in asthma. In a T2-low pattern, a predominance of neutrophils or paucigranulocytic inflammation has been described. Patients with this phenotype are less likely to respond to corticosteroids. In neutrophilic-predominant disease, patients might respond to antibodies that block TNF-α, IL-17, IL-23. Innate lymphoid cells group 1 and group 3 are more predominant in Th2-low disease. These cells produce IFN-γ, IL-17, and IL-22. A T2-high inflammation is suggestive of eosinophilic phenotypes and is more likely to respond to corticosteroids. A multitude of inflammatory cells and cytokines is involved, but targeting specific type 2 cytokines has proven to be an effective strategy, including antagonists of IgE, IL-5, IL-13, and CRTH2. IFN-γ, interferon gamma; ILC1, type 1 innate lymphoid cells; ILC2, group 2 innate lymphoid cells; ILC3, group 3 innate lymphoid cells; NKT, natural killer cells; PGD$_2$, prostaglandin D$_2$; ROS, reactive oxygen species. (*Adapted from* Muraro A, Lemanske RF, Hellings PW, et al. Precision medicine in patients with allergic diseases: airway diseases and atopic dermatitis—PRACTALL document of the European Academy of Allergy and Clinical Immunology and the American Academy of Allergy, Asthma & Immunology. J Allergy Clin Immunol 2016;137(5):1347–58; and Sonnenberg GF, Artis D. Innate lymphoid cells in the initiation, regulation and resolution of inflammation. Nat Med 2015;21(7):698–708.)

neutrophils in sputum, targeting IL-8 by using a CXCR2 blocker reduced the sputum neutrophils but without statistical improvements in forced expiratory volume in 1 second (FEV1) or symptom-control scores.[3] Most attempts at targeting key mediators of neutrophilic inflammation have not proven very effective therapeutically. Furthermore, the lack of reliable biomakers associated with neutrophilic predominant asthma has contributed to the difficulty of identifying these patients for targeted therapy. In the case of paucigranulocytic inflammation, with normal levels of eosinophils and neutrophils in sputum and the airways, using intensive bronchodilator therapy with long-acting muscarinic receptor antagonists and/or long-acting beta-receptor agonists is of some benefit. These patients also are relatively corticosteroid resistant presumably due to the limited airway inflammation. Alternatively, these patients with paucigranulocytic inflammation may be candidates for bronchial thermoplasty to reduce airflow obstruction.[11]

T2-High Asthma

Allergic disease is associated with T2-high inflammation. Typically, patients with childhood-onset asthma before the age of 12 have a history of other atopic diseases. The master regulators IL-33, IL-25, and thymic stromal lymphopoietin (TLSP) stimulate the innate or adaptive immune system to secrete cytokines IL-4, IL-5, and IL-13 (T2-high cytokines) (**Fig. 2**). The accumulation of these type 2 cytokines stimulates key inflammatory cells, such as eosinophils, mast cells, and basophils. In fact, both IL-4 and IL-13, through the activation of the transcription factor GATA3, regulate T2 inflammation. IL-13 and IL-4 are both involved in activation of B-cell isotope switching to produce immunoglobulin E (IgE). IL-5 is central for eosinophilic development, survival, and chemotaxis. Innate lymphoid type 2 cells (ILC2) are also involved in the production of IL-5 and IL-13. Type 2 cytokines also contribute to mucous cell hyperplasia and fibrosis leading to airway remodeling.[2]

Patients with airway eosinophilia typically respond to corticosteroids. However, the degree of response is variable.[12,13] The concept of T2-high disease came from a variety of studies, including those by Haldar and colleagues,[14,15] where they used molecular phenotyping of airway epithelial brushings from corticosteroid-naive

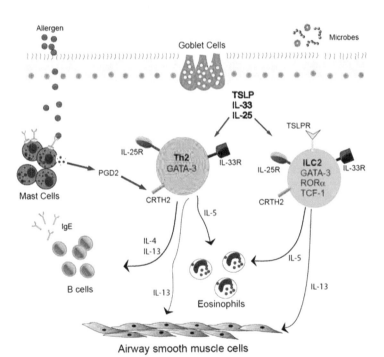

Fig. 2. A very complex interplay of type 2 cytokines and T2-high inflammation. Activation of epithelial cells produces TSLP, IL-25, and IL-33, which stimulates T2 and ILC2. T2 and ILC2s share many features including the expression of transcription factor GATA-3 and production of type 2 cytokines. Secretion of IL-5 from both of these cells stimulates the production of eosinophils in the bone marrow and elicits the migration of eosinophils to the area of inflammation. IL-5 and IL-13 contribute to smooth muscle changes and remodeling changes. IL-4 contributes to IgE class switching in B cells. GATA-3, transcription factor; RoRα, retinoid-related orphan receptor alpha, nuclear receptor; TCF1, T cell factor 1; TSLP, thymic stromal lymphoprotein. (*Adapted from* Lambrecht BN, Hammad H. The immunology of asthma. Nat Immunol 2015;16(1):47.)

asthmatic patients. Subjects defined as having T2-high disease were more apt to have IL-13 and IL-5 messenger RNA, higher number of eosinophils and mast cells, and more atopy compared with T2 low asthma.

T2-related targets that have been examined include IgE, IL-5, IL-13, IL-4, IL-9, IL-4 receptor alpha, chemoattractant receptor homologous molecule on T2 cells (CRTH2), and TLSP.[16] Targeting cytokines and mediators is more successful in appropriately selected patients. In a certain population of patients, clinical benefits have been demonstrated with IgE, IL-5, IL-13, IL-4 receptor alpha, TLSP, and CRTH2 antagonists. The remainder of this review focuses on the discussion of current biologics targeting T2 inflammation and the utility of clinical biomarkers to help guide precision medicine choices (**Table 1**).

Current Biomarkers in T2-High Inflammation

Currently available biomarkers may assist clinicians in the selection of targeted asthma treatments, most of which are specific for T2-high disease. Biomarkers in medicine are divided into 3 categories[17]:

- Type 0, a marker that relates to the natural history of disease;
- Type 1, a marker that reflects drug activity or drug responsiveness;
- Type 2, a marker that acts as a surrogate and defines potential disease process.[17]

With biologics, defining type 1 biomarkers would facilitate selection of patients with severe asthma that would likely respond therapeutically. Current biomarkers unfortunately are not adequate for identifying early-onset asthma nor are they necessarily accessible to clinicians in the outpatient clinics.[5] Nonetheless, T2 inflammation may be recognized by an increase in eosinophils in sputum and/or blood. Indeed, both elevated blood and sputum eosinophils are biomarkers for risk of asthma exacerbations. Many studies have shown better responses to biologics with persistent T2 inflammation despite inhaled or systemic corticosteroids. Clinically, it is difficult to measure eosinophils in the sputum,[18] and blood eosinophils levels are variable. Current research suggests that other markers for eosinophils may be useful. Eosinophil granule proteins, such as eosinophil peroxidase (EPX) in sputum, correlate with respiratory disease activity, including asthma and chronic bronchitis in chronic obstructive pulmonary disease. A strong association has been found with nasal and pharyngeal EPX and sputum-induced eosinophils. Currently, a bioactive paper strip is being developed to use as a point-of-care measure in the clinical setting to measure EPX.[19,20] This quantitative tool could potentially be used as a biomarker to provide better management for poorly controlled patients.

Another marker for T2 inflammation is the concentration of exhaled nitric oxide (fractional exhaled nitric oxide or FeNO). FeNO is a product of the T2-regulated induction of nitric oxide synthase, which generally correlates with eosinophilic inflammation. The American Thoracic and European Respiratory Societies have established parameters for FeNO levels. Normal FeNO is <25 ppb.[17,21] In a study by Mehta and colleagues,[22] in patients with mild to moderate persistent asthma who were treated with mometasone furoate 400 μg/d for 8 weeks, a significant decrease in FeNO was observed as soon as 1 week after the initiation of treatment with Inhaled corticosteroids (ICSs). Patients with high FeNO are more likely to benefit from ICS with change observed as soon as 1 week after the initiation of ICS treatment. If the FeNO values remain at or greater than 50 ppb despite ICS, then corticosteroid resistance or noncompliance should be considered.[17,21,23,24] Similar to eosinophil counts, FeNO is predictive of asthma exacerbations. In fact, particularly in children a FeNO greater than 49 ppb within 4 weeks of discontinuing therapy with ICS was associated with asthma exacerbations.[17,25] An

Table 1
Summary of therapies approved or in clinical trials targeting T2-high severe persistent asthma

Current Therapies	Mechanism of Action	Potential Biomarkers	Effect	FDA Approved	Route	References
Omalizumab	Blocks IgE interaction with FcεRI	Elevated IgE. Patients with higher FeNO and blood eosinophils >300 cells/μL better response	Decrease asthma exacerbations	Yes; ages 6 and older	150–375 mg subcutaneous (SC) every 2–4 wk; frequency based on IgE and body weight Black box warning for anaphylaxis	30,32,33
Mepolizumab	IL-5 antagonist	Peripheral eosinophil count of >150 cells/μL or 300 cells/μL	Decrease in asthma exacerbations and improvement in pre-, postbronchodilator FEV1	Yes; ages 12 and older	100 mg SC every 4 wk; consider shingles vaccine before administration	18,26,34–36
Reslizumab	IL-5 antagonist	Peripheral eosinophil count of >400 cells/μL	Decrease in asthma exacerbations and improvement in FEV1	Yes; 18 and older	3 mg/kg IV every 4 wk Black box warning for anaphylaxis	40,42,43
In clinical trials						
Benralizumab	IL-5 receptor α antagonists targeting both eosinophils and basophils	Elevated peripheral blood eosinophil count	Decreased asthma exacerbations and in small study used in ER visit setting administration contributed to a 50% drop in exacerbation over 12 wk	Phase 3; 12 and older	20–100 mg every 4–8 wk	44–46

Lebrikizumab	IL-13 antagonist	Elevated periostin and DDP-4	Decrease in asthma exacerbations with minimal in improvement in FEV1	Termination of clinical program	N/A	[27,48]
Tralokinumab	IL-13 antagonist	Elevated periostin and DDP-4	Decreased in asthma exacerbations and improvement in FEV1	Phase 2b trials	N/A	[49]
Dupilumab	Inhibits IL-13 and IL-4 by targeting IL-4 α, a common receptor domain for both cytokines	Peripheral eosinophil count of >300 cells/μL or sputum >3% with better response, but improvements in all patients	Decrease in asthma exacerbations and improvement in FEV1	Phase 2b trials	200 mg SC every 2 wk or 300 mg SC every 4 wk; administered at home	[50,51]

increase in FeNO after discontinuation of long-term omalizumab also predicts exacerbations (Ledford D, Busse W, Trzaskoma B, Omachi TA, Rosén K, Chipps BE, et al. A randomized multicenter study evaluating Xolair persistence of response after long-term therapy. Journal of Allergy and Clinical Immunology, In press). Of note, IL-5 antagonists decrease blood eosinophil counts but have little to no effect on the FeNO.[26] FeNO is generally not affected specifically by atopic status.[17] Smoking and obesity are associated with lower FeNO. Men typically have a higher FeNO than women.[17] Although many confounding factors can impact the measured FeNO value, it can nevertheless serve as a clinical biomarker to predict response to T2 therapeutics.

Another marker that is also reflective of T2 inflammation is blood periostin. Periostin is produced by lung epithelial cells and fibroblasts in response to IL-13. Periostin gene expression is increased in airways of subjects with asthma.[21,27] In subjects treated with an IL-13 antagonist, those with higher initial periostin level had a greater improvement in FEV1 than those with lower periostin levels.[27] Hence, this biomarker may identify patients that are more responsive to an IL-13 inhibitor.

Finally, IgE is a biomarker associated with allergic sensitization and asthma. However, it is too nonspecific to be a good predictive therapeutic biomarker. Anti-IgE therapeutics decrease asthma exacerbations and blood eosinophils.

In 2016, some of the biomarkers described are predominantly research tools and not widely used in clinical practice. However, blood eosinophils and FeNO are readily available. It is also important to realize that all of the available biomarkers are reflective of T2 inflammation. The remainder of the discussion focuses on choosing the correct biologics for severe asthmatics that have a T2 high phenotype.

SPECIFIC THERAPIES TARGETING T2-HIGH PATHWAYS
Targeting IgE

Asthma is associated with allergic disease, emphasizing the roles of IgE and the T2 pathway. IgE binds with high affinity to IgE receptors on mast cells, and subsequent to crosslinking by allergen, mast cells release a variety of mediators and cytokines important in inducing airway inflammation. Several approaches have been taken to target the effects of IgE. Decreasing the production of IgE is a novel approach described by Gauvreau and colleagues.[28] Quilizumab, an M1 prime antibody, targeted membrane-expressed IgE-positive cells causing cell death and a decrease in production of IgE. Quilizumab lowered serum IgE levels by about 40% and inhibited both the early and the late allergen-induced asthmatic response. Unfortunately, it did not show clinical efficacy in field trials, halting further development.[29]

Omalizumab, a recombinant, humanized, monoclonal anti-IgE antibody that blocks the interaction between IgE and the high affinity receptor FcεRI, has been on the market more than a decade.[30] Another anti-IgE monoclonal antibody that is currently being studied in severe asthma is ligelizumab, which has 30 to 50 times greater affinity for IgE compared with omalizumab.[31]

Omalizumab has been used for 13 years for asthma, but predictive biomarkers of response were not identified until recently. In a retrospective analysis of the EXTRA study, Hanania and colleagues[32] found that omalizumab was more efficacious in patients with higher levels of FeNO, blood eosinophils, or blood periostin. Busse and colleagues[33] confirmed that patients with eosinophil counts greater than 300 cells/μL responded better to omalizumab with up to a 60% decrease in asthma exacerbations. These data suggest that in patients with higher blood eosinophil levels, omalizumab's effects on exacerbations are similar to those noted for eosinophil-specific IL-5 antagonists (see later discussion). In 2016, the US Food and Drug Administration (FDA) approved omalizumab for use in children ages 6 to 11 years with moderate to severe perennial allergic asthma.

IL-5-based Therapy

IL-5 is a key cytokine for eosinophil growth, differentiation, and migration to the airways. To date, 2 monoclonal antibody approaches have been studied in clinical trials to block the effects of IL-5. The first approach is to bind to IL-5 itself, and the second approach is to bind to a component of the IL-5 receptor, the alpha chain. The latter leads to the enhancement of antibody-dependent, cell-mediated cytotoxicity, and apoptosis of eosinophils and basophils. Mepolizumab and reslizumab are 2 humanized monoclonal antibodies that bind to IL-5 and are US FDA approved for patients with severe, eosinophilic asthma. Benralizumab binds to the IL-5 receptor and is still in clinical development.

Mepolizumab

In an initial double-blinded, placebo-controlled study, Flood-Page and colleagues[34] evaluated patients with uncontrolled, moderate to severe symptomatic asthma despite ICS treatment. Subjects were given 250 or 750 mg mepolizumab intravenously (IV) monthly for 3 months. Compared with placebo, the rate of exacerbations, lung functions, quality-of-life measures, symptoms, and use of short-acting beta agonist were unaffected. However, the number of blood and sputum eosinophil counts decreased significantly in the mepolizumab-treated groups. Subsequent studies targeted patients greater than12 years of age with elevated eosinophil counts on high-dose ICS with a second controller, with or without the use of oral corticosteroids, and a history of severe asthma exacerbations. Two small proof-of-concept studies illustrated that treatment with mepolizumab reduced the risk of asthma exacerbations.[26] Pavord and colleagues[18] in a multicenter, double-blinded, placebo-controlled trial encompassing 81 centers and 13 countries enrolled 621 asthma patients with evidence of eosinophilic asthma. Patients were randomly assigned to placebo or mepolizumab 75 mg, 250 mg, or 750 mg IV every 4 weeks for a total of 13 infusions. The number of clinically significant exacerbations was decreased from 39% to 52% in the treatment groups at all doses. Efficiency of drug was associated with 2 variables: blood eosinophil count and number of exacerbation the previous year. A 2013 meta-analysis of 7 randomized placebo-controlled trials of 1131 patients with eosinophilic asthma treated with mepolizumab showed an improvement in quality-of-life scores and decrease in asthma exacerbations. Lung function was not improved compared with placebo.[35]

In 2014, a randomized, double-blinded study of subjects with recurrent asthma exacerbations and eosinophilic inflammation compared mepolizumab 75 mg IV or 100 mg subcutaneously with placebo administered every 4 weeks for 32 weeks. Study entry required an eosinophil count of 150 cells/μL at screening or greater than 300 cells/μL in the previous year. Both active treatment groups experienced a greater than 50% reduction in asthma exacerbations, approximately 100 mL FEV1 improvement, and better asthma quality-of-life scores compared with placebo.[36] ER visits and hospitalizations were reduced significantly in both mepolizumab groups as well. A predetermined subanalysis of 177 patients with blood eosinophil counts greater than 500 cells/μL treated with 100 mg of mepolizumab subcutaneously showed an 80% reduction in asthma exacerbation and improvement in FEV1 before and after bronchodilator of 132 mL and 222 mL, respectively.

A few studies have investigated the corticosteroid-sparing effect of mepolizumab in subjects with corticosteroid-dependent, eosinophilic asthma. In a small study of 20 subjects on oral corticosteroids for asthma, the addition of 750 mg of IV mepolizumab for 5 months resulted in a reduction of prednisone use by 84% in the active treatment group compared with 48% in patients receiving placebo. Patients in the active treatment group had improvement in lung function and reduction in blood/sputum eosinophil counts up to 8 weeks after the discontinuation of mepolizumab.[37] In a larger study of the corticosteroid-sparing effect of mepolizumab, 135 subjects with severe eosinophilic asthma were treated with 100 mg mepolizumab every 4 weeks for 20 weeks. Mepolizumab resulted in a reduction of corticosteroid use by 50% and also decreased asthma exacerbations and improved symptoms.[38]

Mepolizumab is approved in the United States as add-on maintenance therapy in patients, 12 years and older, with severe asthma of the eosinophilic phenotype. Better responses occur in patients with higher peripheral blood eosinophil counts, but the specific asthma eosinophilic phenotype is not defined in the package insert. Of note, mepolizumab-treated subjects do have an increase in the incidence of *Herpes zoster* outbreaks. Hence, physicians should consider discussion with patients and possibly vaccinate before initiation of treatment. Similar to many of the other biologics, the optimal duration of therapy is undefined, and there is no evidence of treatment-induced asthma remissions. Haldar and colleagues[39] reported that after the cessation of mepolizumab, symptoms recur and serum eosinophil levels increase to the pretreatment levels. Mepolizumab is not currently approved for any other eosinophilic conditions nor is it indicated for acute bronchospasm or status asthmaticus.

Reslizumab

Reslizumab is also a humanized anti-IL-5 monoclonal antibody. This biologic was FDA approved in 2016 for add-on therapy for severe eosinophilic asthma. Initial studies with IV reslizumab 3 mg/kg in poorly controlled, severe asthma patients, unselected for higher blood eosinophils, did not show much clinical benefit. Subjects treated for 16 weeks did have a decrease in sputum and peripheral blood eosinophil counts.[40,42] Castro and colleagues[43] reported 2 simultaneous double-blinded, multicenter studies enrolling patients between the ages of 12 and 75 years with eosinophil counts greater 400 cells/μL. Subjects were randomized to IV reslizumab 3 mg/kg or placebo. The primary endpoint was asthma exacerbations. Enrollment requirements were specified as poorly controlled disease requiring greater than medium-dose ICS plus another controller therapy and with reversibility to short-acting beta-agonist. Study candidates also had at least one asthma exacerbation in the prior year and a blood eosinophil count of 400 cell/μL or greater. The active treatment group demonstrated a significant decrease in asthma exacerbations (relative risk = 0.4–0.5) and a significant improvement in FEV1. Bjermer and colleagues[41] and Corren and colleagues[42] (*Chest*, 2016, in press) showed in a similar patient population significant improvements in lung function, asthma control, and quality-of-life measures. Reslizumab is administered at 3.0 mg/kg IV over 20 to 50 minutes. There is a black box warning for a small (<0.3%) risk of anaphylaxis.

Benralizumab

Benralizumab targets the IL-5 receptor α on eosinophils and basophils and results in apoptosis of these key cells. Similar to the other IL-5 inhibitors, it does result in decreases in sputum and peripheral blood eosinophils.[44] Castro and colleagues[45] in a phase 2b trial in uncontrolled, eosinophilic asthmatics studied the impact of variable doses of benralizumab compared with placebo.[46] Benralizumab was administered every 4 weeks for the first 3 doses and subsequently every 8 weeks for 1 year. A decrease in exacerbations occurred in the 20-mg and 100-mg doses. In the same study, a 1:1 ratio comparison of placebo and 100 mg of benralizumab was examined in a noneosinophilic population. The subjects in the noneosinophilic population did not show benefit in comparison to placebo or those subjects with eosinophils greater than 300 cells/μL, who had an improved FEV1 of 200 mL. Subsequently, Nowak and colleagues[46] showed that asthma exacerbations over 12 weeks were decreased by 50% in patients treated with one dose of benralizumab during an acute asthma flare requiring an ER visit.

IL-13-based Therapy

IL-13 has many roles in T2 inflammation, including IgE synthesis, proliferation of bronchial fibroblasts, induction of airway hyperresponsiveness, enhanced mucus production, and recruitment of eosinophils and basophils.[47] IL-13 stimulates bronchial epithelial cells to produce dipeptidyl peptidase-4 (DPP-4) and periostin. Both periostin and DPP-4 are molecules used as biomarkers to predict response to IL-13 antagonists. Corren and colleagues[27] in 2011 conducted a randomized double-blinded, placebo-controlled study with lebrikizumab, an IL-13 antagonist, in 219 adults with inadequately controlled asthma despite ICS. Patients were treated with 250 mg of subcutaneous lebrikizumab or placebo for 6 months. Subjects receiving lebrikizumab had a 5.5% improvement in FEV1 compared with placebo. Those treated with lebrikizumab who had a higher periostin level had 8.2% improvement in FEV1 compared with 1.6% in subjects with low periostin levels. Subjects with FeNO who were treated with lebrikizumab had a greater improvement in FEV1 as well. However, no improvement was noted in asthma symptoms scores or exacerbations.

In contrast, a phase 2 study looking at the effect of subcutaneous lebrikizumab at 125, 250, and 500 mg monthly in asthmatics not receiving ICS demonstrated no significant improvements in FEV1, peak expiratory flow (PEF), asthma control questionnaire (ACQ) scores or the frequency of albuterol use.

Hanania and colleagues[48] showed that patients with severe asthma who had levels of periostin $\geq$50 ng/mL had a reduction of 80% in asthma exacerbations when treated monthly with 125 or 250 mg of lebrikizumab subcutaneously. These patients also had statistically and clinically meaningful increases in FEV1. On the other hand, patients treated with lebrikizumab who had low periostin did not show improvement in FEV1. Duplicate phase 3 trials have illustrated variable results, with one study showing positive results and the other not, even if enriched with patients having elevated periostin levels. These phase 3 study outcomes resulted in the termination of the asthma program for this agent.

Another IL-13 antagonist, tralokinumab, in phase 2 trials at 150, 300, or 600 mg dosed biweekly for 12 weeks with subsequent 12-week follow-up, failed to demonstrate improvement in asthma symptoms scores. Brightling and colleagues[49] showed treatment with tralokinumab biweekly for 52 weeks did not improve asthma exacerbation rates compared with placebo. However, subjects with elevated periostin or DDP-4 levels or greater airway reversibility did have significantly lower exacerbations and better improvements in FEV1.

Dupilumab is a fully humanized monoclonal antibody that inhibits IL-13 and IL-4. This biologic targets the IL-4 α receptor, which is a common receptor domain for both of these cytokines. In patients with moderate to severe asthma on ICS plus an LABA with elevated peripheral blood eosinophil counts $\geq$300 cells/μL or greater than 3% sputum eosinophils, dupilumab reduced asthma exacerbations compared with placebo. Wenzel and colleagues[50] demonstrated a primary outcome of 87% reduction in asthma exacerbations in patients treated weekly subcutaneously with dupilumab primarily administered at home. Wenzel and colleagues[51] recently showed a biweekly dose of dupilumab administered at home results in improvements in asthma exacerbations and pulmonary function regardless of pretreatment blood eosinophil levels. However, the data were better for patients having a blood eosinophil level greater than 300 cells/μL. Dupilumab is currently being studied in other disease states, including nasal polyposis and atopic dermatitis. It is anticipated that it will be approved for the later disease processes before it achieves an indication for asthma.

Prostaglandin Antagonists

Chemoattractant receptor homologous molecule on T2 cells (CRTH2) is expressed on T2 lymphocytes, ILC2s, eosinophils, and basophils. Prostaglandin D2, which is predominantly secreted by mast cells, binds to CRTH2 and subsequently promotes secretion of IL-5 and IL-13 from ILC2 and Th2 cells, contributing to local airway inflammation.[52] Initial studies with CRTH2 receptor antagonists show variable results. However, CRTH2 receptor antagonists improve FEV1 in patients with blood eosinophil counts greater than 250 cells/uL. Further studies enriching for patients with higher blood eosinophil levels should be considered.

SUMMARY

In summary, all of the biologics currently FDA approved for asthma target T2-high patients. Unfortunately, 50% of patients with severe asthma do not fit this phenotype of disease. Clinicians have access to biomarkers such as total IgE, FeNO, and peripheral blood eosinophils to more appropriately use the current biologics on the market. However, precise biomarkers to predict better responses to specific T2-high asthma therapies are lacking. For example, elevated blood eosinophils track with better responses to all of the T2-targeted therapies and do not allow us to discriminate whether a patient is more likely to respond to one or another. It is important to note that none of the current medications targeting the T2 pathway induce persistent immunomodulation or remission. Once stopped, patient's symptoms and disease manifestations reappear, which is suggestive that the underlying disease process has not been modified. Overall, practicing precision medicine will help decrease associated costs and the burden of disease by using these medications in the most appropriate patients.

DISCLOSURE STATEMENT

T.B. Casale is a research investigator with funds to university employer from Genentech; MedImmune/Astra Zeneca; Novartis; Teva; Sanofi/Regeneron. He is also a consultant with funds to university employer from Novartis; Genentech; Teva; Astra Zeneca; Sanofi/Regeneron. D.K.Ledford has received consultancy fees from AstraZeneca, Boehringer Ingelheim, Genentech, and Novartis; is employed by the VA Administration; has provided expert testimony for Wicker, Smith, O'Hara, McCoy Ford (Latex allergy), Richard Benjamin Wilkes (Drug allergy), and Bradley (Radiocontrast reaction); has received research support from Forest, Circassia, AstraZeneca, and Genentech; has received lecture fees from AstraZeneca, Meda, Teva, Genentech, Novartis, and Merck; receives royalties from UpToDate, CRC Press, and Springer; is on the Chughai Data Safety Monitoring; and receives an editorial stipend from the American Academy of Allergy, Asthma & Immunology for Ask the Expert. F. Tabatabaian has nothing to disclose.

REFERENCES

1. Centers for Disease Control and Prevention: Data, Statistics, and Surveillance. AsthmaStats. 2015. Available from: http://www.cdc.gov/asthma/asthma_stats/default.htm. Accessed February 1, 2017.

2. Fahy JV. Type 2 inflammation in asthma–present in most, absent in many. Nat Rev Immunol 2015;15(1):57–65.

3. Barnes PJ. Therapeutic approaches to asthma-chronic obstructive pulmonary disease overlap syndromes. J Allergy Clin Immunol 2015;136(3):531–45.

4. Muraro A, Lemanske RF Jr, Hellings PW, et al. Precision medicine in patients with allergic diseases: airway diseases and atopic dermatitis—PRACTALL document of the European Academy of Allergy and Clinical Immunology and the American Academy of Allergy, Asthma & Immunology. J Allergy Clin Immunol 2016;137(5): 1347–58.

5. Wenzel SE. Asthma phenotypes: the evolution from clinical to molecular approaches. Nat Med 2012;18(5):716–25.

6. Lambrecht BN, Hammad H. The immunology of asthma. Nat Immunol 2015;16(1): 45–56.

7. Bellini A, Marini MA, Bianchetti L, et al. Interleukin (IL)-4, IL-13, and IL-17A differentially affect the profibrotic and proinflammatory functions of fibrocytes from asthmatic patients. Mucosal Immunol 2012;5(2):140–9.

8. Busse WW, Holgate S, Kerwin E, et al. Randomized, double-blind, placebo-controlled study of brodalumab, a human anti-IL-17 receptor monoclonal antibody, in moderate to severe asthma. Am J Respir Crit Care Med 2013;188(11): 1294–302.

9. Baines KJ, Simpson JL, Wood LG, et al. Transcriptional phenotypes of asthma defined by gene expression profiling of induced sputum samples. J Allergy Clin Immunol 2011;127(1):153–60, 60.e1–9.

10. Wenzel SE, Barnes PJ, Bleecker ER, et al. A randomized, double-blind, placebo-controlled study of tumor necrosis factor-alpha blockade in severe persistent asthma. Am J Respir Crit Care Med 2009;179(7):549–58.

11. Wilhelm CP, Chipps BE. Bronchial thermoplasty: a review of the evidence. Ann Allergy Asthma Immunol 2016;116(2):92–8.

12. Woodruff PG, Boushey HA, Dolganov GM, et al. Genome-wide profiling identifies epithelial cell genes associated with asthma and with treatment response to corticosteroids. Proc Natl Acad Sci U S A 2007;104(40):15858–63.

13. Woodruff PG, Modrek B, Choy DF, et al. T-helper type 2-driven inflammation defines major subphenotypes of asthma. Am J Respir Crit Care Med 2009;180(5): 388–95.

14. Dougherty RH, Sidhu SS, Raman K, et al. Accumulation of intraepithelial mast cells with a unique protease phenotype in T(H)2-high asthma. J Allergy Clin Immunol 2010;125(5):1046–53.e8.

15. Haldar P, Pavord ID, Shaw DE, et al. Cluster analysis and clinical asthma phenotypes. Am J Respir Crit Care Med 2008;178(3):218–24.

16. Fajt ML, Wenzel SE. Asthma phenotypes in adults and clinical implications. Expert Rev Respir Med 2009;3(6):607–25.

17. Berry A, Busse WW. Biomarkers in asthmatic patients: has their time come to direct treatment? J Allergy Clin Immunol 2016;137(5):1317–24.

18. Pavord ID, Korn S, Howarth P, et al. Mepolizumab for severe eosinophilic asthma (DREAM): a multicentre, double-blind, placebo-controlled trial. Lancet 2012; 380(9842):651–9.

19. Rank MA, Ochkur SI, Lewis JC, et al. Nasal and pharyngeal eosinophil peroxidase levels in adults with poorly controlled asthma correlate with sputum eosinophilia. Allergy 2016;71(4):567–70.

20. Wright K. Bioactive paper will revolutionize point-of-care diagnostics 2013. Available from: http://dailynews.mcmaster.ca/article/bioactive-paper-will-revolutionize-point-of-care-diagnostics/. Accessed February 1, 2017.

21. Dweik RA, Boggs PB, Erzurum SC, et al. An official ATS clinical practice guideline: interpretation of exhaled nitric oxide levels (FENO) for clinical applications. Am J Respir Crit Care Med 2011;184(5):602–15.

22. Mehta V, Stokes JR, Berro A, et al. Time-dependent effects of inhaled corticosteroids on lung function, bronchial hyperresponsiveness, and airway inflammation in asthma. Ann Allergy Asthma Immunol 2009;103(1):31–7.

23. Olin AC, Bake B, Toren K. Fraction of exhaled nitric oxide at 50 mL/s: reference values for adult lifelong never-smokers. Chest 2007;131(6):1852–6.

24. Malmberg LP, Petays T, Haahtela T, et al. Exhaled nitric oxide in healthy nonatopic school-age children: determinants and height-adjusted reference values. Pediatr Pulmonol 2006;41(7):635–42.

25. Pijnenburg MW, Bakker EM, Lever S, et al. High fractional concentration of nitric oxide in exhaled air despite steroid treatment in asthmatic children. Clin Exp Allergy 2005;35(7):920–5.

26. Haldar P, Brightling CE, Hargadon B, et al. Mepolizumab and exacerbations of refractory eosinophilic asthma. N Engl J Med 2009;360(10):973–84.

27. Corren J, Lemanske RF, Hanania NA, et al. Lebrikizumab treatment in adults with asthma. N Engl J Med 2011;365(12):1088–98.

28. Gauvreau GM, Harris JM, Boulet LP, et al. Targeting membrane-expressed IgE B cell receptor with an antibody to the M1 prime epitope reduces IgE production. Sci Transl Med 2014;6(243):243ra85.

29. Harris JM, Maciuca R, Bradley MS, et al. A randomized trial of the efficacy and safety of quilizumab in adults with inadequately controlled allergic asthma. Respir Res 2016;17:29.

30. Humbert M, Busse W, Hanania NA, et al. Omalizumab in asthma: an update on recent developments. J Allergy Clin Immunol Pract 2014;2(5):525–36.e1.

31. Arm JP, Bottoli I, Skerjanec A, et al. Pharmacokinetics, pharmacodynamics and safety of QGE031 (ligelizumab), a novel high-affinity anti-IgE antibody, in atopic subjects. Clin Exp Allergy 2014;44(11):1371–85.

32. Hanania NA, Wenzel S, Rosen K, et al. Exploring the effects of omalizumab in allergic asthma: an analysis of biomarkers in the EXTRA study. Am J Respir Crit Care Med 2013;187(8):804–11.

33. Busse W, Spector S, Rosen K, et al. High eosinophil count: a potential biomarker for assessing successful omalizumab treatment effects. J Allergy Clin Immunol 2013;132(2):485–6.e11.

34. Flood-Page P, Swenson C, Faiferman I, et al. A study to evaluate safety and efficacy of mepolizumab in patients with moderate persistent asthma. Am J Respir Crit Care Med 2007;176(11):1062–71.

35. Liu Y, Zhang S, Li DW, et al. Efficacy of anti-interleukin-5 therapy with mepolizumab in patients with asthma: a meta-analysis of randomized placebo-controlled trials. PLoS One 2013;8(3):e59872.

36. Ortega HG, Liu MC, Pavord ID, et al. Mepolizumab treatment in patients with severe eosinophilic asthma. N Engl J Med 2014;371(13):1198–207.

37. Nair P, Pizzichini MM, Kjarsgaard M, et al. Mepolizumab for prednisone-dependent asthma with sputum eosinophilia. N Engl J Med 2009;360(10):985–93.

38. Bel EH, Wenzel SE, Thompson PJ, et al. Oral glucocorticoid-sparing effect of mepolizumab in eosinophilic asthma. N Engl J Med 2014;371(13):1189–97.

39. Haldar P, Brightling CE, Singapuri A, et al. Outcomes after cessation of mepolizu-mab therapy in severe eosinophilic asthma: a 12-month follow-up analysis. J Allergy Clin Immunol 2014;133(3):921–3.
40. Castro M, Mathur S, Hargreave F, et al. Reslizumab for poorly controlled, eosin-ophilic asthma: a randomized, placebo-controlled study. Am J Respir Crit Care Med 2011;184(10):1125–32.
41. Bjermer L, Lemiere C, Maspero J, et al. Reslizumab for Inadequately Controlled Asthma With Elevated Blood Eosinophil Levels: A Randomized Phase 3 Study. Chest 2016;150(4):789–98.
42. Corren J, Weinstein S, Janka L, et al. Phase 3 study of reslizumab in patients with poorly controlled asthma: effects across a broad range of eosinophil counts. Chest 2016;150(4):799–810.
43. Castro M, Zangrilli J, Wechsler ME, et al. Reslizumab for inadequately controlled asthma with elevated blood eosinophil counts: results from two multicentre, par-allel, double-blind, randomised, placebo-controlled, phase 3 trials. Lancet Respir Med 2015;3(5):355–66.
44. Laviolette M, Gossage DL, Gauvreau G, et al. Effects of benralizumab on airway eosinophils in asthmatic patients with sputum eosinophilia. J Allergy Clin Immunol 2013;132(5):1086–96.e5.
45. Castro M, Wenzel SE, Bleecker ER, et al. Benralizumab, an anti-interleukin 5 re-ceptor alpha monoclonal antibody, versus placebo for uncontrolled eosinophilic asthma: a phase 2b randomised dose-ranging study. Lancet Respir Med 2014; 2(11):879–90.
46. Nowak RM, Parker JM, Silverman RA, et al. A randomized trial of benralizumab, an antiinterleukin 5 receptor alpha monoclonal antibody, after acute asthma. Am J Emerg Med 2015;33(1):14–20.
47. Gallelli L, Busceti MT, Vatrella A, et al. Update on anticytokine treatment for asthma. Biomed Res Int 2013;2013:104315.
48. Hanania NA, Noonan M, Corren J, et al. Lebrikizumab in moderate-to-severe asthma: pooled data from two randomised placebo-controlled studies. Thorax 2015;70(8):748–56.
49. Brightling CE, Chanez P, Leigh R, et al. Efficacy and safety of tralokinumab in pa-tients with severe uncontrolled asthma: a randomised, double-blind, placebo-controlled, phase 2b trial. Lancet Respir Med 2015;3(9):692–701.
50. Wenzel S, Ford L, Pearlman D, et al. Dupilumab in persistent asthma with elevated eosinophil levels. N Engl J Med 2013;368(26):2455–66.
51. Wenzel S, Castro M, Corren J, et al. Dupilumab efficacy and safety in adults with uncontrolled persistent asthma despite use of medium-to-high-dose inhaled cor-ticosteroids plus a long-acting beta2 agonist: a randomised double-blind pla-cebo-controlled pivotal phase 2b dose-ranging trial. Lancet 2016;388(10039): 31–44.
52. Kim BS, Wojno ED, Artis D. Innate lymphoid cells and allergic inflammation. Curr Opin Immunol 2013;25(6):738–44.

Biologic Therapy in Chronic Obstructive Pulmonary Disease

Julia W. Tripple, MD[1], Jennifer L. McCracken, MD[1],
William J. Calhoun, MD*

KEYWORDS

- Biologic therapy • COPD • TNF-alpha • IL-5 • Exacerbation

KEY POINTS

- Chronic obstructive pulmonary disease (COPD) has a broader array of mechanisms implicated in its pathogenesis than many other respiratory disorders, including asthma. Accordingly, a broad array of selective biologic agents have been proposed as potential therapies for COPD.
- Antineutrophil approaches have a clear rationale, but the overall experience with strategies that block neutrophil influx and activation has been disappointing. The redundant mechanisms that underlie these critical host defenses may be a partial explanation for these results.
- The more recent understanding of the contribution of eosinophils in COPD, particularly in exacerbation, has raised the possibility that agents that affect eosinophil recruitment and activation may also have a role in COPD, especially in the setting of exacerbation. These studies, although promising, have yet to provide compelling data in support of their use in COPD.

INTRODUCTION

Chronic obstructive pulmonary disease (COPD) is characterized by persistent airflow limitation that is usually progressive and associated with an enhanced chronic inflammatory response in the airways and the lung to noxious particles or gases.[1] It is a global medical problem with a lifetime risk of development estimated to be around 25%.[2] In developed countries, the biggest risk factor for development of COPD is cigarette smoking, whereas indoor pollutants are the major cause in lower-income, developing nations. The economic burden is large, with attributed costs for hospitalizations, loss of productivity, and disability, in addition to chronic medical care. In the

Division of Allergy and Clinical Immunology, University of Texas Medical Branch, 4.116 JSA, 301 University Boulevard, Galveston, TX 77555-0568, USA
[1] These authors contributed equally to this work.
* Corresponding author.
E-mail addresses: william.calhoun@utmb.edu; wjcalhou@utmb.edu

Immunol Allergy Clin N Am 37 (2017) 345–355
http://dx.doi.org/10.1016/j.iac.2017.01.009
0889-8561/17/© 2017 Elsevier Inc. All rights reserved.

United States the estimated direct costs of COPD are $29.5 billion and indirect costs $20.4 billion.[1] Current treatment options are aimed primarily at symptom control with bronchodilation and include long-acting beta agonists and antimuscarinics. Inhaled corticosteroids are indicated in severe COPD (Global initiative for Obstructive Lung Disease (GOLD) stage III and above); however, they are not always effective in controlling symptoms and exacerbations. At present, there are no therapies approved that substantively reduced the inflammatory process and or prevent progression of disease.

The defining characteristic of COPD, chronic airflow limitation, is caused by several mechanisms. Small airway disease is mediated by chronic inflammation leading to airway fibrosis, structural changes, and increased resistance. This process is coupled with parenchymal destruction causing loss of alveolar attachments to the small airways and decrease of lung elastic recoil.[1] Together, these changes diminish the ability of the airway to stay open during expiration, and contribute to dynamic airway collapse. Historically, the inflammation leading to these alterations has been described as type 1 inflammation with neutrophilic predominance; however, recently more evidence has been published about the role of eosinophils in stable COPD.[3] As described in a review by Barnes,[4] inhaled irritants such as cigarette smoke activate airway epithelial cells and macrophages to release tumor necrosis factor (TNF)-α and neutrophil and monocyte chemotactic factors including CC Ligand 2 (CCL2), CXC Ligand 1 (CXCL1), and CXCL8. These mediators attract inflammatory cells, such as Th1 cells, cytotoxic T lymphocytes, and Th17, as well as neutrophils and monocytes, to the site of injury, where they release proteases and other inflammatory mediators and cause elastin degradation leading to emphysema and also increased mucus secretion.[5] The inflammasome also plays a role in the pathogenesis of COPD. Cigarette smoke and microbes can activate pathogen-associated molecular patterns and damage-associated molecular patterns, which activate inflammasomes. This process in turn initiates a cascade of events that result in the recruitment and cleavage of pro–caspase-1 into active caspase-1 molecules, which then mediate the cleavage of pro–interleukin (IL)-1β into its active form IL-1β.[6] IL-1β activates macrophages to secrete inflammatory cytokines and chemokines and the cycle of inflammation and neutrophilic infiltration continues.[4]

Although the role of neutrophilic inflammation is well accepted, emerging evidence suggests a role for eosinophilic or type 2 inflammation in COPD as well. As recently reviewed, eosinophils are recruited to the lung by a multistep process mainly directed by Th2 cytokines.[7] After being released from the bone marrow under the influence of IL-5, eosinophils are directed to the lung via several steps. Lung epithelial cell expression of vascular cell adhesion molecule-1 is induced by local expression of IL-4 and IL-13, which allows for eosinophil binding via VLA-4 and P-selectin. In addition, chemokines, like eotaxin, secreted by airway cells, activate the chemokine receptor CCR3 on eosinophils, further attracting eosinophils into lung tissue. Once present, eosinophil survival in tissue is mediated by local production of IL-5 and granulocyte-macrophage colony-stimulating factor. Release of eosinophilic specific basic proteins, like major basic protein and eosinophilic cationic protein, cause direct injury to lung tissue, and the release of other preformed mediators and proinflammatory cytokines contributes to ongoing inflammation. In addition, IL-33 stimulation of group 2 innate lymphoid cells (ILC2), which are potent producers of IL-5 and IL-13, may contribute to eosinophilic type II inflammation in COPD.[8,9] This article discusses the use of biologic agents to target these inflammatory pathways in the treatment of COPD.

NEUTROPHILIC INFLAMMATION AND POTENTIAL TARGETS FOR THERAPY

TNF-α and several of the other implicated cytokines and chemokines have been studied as potential targets for biologic therapy in the treatment of COPD and are discussed further in this article (**Fig. 1**).

Tumor Necrosis Factor Alpha

TNF-α has been implicated as a key cytokine in the pathogenesis of COPD.[10] It is an important mediator for neutrophil chemotaxis by inducing IL-8 expression as well as increasing endothelial adhesion molecules important in the transmigration of neutrophils.[11] It has also been proved to be at increased levels in peripheral blood and sputum in patients with stable COPD[12] and specifically in those with significant weight loss.[13] Studies have also shown that concentrations of TNF-α increase more than 4-fold during exacerbations compared with stable state.[14] Infliximab and etanercept are monoclonal antibodies that have been developed that bind to TNF-α and neutralize its biological activity. At present they are used successfully for the treatment of rheumatoid arthritis (RA), psoriasis and psoriatic arthritis, and ankylosing spondylitis. Infliximab has additional indications for inflammatory bowel disease.

Suissa and colleagues[15] first published an observational study supporting the use of TNF-α antagonists in the treatment of stable COPD. Patients with both RA and COPD who were being treated with either etanercept or infliximab for their RA were observed for time to first COPD exacerbation and compared with those not on TNF antagonists. Patients on TNF antagonists, specifically etanercept, had a significant reduction in hospitalizations for COPD exacerbations compared with the case controls. However,

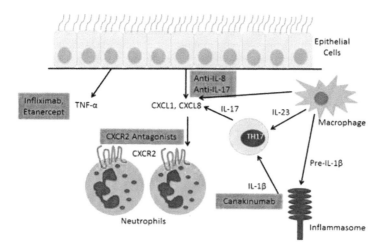

Fig. 1. Targets of biologic therapies to mitigate type 1 inflammation in COPD: neutrophilic inflammation in the airway. Insult to the epithelial cells in the airways leads to production of TNF-α and chemokines important for neutrophil migration. In addition, macrophages are activated and contribute to the inflammatory processes by increasing chemokine and cytokine production. Several biologic therapies have been developed and studied that target different points in the inflammatory process including infliximab, etanercept, anti–IL-8 and IL-17 agents, CXC Receptor 2 (CXCR2) antagonists, and canakinumab. (*Adapted from* Barnes PJ. Therapeutic approaches to asthma-chronic obstructive pulmonary disease overlap syndromes. J Allergy Clin Immunol 2015;136(3):535; with permission.)

several randomized trials have subsequently been conducted that did not support this finding. Van der Vaart and colleagues[11] examined the short-term effects of infliximab on airway inflammation with percentage of sputum neutrophils as their primary end point and, at the end of 8 weeks, found no difference in airway inflammation/neutrophil levels. There was also no difference in the secondary end points, which included quality-of-life indicators, respiratory symptoms, and lung function. This finding was confirmed by a study conducted by Rennard and colleagues,[16] which evaluated the effect of infliximab over 24 weeks. They found no difference in Chronic Respiratory Questionnaire total score, their primary end point, as well as no significant change in secondary measures, including prebronchodilator forced expiratory volume in 1 second (FEV_1), 6-minute walk distance, Sort Form 36 (SF-36) physical score, transition dyspnea index, or moderate to severe COPD exacerbation. Although not statistically significant, more cases of pneumonia and cancer were observed in the infliximab-treated group (n = 9, 5.7%) versus the control group (n = 1, 1.3%). To follow up this finding, a long-term observational study (Remicade Safety Under Long-Term Study in COPD [RESULTS COPD]) was conducted. Malignancy and mortality data were collected for an additional 5 years from patients enrolled in the previously conducted phase 2 studies on infliximab and COPD. Data were analyzed from 107 subjects who participated and a greater proportion of malignancies was observed in those treated with infliximab compared with placebo (5.1% vs 5.2% respectively), and that effect diminished over time.[17]

Another study evaluated the efficacy of TNF-α antagonists in the treatment of acute exacerbations of COPD (AECOPD). As mentioned earlier, TNF-α upregulates adhesion molecules and increases migration of neutrophils into the bronchial mucosa during COPD exacerbations by inducing IL-8 expression as well as stimulating neutrophil degranulation and superoxide production. In a randomized double-blind, double-dummy, placebo-controlled trial, Aaron and colleagues[14] enrolled 81 patients with AECOPD who were either treated with etanercept at randomization and 1 week later or standard therapy with prednisone 40 mg daily for 10 days. Both groups also received levofloxacin and inhaled bronchodilators. Primary end point in this study was change in FEV_1 14 days after randomization. Secondary end points included 90-day treatment failure rates, dyspnea, and quality of life. Etanercept was not more effective than prednisone for treatment of AECOPD because there was no significant difference in the primary end point or any of the secondary end points.[14]

Interleukin-1β

As described earlier, the inflammasome and IL-1 family of cytokines have been implicated in the pathogenesis of COPD. Canakinumab was developed as a human immunoglobulin (Ig) G1 anti–Il-1β monoclonal that binds with high specificity and neutralizes the inflammatory actions of IL-1β.[18] It is currently approved by the US Food and Drug Administration for treatment of cryopyrin-associated periodic syndrome, Muckle-Wells syndrome, and familial cold autoinflammatory syndrome.[19] A phase 1/2 study (NCT00581945) was completed to evaluate the safety, tolerability, and efficacy on pulmonary function in patients with COPD. In this trial, a total of 147 patients were enrolled (74 canakinumab and 73 placebo) and received treatment for 45 weeks with the primary end point of change in pulmonary function. At the completion of the trial, no statistical difference was found in change from baseline in FEV_1, forced vital capacity, Slow vital capacity (SVC), or forced expiratory flow 25% to 75%.[18] Further studies have ceased.

MEDI8968 is a human IgG2 monoclonal antibody that binds to IL-1R1 to inhibit the binding of IL-1α and IL-1β. A phase 2 trial (NCT1448850) was completed in adults with moderate to very severe COPD with the primary end point of moderate/severe acute exacerbations and secondary end points of severe acute exacerbation rate and St George's Respiratory Questionnaire-COPD (SGRQ-C). A total of 324 subjects were enrolled in this randomized, double-blind, placebo-controlled study, which concluded that there was no significant difference in outcomes.[20]

Interleukin-8/CXCR2

IL-8 is a potent chemoattractant for neutrophils and a member of the CXC family of chemokines. It has been evaluated as a possible target for biologic therapy. A fully human monoclonal IgG2 antibody against human IL-8 (ABX-IL8) has been developed and was studied for efficacy and safety in symptomatic patients with COPD who had a component of chronic bronchitis. A pilot study was conducted in 109 patients with dyspnea (measured using the transition dyspnea index) as the primary end point and change in baseline prebronchodilator and postbronchodilator FEV_1, the St George Respiratory Questionnaire (SGRQ), 6-minute walking distance, and use of albuterol as rescue therapy as secondary outcomes. Final results showed a reduced severity of dyspnea in those threated with ABX-IL8, but the difference was only significant at 2 weeks. There was no difference in the secondary end points.[14]

Chemokine receptors have also been studied as possible targets for monoclonal antibodies. Neutrophils have the chemokine receptors CXCR1 and CXCR2, of which CXCR2 is more responsible for chemotaxis and adhesion. MK-7123 (also known as SCH 527123) is a chemokine receptor antagonist with high affinity of CXCR2. It was shown to reduce sputum neutrophils when used in the treatment of ozone-induced airway inflammation.[21] MK-7123 has also been studied in a phase 2 proof-of-concept trial of patients with moderate to severe COPD already on standard therapy. The group was randomized to daily MK-7123 at doses of 10 mg, 30 mg, 50 mg, or placebo. The primary end point of this 6-month trial was change from baseline in postbronchodilator FEV_1. Results showed that only MK-7123 50 mg led to a significant improvement in FEV_1 compared with placebo, although most benefit was seen in current smokers versus ex-smokers. There was also reduced sputum neutrophil count at 3 and 6 months; however, MK-7123 caused a dose-dependent decrease in absolute neutrophil count that led to some subjects' discontinuation of the study.[22]

ADDITIONAL POTENTIAL TARGETS

Several other cytokines have been suggested as potential targets for biologic therapy because of their role in the pathogenesis of COPD. IL-6 amplifies inflammation and increased concentrations have been found in sputum in patients with COPD.[23] An IL-6R–specific antibody (tocilizumab) has been developed and is effective in people with RA but no clinical studies have been conducted in COPD. IL-17 is secreted from T helper 17 (Th17) cells and mediates neutrophilic inflammation by increasing release of CXCL8 (IL-8) from airway epithelial cells. The role of IL-17 in COPD pathogenesis has been supported by the finding of increased concentrations of this cytokine in bronchial biopsy samples and lung and sputum of patients of COPD.[24,25] Several anti–IL-17 monoclonal antibodies have been developed, including ixekizumab, brodalumab, and secukinumab, which are used in the treatment of psoriasis, but no clinical trials have been performed in patients with COPD. There have also been studies evaluating IL-18 involvement in COPD. IL-18 is a proinflammatory cytokine that has been found at increased levels in the serum of patients with severe COPD and had a significant negative correlation between serum level and predicted FEV_1.[26] MEDI2338 is a human IgG1 monoclonal antibody that binds IL-18 and a phase 1 trial was completed in COPD (NCT01322594); however, results are not available.

EOSINOPHILIC CHRONIC OBSTRUCTIVE PULMONARY DISEASE AND POTENTIAL TARGETS FOR THERAPY

Although the inflammatory response in COPD is predominately considered type 1 or neutrophilic predominant there is emerging evidence that type 2 or eosinophilic inflammation also plays a role (**Fig. 2**). Eosinophilic inflammation has been reported in 20% to 40% of induced sputums in patients with stable COPD,[27] and eosinophilic inflammation increases in exacerbations. Bronchial biopsies done during acute exacerbations compared with stable COPD had a 30-fold increase in total number of eosinophils,[28] and blood eosinophilia has been associated with increased mortality in COPD exacerbations.[29] Importantly, strategies designed to reduce eosinophilic airway inflammation are associated with a reduction in severe exacerbations of COPD.[30] COPD exacerbations result in significant morbidity and mortality, and have negative effects on quality of life and high economic burden.[31] Exacerbations also correlate with loss of lung function and progression of disease, and studies have shown that, after exacerbation, FEV_1 does not return to preexacerbation levels.[32] The use of biologic agents that target eosinophilic inflammation in the treatment of asthma has been shown to reduce exacerbation rates,[33–37] thus these agents may prove beneficial in reducing exacerbations with an eosinophilic profile in COPD.

There are several cytokines involved in eosinophilic inflammation, including IL-5, IL-4, and IL-13.

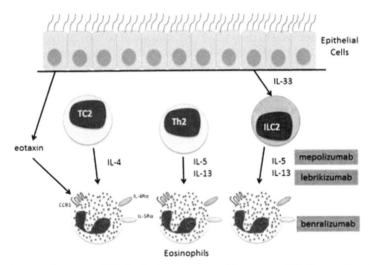

Fig. 2. Schema of targets of biologic therapies to mitigate type 2 inflammation in COPD: eosinophilic inflammation in the airway. Eosinophils are recruited to the lung by local expression of IL-4 and IL-13 inducing eosinophil binding via very-late antigen 4 (VLA-4) and P-selectin. Expression of the chemokine eotaxin by endothelial cells further attracts eosinophils to the lung via binding of its receptor CCR3 on eosinophils. Once in the lung, local production of IL-5 by Th2 cells and ILC2s contributes to the survival of eosinophils in tissue. IL-4 production by CD8+ T cells (Tc2) and IL-13 production by Th2 and ILC2 contribute to the ongoing inflammatory process, fibrosis, and mucus secretion. Monoclonal antibodies targeting IL-5 (mepolizumab), the IL-5Rα (benralizumab), and IL-13 (lebrikizumab) are currently under investigation for their use in COPD. (*Adapted from* Barnes PJ. Therapeutic approaches to asthma-chronic obstructive pulmonary disease overlap syndromes. J Allergy Clin Immunol 2015;136(3):535; with permission.)

Interleukin-5

IL-5 is a proinflammatory cytokine and regulates the differentiation, survival, and activation of eosinophils. It is secreted by T lymphocytes, mast cells, and eosinophils.[38] Although studies are conflicting, patients with eosinophilic COPD have increased IL-5 concentrations in sputum and treatment with systemic steroids leads to reduction in IL-5 level; thus, IL-5 blockade may be a beneficial therapy in COPD with an eosinophilic phenotype.[39,40] Benralizumab is a humanized fucosylated monoclonal antibody that targets the human IL-5 receptor alpha found on eosinophils. A recent study evaluated benralizumab in patients with moderate to severe COPD with sputum eosinophil counts of 3% or more.[41] In this study, benralizumab did not reduce the rate of COPD exacerbations. However, a trend toward improvement in FEV_1 and exacerbations was noted in patients with higher blood eosinophil counts. At present, phase III trials are ongoing to investigate this further. Mepolizumab, a humanized monoclonal antibody against IL-5, was recently approved for the treatment of eosinophilic asthma after it was shown to reduce exacerbations in this population.[33–35] At present, studies are ongoing to evaluate its efficacy in COPD.

Interleukin-4/Interleukin-13

IL-4 and IL-13 are proinflammatory cytokines expressed by T lymphocytes, mast cells, and eosinophils, and are key cytokines in the pathogenesis of type 2 inflammation. There is redundancy in the IL-4/IL-13 pathway resulting from the complex receptor system that shares IL-4 receptor α (IL-4Rα). Receptor binding mediates downstream signaling through signal transducer and activator of transcription factor 6 (STAT-6). IL-4 and IL-13 have been implicated in airway inflammation via eosinophil, macrophage, and dendritic cell activation; stimulation of airway epithelial and goblet cells leading to mucus secretion; and airway fibrosis.[42]

The data on the role of IL-13 and IL-4 are conflicting in COPD. The main evidence for an IL-4/IL-13 pathway in COPD is based on a mouse model of COPD in which mice that overexpressed IL-13 in the lungs spontaneously developed emphysema.[43] However, the role of these cytokines in COPD in humans has been less clear.

IL-13 and IL-4 expression was higher in T lymphocytes from bronchoalveolar lavage fluid from subjects with COPD than from controls,[44] and IL-13 was also found at increased levels in the induced sputum of patients with COPD compared with controls.[45] However, in a conflicting study, IL-13 expression was not increased in induced sputum or bronchial mucosa of patients with COPD compared with control.[46] Studies in stable COPD have shown increased expression of IL-4 from CD8+ T cells in patients with COPD, suggesting that a subset of CD8+ cells (Tc2) may contribute to the expression of these cytokines in COPD.[47] In AECOPD, similar results have suggested a role for Tc2 because increases in CD8+IL-4+ cell levels were seen at the onset of AECOPD in both mild and severe exacerbations.[48,49]

Targeting the IL-4/IL-13 pathway has been an active area of investigation in asthma and benefits have been seen in reducing asthma exacerbation rates.[50–53] Although the data in COPD are mixed, taking from the success of these agents in reducing exacerbations in asthma and the role of eosinophilic inflammation in COPD, targeting IL-4 and IL-13 may prove beneficial in a subgroup of Th2-high patients with COPD, in patients with Asthma/COPD Overlap Syndrome (ACOS), and/or in COPD exacerbations. A phase II trial of lebrikizumab, an IgG4 humanized monoclonal antibody that blocks IL-13, in COPD is currently recruiting participants.

SUMMARY

COPD is a complex disease affecting many people. It carries with it significant morbidity and mortality and a high economic burden. As clinicians gain a better understanding of the inflammatory process underlying COPD, biologic agents may provide targeted treatment options to improve disease control and decrease exacerbation rates. Although promising, biologic agents in COPD have not had the clinical impact that has been seen in asthma. As detailed in this article, many of the biologics studied thus far have failed to provide significant clinical benefit or disease modification. This failure may in part be caused by the lag behind in their application in COPD. In addition, failure to identify specific phenotypes of COPD and target biologics accordingly may have contributed to the lack of efficacy in these studies. Targeting biologics according to particular phenotypes of disease may improve outcomes. Despite these setbacks, biologics have the potential to allow specific inhibition of the inflammatory pathways involved in COPD and provide a means to accomplish personalized treatment of COPD, which warrants further investigation into their therapeutic benefit.

REFERENCES

1. Vestbo J, Hurd SS, Agusti AG, et al. Global strategy for the diagnosis, management, and prevention of chronic obstructive pulmonary disease: GOLD executive summary. Am J Respir Crit Care Med 2013 Feb 15;187(4):347–65.
2. Gershon AS, Warner L, Cascagnette P, et al. Lifetime risk of developing chronic obstructive pulmonary disease: a longitudinal population study. Lancet 2011;378: 991–6.
3. Barker BL, Brightling CE. Phenotyping the heterogeneity of chronic obstructive pulmonary disease. Clin Sci 2013;124:371–87.
4. Barnes PJ. The cytokine network in asthma and chronic obstructive pulmonary disease [review]. J Clin Invest 2008;118:3546–56.
5. Barnes PJ. Immunology of asthma and chronic obstructive pulmonary disease. Nat Rev Immunol 2008;8:183–92.
6. Kim RY, Pinkerton JW, Gibson PG, et al. Inflammasomes in COPD and neutrophilic asthma. Thorax 2015;70(12):1199–201.
7. George L, Brightling CE. Eosinophilic airway inflammation: role in asthma and chronic obstructive pulmonary disease. Ther Adv Chronic Dis 2016;7:34–51.
8. Xia J, Zhao J, Shang J, et al. Increased IL-33 expression in chronic obstructive pulmonary disease. Am J Physiol Lung Cell Mol Physiol 2015;308(7):L619–27.
9. Martinez-Gonzalez I, Steer CA, Takei F. Lung ILC2s link innate and adaptive responses in allergic inflammation. Trends Immunol 2015;36:189–95.
10. Churg A, Wang RD, Tai H, et al. Tumor necrosis factor-α drives 70% of cigarette smoke-induced emphysema in the mouse. Am J Respir Crit Care Med 2004;170: 492–8.
11. Van Der Vaart H, Koëter GH, Postma DS, et al. First study of infliximab treatment in patients with chronic obstructive pulmonary disease. Am J Respir Crit Care Med 2005;172:465–9.
12. Keatings VM, Barnes PJ. Comparison of inflammatory cytokines in chronic obstructive pulmonary disease, asthma and controls. Eur Respir Rev 1997;7:146–50.
13. Di Francia M, Barbier D, Mege JL, et al. Tumor necrosis factor-alpha levels and weight loss in chronic obstructive pulmonary disease. Am J Respir Crit Care Med 1994 Nov;150:1453–5.
14. Aaron SD, Vandemheen KL, Maltais F, et al. TNFα antagonists for acute exacerbations of COPD: a randomised double-blind controlled trial. Thorax 2013;68:142–8.

15. Suissa S, Ernst P, Hudson M. TNF-α antagonists and the prevention of hospitalisation for chronic obstructive pulmonary disease. Pulm Pharmacol Ther 2008; 21:234–8.

16. Rennard SI, Fogarty C, Kelsen S, et al. The safety and efficacy of infliximab in moderate to severe chronic obstructive pulmonary disease. Am J Respir Crit Care Med 2007;175:926–34.

17. Rennard SI, Flavin SK, Agarwal PK, et al. Long-term safety study of infliximab in moderate-to-severe chronic obstructive pulmonary disease. Respir Med 2013; 107:424–32.

18. Rogliani P, Calzetta L, Ora J, et al. Canakinumab for the treatment of chronic obstructive pulmonary disease. Pulm Pharmacol Ther 2015;31:15–27.

19. Dhimolea E. Canakinumab. MAbs 2010;2:3–13.

20. Calverley P, Sethi S, Dawson M, et al. A phase 2 study of MEDI8968, an anti-interleukin-1 receptor I (IL-1RI) monoclonal antibody, in adults with moderate-to-very severe chronic obstructive pulmonary disease (COPD). Am J Respir Crit Care Med 2015;191:A3964.

21. Holz O, Khalilieh S, Ludwig-Sengpiel A, et al. SCH527123, a novel CXCR2 antagonist, inhibits ozone-induced neutrophilia in healthy subjects. Eur Respir J 2010; 35:564–70.

22. Rennard SI, Dale DC, Donohue JF, et al. CXCR2 antagonist MK-7123 a phase 2 proof-of-concept trial for chronic obstructive pulmonary disease. Am J Respir Crit Care Med 2015;191:1001–11.

23. Grubek-Jaworska H, Paplińska M, Hermanowicz-Salamon J, et al. IL-6 and IL-13 in induced sputum of COPD and asthma patients: correlation with respiratory tests. Respiration 2012;84:101–7.

24. Di Stefano A, Caramori G, Gnemmi I, et al. T helper type 17-related cytokine expression is increased in the bronchial mucosa of stable chronic obstructive pulmonary disease patients. Clin Exp Immunol 2009;157:316–24.

25. Doe C, Bafadhel M, Siddiqui S, et al. Expression of the T helper 17-associated cytokines IL-17A and IL-17F in asthma and COPD. Chest 2010;138:1140–7.

26. Imaoka H, Hoshino T, Takei S, et al. Interleukin-18 production and pulmonary function in COPD. Eur Respir J 2008;31:287–97.

27. Saha S. Eosinophilic airway inflammation in COPD. Int J Chron Obstruct Pulmon Dis 2006;1:39–47.

28. Saetta M, Di Stefano A, Maestrelli P, et al. Airway eosinophilia in chronic bronchitis during exacerbations. Am J Respir Crit Care Med 1995;1:1995.

29. Hospers JJ, Schouten JP, Weiss ST, et al. Asthma attacks with eosinophilia predict mortality from chronic obstructive pulmonary disease in a general population sample. Am J Respir Crit Care Med 1999;160:1869–74.

30. Siva R, Green RH, Brightling CE, et al. Eosinophilic airway inflammation and exacerbations of COPD: a randomised controlled trial. Eur Respir J 2007;29:906–13.

31. Seemungal T, Donaldson GC, Paul EA, et al. Effect of exacerbation on quality of life in patients with chronic obstructive pulmonary disease. Am J Respir Crit Care Med 1998;157:1418–22.

32. Donaldson GC, Seemungal TAR, Bhowmik A, et al. Relationship between exacerbation frequency and lung function decline in chronic obstructive pulmonary disease. Thorax 2002;57:847–52.

33. Haldar P, Brightling CE, Hargadon B, et al. Mepolizumab and exacerbations of refractory eosinophilic asthma. N Engl J Med 2009;360:973–84.

34. Pavord ID, Korn S, Howarth P, et al. Mepolizumab for severe eosinophilic asthma (DREAM): a multicentre, double-blind, placebo-controlled trial. Lancet 2012;380: 651–9.

35. Ortega HG, Liu MC, Pavord ID, et al. Mepolizumab treatment in patients with severe eosinophilic asthma. N Engl J Med 2014;371:1198–207.

36. Bel EH, Wenzel SE, Thompson PJ, et al. Oral glucocorticoid-sparing effect of mepolizumab in eosinophilic asthma. N Engl J Med 2014;371:1189–97.

37. Castro M, Zangrilli J, Wechsler ME, et al. Reslizumab for inadequately controlled asthma with elevated blood eosinophil counts: results from two multicentre, parallel, double-blind, randomised, placebo-controlled, phase 3 trials. Lancet Respir Med 2015;3:355–66.

38. Takatsu K, Nakajima H. IL-5 and eosinophilia. Curr Opin Immunol 2008;20: 288–94.

39. Bafadhel M, McCormick M, Saha S, et al. Profiling of sputum inflammatory mediators in asthma and chronic obstructive pulmonary disease. Respiration 2012;83: 36–44.

40. Bafadhel M, Saha S, Siva R, et al. Sputum IL-5 concentration is associated with a sputum eosinophilia and attenuated by corticosteroid therapy in COPD. Respiration 2009;78:256–62.

41. Brightling CE, Bleecker ER, Panettieri RA Jr, et al. Benralizumab for chronic obstructive pulmonary disease and sputum eosinophilia: a randomised, double-blind, placebo-controlled, phase 2a study. Lancet Respir Med 2014;2: 891–901.

42. Oh CK, Geba GP, Molfino N. Investigational therapeutics targeting the IL-4/IL-13/ STAT-6 pathway for the treatment of asthma. Eur Respir Rev 2010;19:46–54.

43. Zheng T, Zhu Z, Wang Z, et al. Inducible targeting of IL-13 to the adult lung causes matrix metalloproteinase- and cathepsin-dependent emphysema. J Clin Invest 2000;106:1081–93.

44. Barceló B, Pons J, Fuster A, et al. Intracellular cytokine profile of T lymphocytes in patients with chronic obstructive pulmonary disease. Clin Exp Immunol 2006;145: 474–9.

45. Eickmeier O, Huebner M, Herrmann E, et al. Sputum biomarker profiles in cystic fibrosis (CF) and chronic obstructive pulmonary disease (COPD) and association between pulmonary function. Cytokine 2010;50:152–7.

46. Saha S, Mistry V, Siva R, et al. Induced sputum and bronchial mucosal expression of interleukin-13 is not increased in chronic obstructive pulmonary disease. Allergy 2008;63:1239–43.

47. Barczyk A, Pierzchała W, Kon OM, et al. Cytokine production by bronchoalveolar lavage T lymphocytes in chronic obstructive pulmonary disease. J Allergy Clin Immunol 2006;117:1484–92.

48. Makris D, Lazarou S, Alexandrakis M, et al. Tc2 response at the onset of COPD exacerbations. Chest 2008;134:483–8.

49. Tsoumakidou M, Tzanakis N, Chrysofakis G, et al. Changes in sputum T-lymphocyte subpopulations at the onset of severe exacerbations of chronic obstructive pulmonary disease. Respir Med 2005;99:572–9.

50. Noonan M, Korenblat P, Mosesova S, et al. Dose-ranging study of lebrikizumab in asthmatic patients not receiving inhaled steroids. J Allergy Clin Immunol 2013; 132:567–74.e12.

51. Piper E, Brightling C, Niven R, et al. A phase II placebo-controlled study of tralokinumab in moderate-to-severe asthma. Eur Respir J 2013;41:330–8.

52. Slager RE, Otulana BA, Hawkins GA, et al. IL-4 receptor polymorphisms predict reduction in asthma exacerbations during response to an anti-IL-4 receptor α antagonist. J Allergy Clin Immunol 2012;130:516–22.e4.
53. Wenzel S, Ford L, Pearlman D, et al. Dupilumab in persistent asthma with elevated eosinophil levels. N Engl J Med 2013;368:2455–66.

Monoclonal Antibodies for the Treatment of Nasal Polyps

Thomas J. Willson, MD[a], Robert M. Naclerio, MD[b],
Stella E. Lee, MD[a],*

KEYWORDS

- Biologics • Chronic rhinosinusitis • Asthma • Nasal polyps • Allergic rhinitis

KEY POINTS

- Biologics are emerging therapeutics that can target immunologic pathways significant in inflammatory disorders, such as nasal polyps and asthma.
- Targets currently under investigation include immunoglobulin E modulation; interleukin 4, 5, and 13; and sialic acid–binding immunoglobulin-type lectins.
- Chronic rhinosinusitis with nasal polyps is a multifactorial inflammatory disorder involving multiple cell signaling pathways and multiple endotypes. Biomarkers are needed to define patient selection and maximal impact.

INTRODUCTION

With the advent of biological therapy, targeted disease and cell-specific therapy have become available for a variety of immune-mediated diseases. These therapeutics derive their utility from being able to intervene directly in dysfunctional immune pathways that remain inaccessible to small molecule–based therapies. Many of these biologics have been initially studied and developed for asthma. The upper airway is often also involved with the lower airway and demonstrates similar pathophysiologic mechanisms lending itself to study and possible concomitant treatment.

Disclosure Statement: Dr S.E. Lee received research support from Sanofi-Aventis (subinvestigator for the phase II study on dupilumab) and from Allakos (principal investigator for the phase II study on AK001, a siglec-8 antibody). Dr R.M. Naclerio is on the advisory boards of TEVA, GSK, Merck, AstraZeneca, and Sanofi. He is participating in an Allakos clinical trial on nasal polyps.
^a Department of Otolaryngology, Head & Neck Surgery, University of Pittsburgh Medical Center, 1400 Locust Street, Suite 2100, Building D, Pittsburgh, PA 15219, USA; ^b Section of Otolaryngology, Head & Neck Surgery, The University of Chicago Medical Center, MC 1035, 5841 South Maryland Avenue, Chicago, IL 60615, USA
* Corresponding author.
E-mail address: lees6@upmc.edu

Immunol Allergy Clin N Am 37 (2017) 357–367
http://dx.doi.org/10.1016/j.iac.2017.01.008
0889-8561/17/© 2017 Elsevier Inc. All rights reserved.

immunology.theclinics.com

Chronic rhinosinusitis (CRS) is a prevalent disease, affecting 12% to 15% of the general population in the United States.[1-3] Mucosal inflammation of the nasal cavity and paranasal sinuses is the hallmark of the disease, which may manifest in several ways. Symptoms include nasal obstruction, nasal discharge, facial pain/pressure, and reduced/lost smell. The most recent international consensus statement requires that 2 of these symptoms be present along with objective findings including a computed tomography (CT) or endoscopic examination with evidence of inflammation and/or purulence to make a diagnosis.[4] The mainstay of treatment consists of nasal saline irrigations in combination with topical intranasal corticosteroids, oral steroids, and surgery for those patients who fail medical therapy.[4,5] Antibiotic therapy in CRS is controversial; although commonly prescribed, the literature bears little substantive support for use in CRS with the exception of the macrolide class, which may have an antiinflammatory effect in certain populations.[4] A variety of preparations, including topical antibiotics, topical decongestants, and leukotriene receptors antagonists, have been trialed; but evidence to support these therapies to effectively treat CRS is scant.

CRS is commonly divided into 2 subsets, with (CRSsNP) and without (CRSwNP) polyps. Those who have polypoid disease (CRSwNP) with comorbid asthma represent a more severe disease variant.[5,6] When compared with the whole, a subset of CRSwNP demonstrate a poorer therapeutic response, with a higher rate of relapse or recurrence following surgical management and/or medical therapy. Based on a few select studies, the ability to control both subjective and objective outcome parameters in patients with CRS has been reported to range from 38% to 51%.[7,8] The mainstay of postsurgical medical therapy has long been a combination of intranasal topical corticosteroid therapy along with intermittent oral corticosteroid therapy based on examination and symptoms. Because of the inability of oral steroids to control the disease in refractory cases and the risks presented by chronic systemic steroid use, there is an increased need for novel therapies.

The most severe nasal polyp patients have comorbid asthma, which may be adult onset and nonatopic. Individuals with CRSwNP are estimated to have comorbid asthma ranging from 20% to 60%.[9-13] Within this subgroup is a unique subset of patients who exhibit exacerbation of respiratory symptoms in association with exposure to cyclooxygenase-1 inhibition. These patients with aspirin-exacerbated respiratory disease (AERD) comprise an important subset of CRSwNP who exhibit increased disease severity. Additional subgroups include allergic fungal rhinosinusitis and eosinophilic mucin rhinosinusitis (EMRS). The former is characterized by type I hypersensitivity, characteristic findings on CT scan, eosinophilic mucin without invasion, nasal polyposis, and a positive fungal stain.[14] This subtype may be found as a unilateral or bilateral process and generally exhibits fungal debris and polyps. Over time, the disease progression may cause bony remodeling and/or erosion. EMRS, on the other hand, is an inflammatory disease presenting with diffuse bilateral polyps, with the hallmark of thick and tenacious eosinophilic mucin, but without fungal elements on staining and no fungal hypersensitivity.[15]

PATHOPHYSIOLOGY

CRS is conceptualized as a dysfunctional host response that elicits and propagates uncontrolled inflammation. The interplay between external triggers, modifiers, the innate and adaptive host immune system, anatomic and genetic predisposition likely contributes to the phenotype that is recognized as CRS. At present there is no singular theory that explains the entire range of CRS, which exists on a spectrum of many subtypes defined by diverse clinically observed features, responses to therapy, and pathophysiology. Broadly, CRS may be subdivided by both phenotype, whether with or without polyps or comorbid asthma, or by endotype. Endotypes signify the specific biological pathways driving the disease process and in this case may be attributed to mechanisms surrounding the T-helper cells that drive the inflammatory process. This variation in immunologic drivers of disease explains why there is corresponding variation in the responsiveness of the disease to any given therapy. This variation is akin to the pathogenesis observed in asthma, whereby considerable effort has been placed into developing adjuvant therapies for refractory subtypes. Defining the *endotype* is critical in the understanding of the immunologic processes involved in the disease progression and, thus, informs the therapeutic strategies that may effectively treat the disease.

Although an oversimplification, immunologically, CRSsNP is generally associated with a T-helper 1 (Th1) inflammatory pattern, demonstrating Th1 and Th17 cytokine patterns. This type 1 inflammatory pattern demonstrates relative neutrophilia (eosinophils are still present but in lower levels)[5] and elevated type 1 cytokines including interferon-γ.

In stark contrast to the Th-1 pattern, Th-2 inflammation demonstrates predominance of eosinophilia, mast cells, and basophils as well as T-helper 2 (Th2) cells. Here, type 2 cytokines predominate, including interleukin (IL) 4, 5, and 13. Interestingly, innate lymphoid cells (ILCs) are also capable of secreting Th2 cytokines and driving inflammation. In Th2 inflammation, IL-4 binds its receptor on the surface of naïve Th0 lymphocytes inducing maturation into Th2 cells. Via the IL-4 receptor, immunoglobulin E (IgE) isotype switching is induced and transcription activated.[16] IL-4 also increases the IgE-mediated immune response, upregulating IgE receptors in the surface of basophils, mast cells, B cells, and monocytes. There is a concomitant notable increase in leukotriene levels and their receptors in response to IL-4. IL-4 also causes immune cellular chemotaxis toward the site of inflammation by interaction with vascular cell adhesion molecule-1. Interestingly, this may be the mechanism by which local eosinophilia occurs pathologically in CRSwNP. In contrast, IL-5 does not play a significant role in chemotaxis but binds to its receptor on basophils, eosinophils, and mast cells. Working from within the bone marrow it drives several functions in eosinophils, including maturation, differentiation, migration, activation, and survival. This cytokine is notably elevated in comorbid asthmatic patients as well as in AERD.[17] IL-13 plays many similar roles to IL-4, regulating IgE production, and induces production of matrix metalloproteases but does not exert effect on T-cell maturation. Along with IL-4, it exerts effect on B cells to switch isotypes from IgM to IgE as seen in allergy and allergic asthma.

Studies have investigated cytokine levels in CRSwNP, and the cytokine profiles seem to vary in differing populations.[18] In approximately 80% to 85% of Western (United States and Europe) CRSwNP, Th2-type inflammation with eosinophils and elevated IL-4, 5, and 13 predominates.[19] In the Asian population, CRSwNP seems to have a mixed inflammatory pattern, which may present different therapeutic implications.[18]

The mucosal epithelium not only serves as a mechanical barrier preventing entry from the outside environment but also serves to stimulate host innate immune response via cytokine production. These include thymic stromal lymphopoietin (TSLP), IL-33, and IL-25 and have the capacity to activate type 2 ILCs (ILC2s), which is a unique subset of cells that synthesize and release type 2 cytokines, including IL-5 and IL-13.[20–22] TSLP is produced in various organ systems and is linked to many inflammatory disorders, including atopic dermatitis, eosinophilic esophagitis, and asthma. It upregulates surface expression of the OX40 ligand on dendritic cells, which subsequently, by interaction with its receptor expressed on CD4+ T-cells, mediates differentiation to Th2 variety. Similarly, IL-33 is released by epithelial cells in response to pathogen-related or stress-related injury at the surface interface along the respiratory tract, skin, and gastrointestinal tract.[23] Once released IL-33 activates and recruits immune cells including Th2 cells, mast cells, and basophils. Importantly, IL-33 also activates ILC2s and enhances the production of IL-13 one of the key mediators of the Th2 inflammatory response.[20]

IMMUNOGLOBULIN E TARGETED THERAPIES
Omalizumab

One of the earliest promising biological therapies for CRS has been omalizumab, which is currently an approved treatment in the United States and Europe for patients with severe allergic asthma. Omalizumab is a human anti-IgE monoclonal antibody (mAb) that lowers circulating IgE levels, binding the third constant domain of the IgE molecule. This binding prevents the interaction of the ligand with its receptor, which can lead to a reduction in circulating levels of free IgE and downregulation of FcεRI surface expression. Reduced free IgE lowers the rate of IgE binding to the high-affinity IgE receptor on basophils and mast cells. Thus, allergen-induced degranulation is inhibited, preventing the release of cytokines and inflammatory mediators. Over time, treatment with omalizumab causes the downregulation of the high-affinity IgE receptor on mast cells, dendritic cells, and basophils.[24,25] Several studies have investigated the clinical efficacy of omalizumab therapy in the setting of nasal polyposis and/or asthma. Patients in a cohort with severe asthma showed a reduction in the number of asthma exacerbations, reduced symptom scores, and increased quality-of-life (QOL) scores.[26] Pinto and colleagues[27] studied omalizumab in a cohort of subjects with CRS in a double-blind, randomized, placebo-controlled trial. All subjects had prior sinus surgery, most presenting with polyps (12 of 14), and were randomized to either placebo or monthly injections of omalizumab for 6 months. Subjects were allowed to continue their current medication regimen throughout the study, in effect making this an assessment of add-on therapy. QOL data were collected throughout the study, and pretreatment and posttreatment CT scans were performed. In the treatment group there was a statistically significant decrease in sinus inflammation as assessed by CT scan, which was not seen in the placebo group. However, when the magnitude of change was compared across groups, significance was not shown. The treatment group did show a reduced need for steroid therapy; however, none of the remaining secondary outcomes demonstrated statistically significant differences between groups. In a second randomized, double-blind, placebo-controlled study, Gevaert and colleagues[28] investigated the effect of omalizumab on endoscopic polyp scores in 24 subjects with CRS and comorbid asthma. Subjects were subdivided into allergic versus nonallergic groups by skin prick testing at the study outset. The treatment arm (n = 16) received 4 to 8 injections of omalizumab and was assessed endoscopically at the 16-week end point for changes in polyp scores. Importantly, the subjects were not allowed to use systemic or inhaled corticosteroids, nasal decongestants, antibiotics, or leukotriene receptor antagonists. The investigators noted a statistically significant decrease in the endoscopic polyps scores of allergic subjects, which was confirmed on CT scoring. Interestingly, the response was similar in the nonallergic subjects. Further, there was a beneficial effect on secondary outcomes, including airway and QOL measures. Chandra and colleagues[29] retrospectively investigated the effect of omalizumab on a cohort of subjects with CRS and comorbid asthma. Pretreatment and posttreatment antibiotic and steroid use was evaluated in 25 subjects. Subjects were treated with omalizumab via subcutaneous injection at 2- or 4-week intervals depending on IgE levels. Four subjects with significantly elevated IgE (>700 IU/mL) were given maximum dosing. Omalizumab reduced use of antibiotics in this cohort and decreased steroid use within a specific subset of their cohort. The investigators noted that the responders were composed mostly (87%) of female subjects, but they were unable to categorize the group further secondary to sample size. Those subjects with higher mean baseline IgE tended to respond in a lesser degree with regard to the stated outcome measures. The observed decrease in steroid use did not reach statistical significance. There was an observed statistically significant reduction in the use of antibiotics in the cohort after initiating therapy with omalizumab, though this was on retrospective review and therapy was not standardized.[29]

Side effects related to omalizumab therapy have been studied, and the Omalizumab Joint Task Force (OJTF) reported an overall 0.09% rate of anaphylaxis following injection. In their report, 61% of these reactions occurred within the first 2 hours after injection, after the first 3 injections and 14% occurred within 0.5 hours after the fourth or later injection.[30] Based on these findings and review of more than 100 cases of reported anaphylaxis, the OJTF made the following recommendations: informed consent should be obtained; anaphylaxis education should be performed; an epinephrine autoinjector should be provided; a preinjection health assessment should be performed; a waiting period of 30 minutes should be observed after each injection and extended to 2 hours once the first 3 injections have been given.[30,31] Concern has been raised regarding the risk of malignancy in those treated with omalizumab. A large prospective study, Evaluating Clinical Effectiveness and Long-Term Safety in Patients with Moderate to Severe Asthma, evaluated the risk of developing malignancy in individuals with allergic asthma and a high cancer risk profile. About two-thirds of the cohort were treated with omalizumab at baseline (n = 2696) and the remainder (n = 1689) were not. The investigators were able to conclude after a follow-up period up to 5 years that there was no increased risk of malignancy attributable to omalizumab therapy.[32]

INTERLEUKIN 5 TARGETED THERAPY

IL-5 plays a key role in chemotaxis, differentiation, chemotaxis, and survival of eosinophils. Because local and systemic eosinophilia have been observed in patients with Th2-skewed inflammation, anti–IL-5 therapeutics have been developed to target this pathway.

Mepolizumab

Mepolizumab is a humanized mAb also with affinity for IL-5 and was approved by the Food and Drug Administration for the treatment of severe refractory asthma in the fall of 2015. Mepolizumab was trialed in a cohort of 30 patients with CRSwNP refractory to topical glucocorticoid therapy following surgery.[33] Patients were randomized in a double-blinded fashion to receive either mepolizumab (2 injections 28 days apart) or placebo. Nasal polyp scores were assessed until 1 month after the therapy period was completed. Sixty percent in the treated arm were noted to have improved polyp scores and CT scores versus 10% in the placebo group. There are no other published data sets regarding the use of mepolizumab in rhinosinusitis. However, search of ongoing clinical trials revealed a recent trial evaluating the utility of mepolizumab to reduce the need for surgery in patients with nasal polyps. Forty-one total eligible patients completed this double-blind, randomized, placebo-controlled study which seems to show a reduction in the need for surgery in the treatment arm versus placebo as well as reduced SinoNasal Outcome Test (SNOT-22) scores.[34] Full statistical analysis is not yet available.

Reslizumab

Reslizumab is a human mAb with affinity for free IL-5. In a 24-subject pilot study featuring reslizumab, a single dose of therapy demonstrated a significant reduction in polyp size after a single intravenous injection dosed at 1 mg/kg. Post hoc analysis showed that elevated levels of IL-5 in the nasal secretions predicted whether subjects would be responders or nonresponders to the medication.[17]

Investigators were able to monitored the disease state by IL-5 levels in subjects. Interestingly, there was regrowth of polyps after discontinuation of the drug associated with increasing and suprabaseline eosinophilia in the treatment group. The findings in this initial study helped provide insight into IL-5 antagonism and its role in the treatment of eosinophilic nasal polyps.

Benralizumab

Benralizumab is a humanized afucosylated mAb targeting the IL-5 receptor as opposed to free IL-5. The IL-5 receptor is expressed on the surface of both eosinophils and basophils. Benralizumab is able to competitively inhibit IL-5 interaction with its receptor and also causes antibody-dependent, cell-mediated cytotoxicity.[35] There is currently a single phase II study to evaluate the utility of this drug in the therapy for eosinophilic rhinosinusitis. The study is designed as a double-blind, randomized, placebo-controlled trial and recently began recruiting patients. There are no further available studies detailing its use in rhinosinusitis; however, this drug targets not only eosinophils but also basophils, which are also elevated in CRSwNP.

THE INTERLEUKIN 4 AND INTERLEUKIN 13 PATHWAY

As in asthma, IL-4 and IL-13 are important drivers of Th2 differentiation activating type 2 inflammatory responses via IgE synthesis and related cell types.

IL-4 and IL-13 share the IL-4Rα as a common receptor. Dupilumab, a fully human mAb, is directed against the IL-4Rα. In a phase II multinational, multicenter, randomized, double-blind, placebo-controlled study, dupilumab was evaluated for effect on patients with CRSwNP refractory to intranasal corticosteroids. Over the course of 16 weeks, patients received subcutaneous injection on a weekly basis and used intranasal mometasone furoate daily. Sixty patients were randomized to either treatment or placebo arms, and 51 completed the study. The primary end point assessed was a decrease in the polyp burden based on endoscopic score from baseline to week 16. Secondarily the study sought to assess change in SNOT-22 symptom scores, Lund-McKay (CT) scores, olfaction (based on University of Pennsylvania Smell Identification Test), nasal peak inspiratory flows, and polyp scores in a subgroup of CRSwNP and comorbid asthma.[36,37] With regard to the primary outcome, the dupilumab group experienced a significant reduction in polyp burden that became noticeable clinically as early as the fourth treatment week. Further, there was significant improvement favoring the dupilumab group over placebo for all secondary outcome measures.[37] Of the inflammatory markers measured during the study, there was a statistically significant decrease in both IgE and eotaxin favoring dupilumab versus placebo.[37] This study provided insight into the importance of the IL-4/IL-13 pathway in the pathogenesis of CRSwNP and showed marked improvement in multiple parameters when this pathway can be inhibited.

AMG 317 is a fully human IgG2 mAb with high affinity for IL-4Rα, inhibiting IL-4 and IL-13 interaction.

AMG 282

AMG 282 is a novel mAb that inhibits binding of IL-33 to the ST2 receptor. Although there are currently no results available, a study is complete assessing the safety and tolerability of AMG 282 in "healthy volunteers" with CRSwNP.[38] The primary outcome measures of the study are to assess the safety and immunogenicity of the drug; however, if the therapy shows promise, there will likely be continued investigation for use as therapy in CRSwNP.

SIALIC ACID IMMUNOGLOBULIN-LIKE LECTINS

Sialic acid immunoglobulin-like lectins (siglecs) are members of the immunoglobulin gene family and are cell surface proteins found predominantly on cells of the immune system. Among this family, siglec-8 is distinctively expressed by eosinophils, mast cells, and basophils.[39] This unique expression provides the opportunity to selectively target these cell types in asthma, rhinosinusitis, and potentially other Th2-skewed immunologic disorders. Laboratory data have shown that when these cell surface proteins on eosinophils are bound by antibody, the targeted cell undergoes apoptosis.[39] When incubated with mast cells it does not have the same effect, however; the release of proinflammatory mediators is attenuated.[39] These properties make siglecs an interesting target for biological therapies. Currently there is one phase II trial actively recruiting patients.

DISCUSSION

The use of biologics in the treatment of nasal polyposis shows promise as an alternative therapy to severe chronic sinusitis with nasal polyps refractory to conventional therapies and surgery (**Fig. 1**). This strategy, however, is not without cost; utilization of biological therapies is quite expensive versus current management. Rudmik and colleagues investigated the economic benefit of surgery versus conventional medical therapy for the treatment of CRS.[40] Using non–biological-based therapy in their computations, they estimated that surgical intervention began to become more cost-effective than medical therapy alone at a 3-year time horizon after initial surgery. Insurers may be unlikely to cover an expensive long-term therapy for a condition that is not necessarily life threatening in spite of the fact that it may be life altering. The decision algorithm of which patients should be routed toward biological therapy has yet to be elucidated. It is reasonable that patients with concomitant asthma unresponsive to standard therapies would be candidates for these medications. Given that current medical and surgical therapy may not be acceptable or effective for some patients, biological therapy offers an alternative. Further, there may be instances in which use of biological therapy presents an advantage either from a standpoint of disease-specific factors, such as asthma or economic utility. Now many studies evaluate reducing dependence on standard medical therapies, but little investigation has been performed to assess the ability of a biological therapy to dovetail into or precede a medical therapy. There also may be utility in intermittent use of biological therapy to prolong the need for revision surgical intervention or steroid therapy. Comparative efficacy of these interventions needs to be studied further. Finally, long-term side effects of these biologics are currently unknown; the potential for dysregulation of the immune

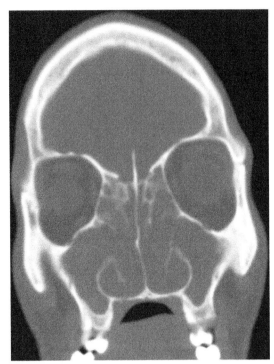

Fig. 1. A case of severe nasal polyposis with pansinusitis, unlikely to be well controlled by current therapies.

system due to modification of these specific pathways awaits investigation. It is important to realize that these biologics do not offer a cure for the underlying chronic inflammatory disease process; therefore, the understanding of the pathogenesis of disease still remains the most relevant question. As biologics continue to grow in popularity and become approved for use, however, they must be considered relevant to the changing landscape of CRS therapy. Studies must not be done versus placebo but rather against maximal medical management.

SUMMARY

In CRS there are a variety of immunologic and pathophysiologic mechanisms that initiate inflammation and propagate its course. Improved understanding of these mechanisms expands the potential to specifically target, mediate, or ameliorate disease progression. Current studies have highlighted the importance of certain cytokines and cells in nasal polyps. Further investigation of biological therapies, including those targeting the IgE, IL-5, IL-4/IL-13, and epithelial cell-derived cytokine pathways, will continue to change the paradigm of how CRS is understood and ultimately treated. The progress made with the current repertoire of targeted therapies has already opened the door to a shift in the management of CRS and in particular CRSwNP.

REFERENCES

1. Bhattacharyya N. Contemporary assessment of the disease burden of sinusitis. Am J Rhinol Allergy 2009;23(4):392–5.

2. Blackwell DL, Lucas JW, Clarke TC. Summary health statistics for U.S. adults: national health interview survey, 2012. Vital Health Stat 10 2014;260:1–161.
3. Hamilos DL. Chronic rhinosinusitis: epidemiology and medical management. J Allergy Clin Immunol 2011;128(4):693–707 [quiz: 708–9].
4. Orlandi RR, Kingdom TT, Hwang PH, et al. International consensus statement on allergy and rhinology: rhinosinusitis. Int Forum Allergy Rhinol 2016;6(Suppl 1): S22–209.
5. Fokkens WJ, Lund VJ, Mullol J, et al. EPOS 2012: European position paper on rhinosinusitis and nasal polyps 2012. A summary for otorhinolaryngologists. Rhinology 2012;50(1):1–12.
6. Bachert C, Zhang N, Holtappels G, et al. Presence of IL-5 protein and IgE antibodies to staphylococcal enterotoxins in nasal polyps is associated with comorbid asthma. J Allergy Clin Immunol 2010;126(5):962–8, 968.e1–6.
7. Baguley C, Brownlow A, Yeung K, et al. The fate of chronic rhinosinusitis sufferers after maximal medical therapy. Int Forum Allergy Rhinol 2014;4(7):525–32.
8. Lal D, Scianna JM, Stankiewicz JA. Efficacy of targeted medical therapy in chronic rhinosinusitis, and predictors of failure. Am J Rhinol Allergy 2009;23(4): 396–400.
9. Bachert C, Pawankar R, Zhang L, et al. ICON: chronic rhinosinusitis. World Allergy Organ J 2014;7(1):25.
10. Batra PS, Tong L, Citardi MJ. Analysis of comorbidities and objective parameters in refractory chronic rhinosinusitis. Laryngoscope 2013;123(Suppl 7):S1–11.
11. Hakansson K, Bachert C, Konge L, et al. Airway inflammation in chronic rhinosinusitis with nasal polyps and asthma: the united airways concept further supported. PLoS One 2015;10(7):e0127228.
12. Larsen K. The clinical relationship of nasal polyps to asthma. Allergy Asthma Proc 1996;17(5):243–9.
13. Promsopa C, Kansara S, Citardi MJ, et al. Prevalence of confirmed asthma varies in chronic rhinosinusitis subtypes. Int Forum Allergy Rhinol 2016;6(4):373–7.
14. Bent JP 3rd, Kuhn FA. Diagnosis of allergic fungal sinusitis. Otolaryngol Head Neck Surg 1994;111(5):580–8.
15. Ferguson BJ. Eosinophilic mucin rhinosinusitis: a distinct clinicopathological entity. Laryngoscope 2000;110(5 Pt 1):799–813.
16. Stone KD, Prussin C, Metcalfe DD. IgE, mast cells, basophils, and eosinophils. J Allergy Clin Immunol 2010;125(2 Suppl 2):S73–80.
17. Gevaert P, Lang-Loidolt D, Lackner A, et al. Nasal IL-5 levels determine the response to anti-IL-5 treatment in patients with nasal polyps. J Allergy Clin Immunol 2006;118(5):1133–41.
18. Kashani S, Carr TF, Grammer LC, et al. Clinical characteristics of adults with chronic rhinosinusitis and specific antibody deficiency. J Allergy Clin Immunol Pract 2015;3(2):236–42.
19. Bachert C, Zhang L, Gevaert P. Current and future treatment options for adult chronic rhinosinusitis: focus on nasal polyposis. J Allergy Clin Immunol 2015; 136(6):1431–40 [quiz: 1441].
20. Shaw JL, Fakhri S, Citardi MJ, et al. IL-33-responsive innate lymphoid cells are an important source of IL-13 in chronic rhinosinusitis with nasal polyps. Am J Respir Crit Care Med 2013;188(4):432–9.
21. Nagarkar DR, Poposki JA, Tan BK, et al. Thymic stromal lymphopoietin activity is increased in nasal polyps of patients with chronic rhinosinusitis. J Allergy Clin Immunol 2013;132(3):593–600.e12.

22. Artis D, Spits H. The biology of innate lymphoid cells. Nature 2015;517(7534): 293–301.
23. Saluja R, Khan M, Church MK, et al. The role of IL-33 and mast cells in allergy and inflammation. Clin Transl Allergy 2015;5:33.
24. D'Amato G, Stanziola A, Sanduzzi A, et al. Treating severe allergic asthma with anti-IgE monoclonal antibody (omalizumab): a review. Multidiscip Respir Med 2014;9(1):23.
25. Prussin C, Griffith DT, Boesel KM, et al. Omalizumab treatment downregulates dendritic cell FcepsilonRI expression. J Allergy Clin Immunol 2003;112(6): 1147–54.
26. Verma P, Randhawa I, Klaustermeyer WB. Clinical efficacy of omalizumab in an elderly veteran population with severe asthma. Allergy Asthma Proc 2011; 32(5):346–50.
27. Pinto JM, Mehta N, DiTineo M, et al. A randomized, double-blind, placebo-controlled trial of anti-IgE for chronic rhinosinusitis. Rhinology 2010;48(3):318–24.
28. Gevaert P, Calus L, Van Zele T, et al. Omalizumab is effective in allergic and nonallergic patients with nasal polyps and asthma. J Allergy Clin Immunol 2013;131(1):110–6.e1.
29. Chandra RK, Clavenna M, Samuelson M, et al. Impact of omalizumab therapy on medication requirements for chronic rhinosinusitis. Int Forum Allergy Rhinol 2016; 6(5):472–7.
30. Cox L, Platts-Mills TA, Finegold I, et al. American Academy of Allergy, Asthma & Immunology/American College of Allergy, Asthma and Immunology Joint Task Force Report on omalizumab-associated anaphylaxis. J Allergy Clin Immunol 2007;120(6):1373–7.
31. Cox L, Lieberman P, Wallace D, et al. American Academy of Allergy, Asthma & Immunology/American College of Allergy, Asthma & Immunology Omalizumab-Associated Anaphylaxis Joint Task Force follow-up report. J Allergy Clin Immunol 2011;128(1):210–2.
32. Long A, Rahmaoui A, Rothman KJ, et al. Incidence of malignancy in patients with moderate-to-severe asthma treated with or without omalizumab. J Allergy Clin Immunol 2014;134(3):560–7.e4.
33. Gevaert P, Van Bruaene N, Cattaert T, et al. Mepolizumab, a humanized anti-IL-5 mAb, as a treatment option for severe nasal polyposis. J Allergy Clin Immunol 2011;128(5):989–95.e1–e8.
34. GSK Clinical Trials. A two-part, randomised, double-blind, placebo controlled, multi-center study to investigate the use of mepolizumab (Sb-240563) in reducing the need for surgery in subjects with severe bilateral nasal polyposis. In: ClinicalTrials.gov [internet]. Bethesda (MD): National Library of Medicine (US); 2011. Available at: https://clinicaltrials.gov/ct2/show/NCT01362244. NLM Identifier: NCT01362244. Accessed 6 June, 2016.
35. Kolbeck R, Kozhich A, Koike M, et al. MEDI-563, a humanized anti-IL-5 receptor alpha mAb with enhanced antibody-dependent cell-mediated cytotoxicity function. J Allergy Clin Immunol 2010;125(6):1344–53.e2.
36. Sanofi. An evaluation of dupilumab in patients with nasal polyposis and chronic symptoms of sinusitis. In: ClinicalTrials.gov [Internet]. Bethesda (MD): National Library of Medicine (US); 2013. Available at: https://clinicaltrials.gov/ct2/show/ NCT01920893. NLM Identifier: NCT01920893. Accessed June 14, 2016.
37. Bachert C, Mannent L, Naclerio RM, et al. Effect of subcutaneous dupilumab on nasal polyp burden in patients with chronic sinusitis and nasal polyposis: a randomized clinical trial. JAMA 2016;315(5):469–79.

38. Amgen A. Study to evaluate the safety, tolerability, pharmacokinetics, and pharmacodynamics of AMG 282 in healthy subjects and subjects with chronic rhinosinusitis with nasal polyps. In: ClinicalTrials.gov [internet]. Bethesda (MD): National Library of Medicine (US); 2014. Available at: https://clinicaltrials.gov/ct2/show/NCT02170337. NLM Identifier: NCT02170337. Accessed June 14, 2016.
39. Kiwamoto T, Kawasaki N, Paulson JC, et al. Siglec-8 as a drugable target to treat eosinophil and mast cell-associated conditions. Pharmacol Ther 2012;135(3): 327–36.
40. Rudmik L, Soler ZM, Mace JC, et al. Economic evaluation of endoscopic sinus surgery versus continued medical therapy for refractory chronic rhinosinusitis. Laryngoscope 2015;125(1):25–32.

Biologic Therapies for Immunoglobulin E–mediated Food Allergy and Eosinophilic Esophagitis

Iris M. Otani, MD*, Kari C. Nadeau, MD, PhD[1]

KEYWORDS

- Food allergy • Eosinophilic esophagitis • Anti-IgE • Anti–IL-5 • Anti–IL-13 • QAX576
- OC000459

KEY POINTS

- Immunoglobulin (Ig) E–mediated food allergy and eosinophilic esophagitis (EoE) are chronic, allergen-mediated disorders.
- Investigation of biologic therapies in IgE-mediated food allergy and EoE have provided insights into the pathophysiology and treatment of these disorders.
- In IgE-mediated food allergy, anti-IgE therapy seems to increase tolerability of food allergens and safety of oral desensitization protocols, although further larger studies are necessary to further elucidate the most safe and effective use of anti-IgE.
- In EoE, the use of biologics targeting interleukin (IL)-5, IL-13, IgE, and the CRTH2 receptors, have had mixed results. Decreases in esophageal eosinophilia were not necessarily accompanied by symptomatic remission.
- Identification of EoE phenotypes that are responsive to biologics and investigation of biologics in combination with other therapies may help elucidate a role for biologic therapy in EoE.

INTRODUCTION

Food allergy is defined as an aberrant immune response to food proteins leading to mucocutaneous, gastrointestinal, and/or respiratory symptoms. Food allergy can encompass purely IgE-mediated food allergy as well as mixed IgE-mediated and non–IgE-mediated disease, such as eosinophilic esophagitis (EoE).[1] The development

Disclosure: The authors have nothing to disclose.
Department of Medicine, Sean N. Parker Center for Allergy and Asthma Research, Stanford University, Palo Alto, CA, USA
[1] Present address: CCSR 3215c, 269 Campus Drive, Stanford, CA 94305.
* Corresponding author. H3143, 300 Pasteur Drive, Stanford, CA 94305-5236.
E-mail address: kagome@stanford.edu

Immunol Allergy Clin N Am 37 (2017) 369–396
http://dx.doi.org/10.1016/j.iac.2017.01.010
0889-8561/17/© 2017 Elsevier Inc. All rights reserved.

immunology.theclinics.com

and investigation of biologics for the treatment of IgE-mediated food allergy and EoE have provided further insight into the pathophysiology and management of these disorders. This article provides an overview of biologic therapies that are being investigated or have potential as treatments for IgE-mediated food allergy and EoE.

IMMUNOGLOBULIN E–MEDIATED FOOD ALLERGY

The prevalence of food allergy has been estimated at 8% in children and 5% in adults.[2] Although the incidence of food allergy continues to increase,[3] allergen avoidance and treatment of accidental ingestion with epinephrine remain the only US Food and Drug Administration (FDA)–approved treatments.[4] Allergen avoidance and fear of accidental ingestion are associated with stress and anxiety that significantly impair quality of life for affected children and their caregivers.[5]

Food allergen immunotherapy via oral, sublingual, and epicutaneous routes is being actively investigated as a treatment of IgE-mediated food allergy. Gradually increasing exposure to food allergens can lead to desensitization and induce immune tolerance to food allergens. The safety and efficacy of immunotherapy for food allergy remain unclear, because adverse reactions can occur and tolerance has been shown to wane after active immunotherapy is discontinued.[6,7]

Anti–Immunoglobulin E for Immunoglobulin E–Mediated Food Allergy

IgE-mediated food allergy reactions occur when mast cells and basophils are activated after allergen exposure through cross-linking of preformed allergen-specific IgE on the cell surface.[8] Anti-IgE is under investigation both as a stand-alone therapy and an adjunctive treatment that could potentially improve the safety and efficacy of allergen immunotherapy (**Table 1**).

Omalizumab

Omalizumab (Xolair; Genentech, South San Francisco, CA) is a humanized IgG_1 monoclonal antibody (mAb) that binds the Fc region of IgE and blocks the binding of IgE to its high-affinity FcεRI on mast cells, basophils, and dendritic cells, thereby interrupting the allergic cascade.[18] It is administered subcutaneously and is FDA approved for moderate to severe persistent allergic asthma inadequately controlled with inhaled corticosteroids in patients 12 years of age or older.[19] Omalizumab is also FDA approved for chronic idiopathic urticaria inadequately controlled with H1 antihistamines in patients 12 years of age or older.[20]

For allergic asthma, dosing is calculated based on pretreatment serum IgE levels and body weight, with dosages ranging between 150 to 375 mg administered subcutaneously every 2 to 4 weeks.[19] For chronic idiopathic urticaria, the dosage is between 150 to 300 mg administered subcutaneously every 4 weeks, independent of serum IgE level or body weight.[20]

Omalizumab can exert several biological effects in allergic disease. It can significantly reduce FcεRI expression on basophils and plasmacytoid dendritic cells,[21–24] decrease serum IgE levels,[25,26] and decrease allergen-specific basophil reactivity[27] and histamine release.[28,29] It has been investigated both as a stand-alone and adjunctive therapy to allergen immunotherapy in allergic rhinitis and as a therapy for atopic dermatitis, with mixed results.[20]

Talizumab

Talizumab (TNX-901; Tanox, Houston, TX) is a humanized IgG_1 mAb administered subcutaneously. Like omalizumab, talizumab binds the Fc region of IgE, blocking IgE binding to FcεRI.[18]

Table 1
Published clinical trials and case series investigating anti–immunoglobulin E as a therapy for immunoglobulin E–mediated food allergy

First Author, Year	Allergen	Patient Groups	Design/Doses	Clinical Results	AEs
OMA as Stand-alone Therapy to Improve Food Allergy Tolerance					
Leung et al,[9] 2003	Peanut	Placebo (n = 23) 150 mg (n = 19) 300 mg (n = 19) 450 mg (n = 19)	Randomized, double-blind, placebo-controlled, dose-ranging Age: 13–59 y Screening: DBPCFC Drug: 150 mg, 300 mg, or 450 mg of TNX-901 or placebo SQ every 4 wk for 4 doses OFC: 2–4 wk after the fourth dose of TNX-901 or placebo	Clinical results: Increase from baseline in the mean threshold dose that induced hypersensitivity to peanut flour: increase of 2627 mg in the group given 450 mg of TNX-901 ($P<.001$) Immune changes: Significant decreases in serum IgE levels at all 3 dosing levels compared with placebo	Number of systemic AEs (45–50 per group) and number of patients who had AEs (15–19 per group) similar among the 4 groups Diarrhea, nausea, vomiting, fatigue, fever, food allergy unrelated to OFC, upper respiratory tract infection, headache, arthralgia
Rafi et al,[10] 2010	Fish Shellfish Peanut Tree Nuts Egg Soybean Wheat Multiple other	22 patients with persistent asthma and IgE-mediated food allergy	Prospective pilot Age: 4–66 y Drug: OMA 150–300 mg every 2–4 wk for 6 doses	Clinical results: Decreases (improvements) in food-induced symptoms (atopic dermatitis, n = 8; lower respiratory symptoms, n = 13; upper respiratory symptoms, n = 8; urticaria, n = 3; angioedema, n = 9)	No AE caused by OMA use

(continued on next page)

Table 1
(continued)

First Author, Year	Allergen	Patient Groups	Design/Doses	Clinical Results	AEs
Sampson et al,[11] 2011	Peanut	Placebo (n = 5) OMA (n = 9)	Multicenter, randomized, double-blind, placebo-controlled, parallel-group Age: Placebo, mean 26.6 y; OMA, mean 16.3 y Screening: DBPCFC Drug: placebo or OMA (minimum of 0.016 IU/mL every 4 wk; doses >300 mg received divided dose every 2 wk) for 24 wk Week 24: second double-blind OFC	Clinical results: 4 (44.4%) OMA-treated subjects vs 1 (20%) placebo-treated subject tolerated ≥1000 mg peanut flour during OFC after 24 wk of treatment with study drug (P = .324)	Study stopped early because of severity of 2 anaphylactic reactions during screening OFCs
Savage et al,[12] 2012	Peanut	n = 14	6-mo open-label study Age: 18–44 y 6 mo of OMA OFC1 during screening OFC2 between weeks 2–8 once Pn-BHR (decreased to <20% baseline) OFC 3 at 6 mo	Clinical results: OFC2: significant increase in the threshold dose of peanut inducing allergic symptoms (80–6500 mg, P<.01); OFC3: no further increases in the OFC threshold dose Immune changes: By week 8 of OMA therapy, 5 patients had near-complete suppression of Pn-BHR and 9 patients had a 10-fold increase in the amount of allergen required to achieve maximal BHR	—

OMA as Adjunctive Therapy to Increase Safety of Desensitization

Nadeau et al,[13] 2011; Bedoret et al,[14] 2012	CM	n = 11	Pilot study Age: 7–17 y CM OIT performed in combination with 16 wk of OMA OMA treatment started at week 0, and CM OIT started at week 9 DBPCFC performed 8 wk later (week 24 of the study)	Clinical results: 9 of 10 subjects reached the maximum daily dose of 2000 mg milk (the primary end point of the study). 9 patients who had reached a daily dose of 2000 mg passed DBPCFC and open challenge. 9 patients continued with daily milk ingestion >8000 mg daily Immune changes: Post-hoc subanalysis of blood drawn at weeks 0, 9, 10, 12, 14, 16, 24, 30, 36, and 52 in 5 subjects. Decrease in milk-specific CD4+ T-cell proliferation 1 wk into desensitization protocol. Milk-specific CD4+ T-cell proliferation returned with shift from IL-4 to IFN-γ production, whereas the subjects remained on high doses of daily oral milk over the following 3 mo. Decrease in milk-specific IgE and a 15-fold increase in milk-specific IgG4	One subject voluntarily discontinued the study because of abdominal migraines 2 reactions required epinephrine

(continued on next page)

Table 1
(continued)

First Author, Year	Allergen	Patient Groups	Design/Doses	Clinical Results	AEs
Schneider et al,[15] 2013	Peanut	n = 13	Age: 8–15 y Week 0–12: pretreatment with OMA Week 12: initiation of oral desensitization (11 doses of 0.1, 0.5, 1.5, 3, 7, 15, 30, 60, 125, 250, and 500 mg; cumulative dose, 992 mg peanut flour; administered over 6 h) Week 12–20: weekly increase in the daily oral dose to 4000 mg peanut flour (750, 1000, 1250, 1600, 2000, 2600, 3250, and 4000 mg) Week 20: OMA discontinued after subjects reached 4000 mg daily dose. Daily peanut dosing continued Week 30–32: DBPCFC followed by open peanut challenge (8000 mg)	Clinical results: 13 subjects tolerated initial desensitization on the first day (maximum dose, 500 mg peanut flour; cumulative dose, 992 mg). 12 subjects reached maximum maintenance dose of 4000 mg peanut flour per day in a median time of 8 wk. 12 subjects continued 4000 mg peanut flour daily dosing and subsequently tolerated OFC with 8000 mg peanut flour (about 20 peanuts)	Total of 72 reactions during the study First day of desensitization: 6 of 13 grade 1 allergic reactions requiring no treatment or antihistamines Up-dosing phase: 1 of 13 with history of supraventricular tachycardia required epinephrine for nausea, light-headedness, hypersalivation after a 1250-mg dose. 1 of 13 withdrew from study because of persistent nausea, vomiting, and hypersalivation after reaching 1250-mg dose. 6-mo maintenance phase: 1 of 13 required epinephrine for vomiting, diarrhea, and wheezing. 1 of 13 received epinephrine 3 times for coughing, hives, and wheezing (possibly food-dependent exercise-induced anaphylaxis) and withdraw from study

Study	Allergen	n	Study design	Clinical results	Outcome
Wood et al,[16] 2016	CM	n = 57	Randomized, double-blind, placebo-controlled Age: 7–32 y Screening DBPCFC with 2 g milk First 16 mo: Treatment with OMA or placebo After 4 mo of study drug: Open-label MOIT initiated with escalation to maintenance over 22–40 wk to at least 520 mg (goal 3800 mg), followed by daily maintenance dosing through month 28 Month 16: treatment unblinded; OMA continued for 12 mo; placebo injections discontinued Month 28: OMA discontinued, patients underwent 10 g OFC Month 28–32: subjects who passed OFC continued milk maintenance dose for 8 wk and then stopped milk OIT for 8 wk Month 32: rechallenge with 10 g OFC to assess sustained unresponsiveness	Clinical results: No significant differences in subjects who passed 10 g desensitization OFC (88.9% in OMA group vs 71.5% in placebo-treated group) or achieved SU (48.1% in the OMA group vs 35.7% in the placebo group) Immune changes: Milk and casein IgE levels significantly increased in OMA group and significantly reduced in placebo group at month 4. Casein and β-lactoglobulin IgG4 levels, IgG levels, and IgG4/IgE ratios increased in both OMA and placebo groups. Basophil activation to milk stimulation lower in the OMA group compared with placebo	Percentage of symptom-free doses during escalation significantly greater in OMA group compared with placebo (91.5% vs 73.9%; P<.0001). Median dose-related reactions requiring treatment significantly fewer in OMA group (0.0% vs 3.8% of doses per subject; P = .0008). Severity grade of allergic reactions significantly milder in OMA group (mild: median, 0.5% vs 7.9% doses per subject, P = .0001; moderate: median, 0.0% vs 0.5% doses per subject, P = .0005)
Martorell-Calatayud et al,[17] 2016	CM Egg	CM (n = 5) Egg (n = 9)	Case series Age: 3–13 y CM or egg OIT with OMA given as pretreatment for 9 wk and in conjunction with OIT until 2 mo after the maintenance dose was reached (6.6 g milk, 1.8 g egg)	Patients who could not tolerate the same OIT protocol without OMA were able to reach goal maintenance dose with OMA as pretreatment and concurrent therapy	4 patients (28%) developed mild allergic reactions during the induction phase of OIT

Abbreviations: AE, adverse events; BHR, basophil histamine release; CM, cow's milk; DBPCFC, double-blind placebo-controlled food challenge; IFN, interferon; OFC, oral food challenge; OIT, oral immunotherapy; OMA, omalizumab; Pn-BHR, peanut-induced basophil histamine release; SQ, subcutaneous; TNX-901, talizumab.

Clinical Trials in Food Allergy

Anti–immunoglobulin E as stand-alone therapy to decrease food allergy symptoms

Leung and colleagues, 2003 The first trial of anti-IgE for treatment of food allergy was performed with talizumab in 2003.[9] This randomized, double-blind, placebo-controlled, dose-ranging study included 84 patients aged 12 to 60 years with a history of immediate hypersensitivity to peanut, total serum IgE levels between 30 and 1000 IU/mL, a positive SPT to peanut, and reactivity to peanut confirmed by a double-blind, placebo-controlled oral food challenge (DBPCFC). These patients were randomly assigned to talizumab (150, 300, or 450 mg) or placebo subcutaneously every 4 weeks for 4 doses. All 3 dosages increased the threshold of reactivity to peanut during an oral food challenge performed 2 to 4 weeks after the last administered dose of anti-IgE. This change was statistically significant in the group receiving the highest dose of talizumab. In this 450-mg dose group, the threshold increased from 178 mg of peanut (approximately one-half of a peanut) to 2805 mg (almost 9 peanuts).

Talizumab was taken off the market because of legal difficulties, and subsequent studies with anti-IgE in IgE-mediated food allergy have been performed with omalizumab.

Rafi and colleagues, 2010 This publication reported that 22 patients treated with omalizumab for allergic asthma with concomitant food allergy (history of allergic food reaction and skin prick test positive to food) had decreased or absent clinical symptoms on accidental or intentional (but not medically recommended) ingestion.[10] These clinical improvements were seen by the sixth dose of omalizumab. The reported improvements in food-induced symptoms (atopic dermatitis, n = 8; lower respiratory symptoms, n = 13; upper respiratory symptoms, n = 8; urticaria, n = 3; angioedema, n = 9) and doses of ingested food were variable, making the results subject to interpretation.

Sampson and colleagues, 2011 A phase II, multicenter, randomized, double-blind, placebo-controlled, parallel-group trial investigated whether omalizumab (at a dose of 0.016 mg/kg/IgE) would be effective, similar to talizumab, at preventing allergic reactions after peanut ingestion in peanut-allergic children 6 years of age or older.[11] The study was stopped early because of the severity of 2 anaphylactic reactions that occurred during the screening oral food challenges. Therefore, only 14 subjects reached the primary end point of DBPCFC after treatment with the study drug omalizumab or placebo. However, even the limited data suggested an increase in tolerability to peanut with omalizumab: 44% (4 out of 9) of the omalizumab-treated subjects compared with 20% (1 out of 5) of the placebo-treated subjects were able to tolerate greater than or equal to 1000 mg of peanut flour during an oral food challenge after 24 weeks of treatment.

Savage and colleagues, 2012 A 6-month open-label study showed that the mean tolerated dose of peanut protein increased from 80 mg to 6500 mg after 2 to 8 weeks and 5080 mg after 6 months of omalizumab therapy in 14 subjects with peanut allergy.[12] By week 8 of omalizumab therapy, 5 patients had near-complete suppression of peanut-induced basophil histamine release and 9 patients had a 10-fold increase in the amount of allergen required to achieve maximal basophil histamine release.

Taken together, these data suggest the possibility of using anti-IgE as a means to increase threshold tolerance levels and offer a degree of protection for patients in cases of accidental ingestions.

Anti–immunoglobulin E as an adjunctive therapy for oral immunotherapy

Omalizumab has also been investigated as a potential adjunctive therapy that could decrease the immediate adverse reactions that occur during oral immunotherapy (OIT) and possibly enhance the development of tolerance.

Nadeau and colleagues, 2011 In the first study of omalizumab in combination with OIT, omalizumab seemed to be safe and efficacious at enhancing the development of tolerance. In this pilot, phase I study, 11 children (7–17 years of age) with cow's milk allergy were pretreated with omalizumab for 9 weeks before undergoing rush desensitization to milk.[13] Oral milk doses were increased from 0.1 to 1000 mg over 6 hours and then to 2000 mg over 7 to 11 weeks. Subjects remained on omalizumab throughout the dose escalation phase. One subject discontinued the study because of nonallergic abdominal migraines. Of the remaining 10 patients, 9 reached the maximum daily dose of 2000 mg of milk and passed a DBPCFC (cumulative dose of 7250 mg, or 220 mL, of milk) and an additional open challenge of 4000 mg (120 mL) of milk. The tenth patient tolerated a maximum dose of 500 mg of milk during the DBPCFC (total cumulative dose, 1000 mg, 30 mL). All patients in the study experienced allergic reactions, although most were mild and did not require treatment. One subject required epinephrine for rhinitis and urticaria after the 1000-mg dose of rush desensitization. Two other subjects received epinephrine at home by their caregivers during the maintenance phase, one for upper lip swelling and urticaria on the left leg, and one for urticaria on the right arm. There were no adverse reactions reported to the omalizumab injections.

Bedoret and colleagues, 2012 A post-hoc analysis of 5 patients who were enrolled in this study showed a marked decrease in milk-specific CD4+ T-cell proliferation 1 week after initiation of desensitization.[14] This decrease persisted during the dose escalation phase. However, milk-specific CD4+ T-cell proliferation subsequently returned while patients remained on daily oral milk. T-regulatory cells did not seem to be involved in the reduction of milk-specific CD4+ T-cell proliferation. Rather, anergy of the milk-specific CD4+ T cells was implicated as a possible explanation.

Schneider and colleagues, 2013 Omalizumab was also shown to possibly be safe and efficacious as an adjunctive treatment to facilitate rapid and successful oral desensitization in peanut allergy.[15] Thirteen patients with peanut allergy were treated with omalizumab for 12 weeks before starting OIT with peanut. All patients were able to reach a dose of 500 mg of peanut on the first day (cumulative dose of 992 mg). Twelve patients were able to reach the maintenance dose of 4000 mg of peanut, after which omalizumab treatment was discontinued. These patients were able to tolerate a cumulative dose of 8000 mg of peanut flour during a DBPCFC or an open challenge greater than or equal to 12 weeks after omalizumab was discontinued. In terms of safety, there were 2 patients who received epinephrine at home during the maintenance phase. One patient received epinephrine for vomiting, diarrhea, and wheezing that occurred 2.5 hours after peanut dosing. The other patient received epinephrine 3 times for coughing, hives, and wheezing, for what could have been food-dependent exercise-induced anaphylaxis.

Wood and colleagues, 2016 The first double-blind placebo-controlled trial comparing omalizumab with placebo as adjunctive therapy for cow's milk OIT in 57 subjects with severe milk allergy was recently published.[16] Patients received 4 months of omalizumab or placebo pretreatment before initiation and dose escalation of milk OIT over 22 to 40 weeks followed by a maintenance phase through month 28, after which omalizumab/placebo was discontinued. Patients who passed an oral food challenge at month 28 continued maintenance dosing for 8 weeks, followed by a period of discontinuation before rechallenge at month 32 to assess sustained unresponsiveness. There was no difference in rates of desensitization (proportion of patients who passed a 10-g oral food challenge at month 28) or sustained unresponsiveness (proportion of patients who passed the rechallenge at month 32). However, there were significantly fewer adverse reactions during dose escalation and fewer doses were required to achieve maintenance in the omalizumab-treated subjects. Significantly fewer reactions requiring epinephrine occurred in the omalizumab-treated group (2 doses in the omalizumab-treated group vs 18 doses in the placebo-treated group). This finding suggests that the primary advantage of omalizumab possibly lies in its ability to significantly improve the safety of OIT.

Martorell-Calatayud et al, 2016 Subsequently, a case series was published of 14 egg-allergic and cow's milk–allergic patients who had previously failed OIT because of grade 3 to 4 allergic reactions, but were able to tolerate OIT with only mild allergic reactions when omalizumab was given as pretreatment for 9 weeks and in conjunction with OIT until 2 months after the maintenance dose was reached.[17]

Summary
Omalizumab has been trialed as a stand-alone therapy to decrease food allergy symptoms and as an adjunct therapy in OIT trials. Initial results suggested that omalizumab increased tolerability of peanut in peanut-allergic patients[11,12] and possibly increased tolerability of OIT in peanut-allergic and cow's milk–allergic patients.[13,15] The most recent double-blind placebo-controlled trial for omalizumab with OIT suggests that omalizumab may allow for safer desensitization by increasing the tolerance threshold, although it may not affect efficacy outcomes such as desensitization and sustained unresponsiveness.[16] Further information is needed about safety issues surrounding the use of omalizumab with OIT because allergic reactions requiring the use of epinephrine still occurred during these trials. Larger studies evaluating omalizumab with OIT for peanut allergy are currently ongoing.[7]

EOSINOPHILIC ESOPHAGITIS

EoE is a chronic, antigen-mediated immune disease characterized by esophageal remodeling and dysmotility leading to food impactions and strictures and symptoms of chronic pain, feeding intolerance, and dysphagia. Diagnostic criteria are esophageal eosinophilia of greater than or equal to 15 eosinophils per high-power field (HPF) despite adequate acid blockade with proton pump inhibitor therapy.

Successful therapeutic interventions in patients with EoE include elimination diets, topical steroids, and amino acid.[30]

The T_H2 pathway has been implicated in EoE pathogenesis. As such, biologic therapies targeting IL-5, IL-13, and IgE have been investigated as potential treatments for EoE. The results of these studies and other potential biologic agents that could be useful for EoE treatment are reviewed later (**Table 2**).

Anti–Interleukin-5

IL-5 has a critical role in eosinophil expansion, differentiation, activation, migration, and tissue survival.[43] Antibodies targeting the cytokine IL-5 (mepolizumab, reslizumab) or the IL-5 receptor (benralizumab) have been developed. Out of the developed anti–IL-5 therapies, mepolizumab has been investigated most extensively as a treatment of various allergic and/or eosinophil-driven disorders, including asthma, atopic dermatitis, hypereosinophilic syndrome, eosinophilic granulomatosis with polyangiitis, and nasal polyposis.[44–52]

In severe asthmatics with blood and sputum eosinophilia, mepolizumab was shown to decrease peripheral eosinophilia, reduce the number of clinically significant exacerbations, improve forced expiratory volume in 1 second (FEV_1) before and after

Table 2
Summary of clinical trials and studies investigating the use of biologics as potential treatment of eosinophilic esophagitis

First Author, Year	Study Design and Dose	Follow-up EGD* (wk)	Age (y)	Patient Groups	Clinical Results	Immune Changes	Adverse Events
Mepolizumab							
Stein et al,[31] 2006	Open-label phase I/II safety and efficacy study 10 mg/kg (maximum, 750 mg) at week 8, 12, and 16	8 and 20	18–41	n = 4	Improvement of SF-36 quality-of-life scores (P = .03)	Significant decrease in blood eosinophil counts and percentage of CCR3+ cells Significant decrease in mean, median, and maximum esophageal eosinophil counts	Mild, including headache, URI symptoms, and 1 episode of hypotension
Stein et al,[32] 2008	Open-label phase I/II 10 mg/kg (maximum, 750 mg) at week 8, 12, and 16 Cohort A (n = 14): No change in immunosuppressant or antieosinophil medications Cohort B (n = 6): Decrease immunosuppressant or antieosinophil medications by 25% after the second mepolizumab infusion at week 12 Cohort C (n = 5): Decrease immunosuppressant or antieosinophil medications by 50% after the second mepolizumab infusion at week 12	Blood drawn at weeks 8 and 20	18–57	HES (n = 18) EoE (n = 6) EGID (n = 1)	—	Decreased blood eosinophil counts in 23 of 25 subjects Decreased percentage of CCR3+ cells Increased IL-5Rα expressed in eosinophils Increased number of IL-5 producing CD8+ cells	Mild, including headache, and 1 episode of hypotension

(continued on next page)

Table 2
(continued)

First Author, Year	Study Design and Dose	Follow-up EGD* (wk)	Age (y)	Patient Groups	Clinical Results	Immune Changes	Adverse Events
Straumann et al,[33] 2010	Randomized, double-blind, placebo-controlled phase I/II 750 mg at weeks 0 and 1 Nonresponders by week 4 also received 1500 mg at weeks 5 and 9	4 and 13	M: mean 32 P: mean 34	M (n = 5) P (n = 6)	M: >20% improvement in proportion of days subjects reported dysphagia between weeks 9 and 13, which increased up to ~30% compared with baseline between weeks 13 and 17 P: 20% and 18%, respectively	Following changes seen after treatment in M group but not P group: 1. Decreased peak and mean esophageal eosinophil counts, although primary end point (<5 eosinophils per HPF) was not met 2. Decreased blood eosinophil counts 3. Decreased extracellular EDN deposition in the esophagus 4. Decreased esophageal EDN-positive eosinophils, eotaxin-1 positive cells, eotaxin-2 positive cells, eotaxin-3 positive eosinophils, IL-5–positive cells 5. Decreased TGFβ1 and tenascin C expression by epithelial cells 6. Decreased blood ECP and EDN levels	Mild, including fatigue, URI symptoms

Conus et al,[34] 2009	Subanalysis of Straumann 2010[33]	4 and 13	M: mean 32 P: mean 34	M (n = 5) P (n = 6)	—	No changes in IL-5Rα expressed in eosinophils	—
Conus et al,[35] 2010	Post-hoc analysis of Straumann 2010	4 and 13	M: mean 32 P: mean 34	M (n = 5) P (n = 6)	—	Mepolizumab did not alter levels of eosinophils, T cells, and mast cells in the duodenal mucosa	—
Assa'ad et al,[36] 2011	International, multicenter, double-blind, randomized, prospective trial 0.55, 2.5, or 10 mg/kg every 4 wk for 3 doses (week 0, 4, 8)	12 and 24	2–17	0.55 mg/kg (n = 19) 2.5 mg/kg (n = 20) 10 mg/kg (n = 20)	No significant improvement in clinical symptoms using pediatric-specific EoE questionnaire. Of note, 11 of 59 subjects were already symptom free during screening period	5 of 57 subjects reached primary end point of peak esophageal intraepithelial eosinophil count of <5 per HPF at week 12 Significant decrease in peak and mean esophageal intraepithelial eosinophil counts at week 12 Higher baseline esophageal intraepithelial eosinophil counts associated with greater response to study drug Resolution of most eosinophil microabscesses and aggregations by week 12 Decreased blood eosinophil counts 24 h after first injection and low until week 12	51 of 59 subjects had AE, including (in order of decreasing frequency) vomiting, diarrhea, and upper abdominal pain 3 serious AE (chest pain, food impaction, esophageal injury caused by endoscopy)

(continued on next page)

Table 2
(continued)

First Author, Year	Study Design and Dose	Follow-up EGD* (wk)	Age (y)	Patient Groups	Clinical Results	Immune Changes	Adverse Events
Otani et al,[37] 2013	Post-hoc analysis of Assa'ad 2011	12 and 24	2–17	0.55 mg/kg (n = 19) 2.5 mg/kg (n = 20) 10 mg/kg (n = 20)	Esophageal mast cell numbers correlated with EoE symptom severity in subjects who had a >70% decrease in esophageal mast cell numbers after mepolizumab treatment	Intraepithelial mast cells were significantly decreased at week 12, particularly in subjects whose intraepithelial eosinophil count decreased to <15 eosinophils per HPF (defined in the study as responders) Mast cells were found in proximity to eosinophils in the esophagus, and mast cell/eosinophil couplets decreased significantly in responders IL-9-positive cells decreased by week 12 and correlated with mast cell numbers in responders	—
Reslizumab							
Spergel et al,[38] 2012	Prospective, randomized, placebo-controlled 1, 2, or 3 mg/kg at weeks 0, 4, 8, and 12	End of therapy or early withdrawal	5–18	1 mg/kg (n = 55) 2 mg/kg (n = 57) 3 mg/kg (n = 57)	No significant differences in the physician's EoE global assessment scores, patient's EoE predominant symptom	Peak esophageal eosinophil counts were reduced significantly more in treatment groups	Mild AE: headache, cough No serious AE related to study drug

				Placebo (n = 57)	assessment scores, and Children's Health Questionnaire scores between the treatment and placebo groups and the placebo group	
QAX576						
Rothenberg et al,[39] 2015	Prospective, randomized, placebo controlled 6 mg/kg at weeks 0, 4, and 8 with option for responders who relapsed to receive open-label extension of 3 more monthly doses	12 and 33	18–48	Completed to week 12: QAX576 (n = 15) Placebo (n = 8)	No significant difference between change in Mayo Dysphagia Questionnaire score between QAX576 and placebo group	No significant difference in proportion of responders (subjects who had ≥75% in peak eosinophil count per HPF from baseline to week 12) between QAX576 and placebo group / Mean esophageal eosinophil count decreased by 60% in Q group vs 23.3% in the P group / QAX576 lead to normalization of EoE-related gene expression, including eotaxin-3, periostin, carboxypeptidase A3, and desmoglein-1 CXCL1, CXCL6, and DHRS9 expression was significantly different at baseline between nonresponders and responders / Mild AE: cough, reflux

(continued on next page)

Table 2
(continued)

First Author, Year	Study Design and Dose	Follow-up EGD* (wk)	Age (y)	Patient Groups	Clinical Results	Immune Changes	Adverse Events
OC000459							
Straumann et al,[33] 2013	Randomized, placebo-controlled, parallel-group, single-center trial 100-mg OC000459 tablets, twice daily after meals for 8 wk	8 and 20 (or when symptoms reappeared between weeks 8 and 20 in subjects who had achieved remission)	22–69	OC000459 (n = 14) Placebo (n = 12)	Physician's global assessment of disease activity improved significantly only in the OC000459 group Patient-reported outcomes (measured by visual dysphagia questionnaire and pain questionnaire) improved significantly in both the OC000459 and placebo groups	In OC000459 treatment group: Significant decrease in mean eosinophil number measured in a total of 40 HPF from 294 biopsies taken from the proximal and distal esophagus Number of MCs and CD3+ T cells unchanged Epithelial expression of TSLP unchanged Significant increase in TGFβ1 expression by epithelial cells Reduced extracellular deposits of eosinophil peroxidase and tenascin C	1 severe AE unrelated to study drug: appendicitis
Omalizumab							
Foroughi et al,[40] 2007	Single-center open-label trial 0.0073–0.025 mg/kg/IU/mL every 2 wk for 8 doses	16	33–60	EGID (n = 9)	Symptom scores (using EGID scoring system modified from Crohn Disease Activity Index) improved significantly by	Absolute eosinophil count decreased significantly by week 16 Tissue eosinophil counts decreased in the duodenum and gastric	No severe AE

Study	Study design and dosing				Subjects	Time of evaluation	Symptoms	Other outcomes
Clayton et al,[41] 2014	Prospective, double-blind, randomized, placebo-controlled trial 0.016 IU/mL every 2–4 wk for 16 wk	—	16	16–20	12–35 / OMA (n = 16) Placebo (n = 14)	week 7–8 and week 15–16	No decrease in symptoms compared with placebo	antrum but trended upward in the esophagus. Basophil and dendritic cell FcεRI expression and free IgE levels decreased significantly. No significant decrease in esophageal eosinophil counts compared with placebo. Significant decrease in serum IgE levels compared with placebo —
Loizou et al,[42] 2015	Open-label, single arm, unblinded trial 150–375 mg every 4 wk for 12 wk				n = 15		Symptom scores (using EGID scoring system modified from Crohn Disease Activity Index)	5 of 15 subjects achieved full remission (<15 eosinophils per HPF in esophagus). Numbers of esophageal eosinophil, mast cells, and IgE significantly decreased —

Abbreviations: ECP, eosinophil cationic protein; EDN, eosinophil-derived neurotoxin; EGD, esophagogastroduodenoscopy; EGID, esophageal gastrointestinal disorder; HES, hypereosinophilic syndrome; HPF, high-power field; M, mepolizumab; P, placebo; TGF, transforming growth factor; TSLP, thymic stromal lymphopoietin.

bronchodilation, improve quality-of-life scores, and improve ACQ5 scores.[45,53] Furthermore, in severe steroid-dependent eosinophilic asthmatics, mepolizumab had significant steroid-sparing effects.[44] Mepolizumab 100 mg administered subcutaneously every 4 weeks was recently FDA approved as a maintenance therapy for severe eosinophilic asthma in patients greater than or equal to 12 years of age.[54]

IL-5 has been repeatedly implicated in atopic dermatitis pathogenesis, with atopic dermatitis being associated with blood[55] and skin eosinophilia,[56] and increased numbers of IL-5–producing cells in lesional skin biopsies.[57] A pathogenic IL-5–producing CCR8+ Th2 cell population has been reported to play a role in the chronic phase of eosinophilic atopic dermatitis.[58] However, mepolizumab did not show clinical efficacy in atopic dermatitis.[49] It has been hypothesized that the lack of clinical efficacy was caused by the inability to block tissue eosinophilia because tissue eosinophil counts were similar in mepolizumab-treated and placebo groups after atopy patch testing.[59]

Mepolizumab has also been shown to be well tolerated, reduce blood eosinophil counts, and have steroid-sparing effects in hypereosinophilic syndrome.[32,46,60–62] In addition, mepolizumab has shown promise as a potential steroid-sparing agent in 2 small (7 and 10 subjects), uncontrolled trials in patients with eosinophilic granulomatosis with polyangiitis, albeit at higher doses (750 mg) than the approved 100-mg dose for eosinophilic asthma.[47,48] Mepolizumab was granted orphan drug status by the FDA for hypereosinophilic syndrome in 2004 and for eosinophilic granulomatosis with polyangiitis in 2011.[54]

Clinical trials in adult eosinophilic esophagitis

Stein and colleagues, 2006 Mepolizumab was first investigated as a potential treatment of EoE by Stein and colleagues.[31] In an open-label phase I/II safety and efficacy study, 4 adult patients with EoE were treated with mepolizumab intravenously at 10 mg/kg (maximum 750 mg) at weeks 8, 12, and 16. Peripheral blood eosinophilia and percentage of CCR3+ cells decreased, as well as mean and maximum esophageal eosinophil counts. Clinically, mepolizumab was well tolerated and patients reported an improved quality of life.

Stein and colleagues, 2008 Results from another open-label phase I/II study with mepolizumab administered intravenously at 10 mg/kg (maximum 750 mg) at weeks 8, 12, and 16, this time for patients with hypereosinophilic syndrome (n = 18), EoE (n = 6), and eosinophilic gastrointestinal disorder (n = 1), was published in 2008.[32] This study again found that mepolizumab decreased serum eosinophil counts, CCR3+ cells, but not peripheral blood leukocyte, total lymphocyte, or lymphocyte subset counts. These investigators also reported that IL-5 and IL-5-Rα levels seemed to increase on mepolizumab therapy. Subsequent investigation into this phenomenon found that in patients with EoE treated with mepolizumab 750 mg at weeks 0 and 1 and 1500 mg at weeks 5 and 9, IL-5-Rα expression was not increased on eosinophils.[34]

Straumann and colleagues, 2010 In the first randomized, double-blind, placebo-controlled trial, mepolizumab 750 mg or placebo was administered intravenously every week for 2 doses.[33] If remission (defined as <5 eosinophils per HPF) was not observed following the first 2 doses in the treatment arm, mepolizumab 1500 mg was administered intravenously every week for 4 weeks for 2 doses. Significant decreases in serum, and peak and mean esophageal eosinophil counts were seen, although the primary end point of less than 5 peak eosinophils per HPF was not reached. In esophageal tissue, extracellular eosinophil-derived neurotoxin (EDN) deposition and EDN-positive cell numbers decreased, as did eotaxin-1, eotaxin-2, eotaxin-3, and IL-5 levels. The number of mast cells and CD3+ T cells did not change following treatment. Reductions in epithelial cell expression of transforming growth factor (TGF) β1 and tenascin C were also observed in the mepolizumab group. Serum eotaxin, eosinophil cationic protein, and EDN levels decreased in the mepolizumab group only. IL-5-Rα expression on blood eosinophils did not change.

Clinically, mepolizumab had an acceptable safety profile. Investigators evaluated clinical symptoms by measuring the proportion of days on which subjects reported dysphagia during the 7 days before a clinic visit, and by asking subjects whether they had global changes in EoE symptoms compared with baseline. Subjects treated with mepolizumab had greater improvement in the proportion of days with reported dysphagia and had slightly more improvement in global change of EoE symptoms. However, these changes were minimal and not clinical significant.

Although mepolizumab decreases aberrantly increased eosinophil counts in the esophagus, it has also been shown that mepolizumab does not affect physiologically normal numbers of eosinophils, T cells, and mast cells in the duodenum.[35]

Clinical trials in pediatric eosinophilic esophagitis

Assa'ad et al, 2011 This international, multicenter, double-blind, randomized, stratified, parallel-group study was the first to investigate the effects of mepolizumab in pediatric EoE (2–17 years of age).[36] Pediatric patients resistant to previous EoE treatment were randomized to one of 3 treatment arms (no placebo arm): 0.55, 2.5, or 10 mg/kg of mepolizumab. Significant decreases in the mean and peak esophageal eosinophil count were seen with mepolizumab. Higher baseline intraesophageal eosinophil counts were predictive of histologic response.

Although mepolizumab led to histologic improvements and had an acceptable safety profile, significant improvements in clinical symptoms were not seen. Symptom assessment was performed using a pediatric EoE-specific questionnaire that assessed the presence and severity of abdominal/chest/throat pain, regurgitation, vomiting, and dysphagia.[63]

Spergel and colleagues, 2012 Spergel and colleagues[38] were the first to investigate reslizumab in a large prospective, randomized, placebo-controlled trial. Children and adolescents (n = 262; 5–18 years of age) with greater than or equal to 24 eosinophils per HPF, a history of EoE symptoms, and failure to respond to at least 4 weeks of proton pump inhibitor therapy, were randomly assigned to treatment with reslizumab 1, 2, or 3 mg/kg, or placebo. Similar to prior studies, histologic improvement was seen with anti–IL-5 therapy, with a significant decrease in peak esophageal eosinophil counts. However, histologic improvement was not accompanied by clinical improvement as assessed by physician's EoE global assessments, patient's EoE predominant symptom assessments, and the Children's Health Questionnaire.

Summary
Because tissue eosinophilia is a hallmark of EoE, it follows that IL-5, a key cytokine for eosinophil activation and survival, likely plays a major role in EoE pathogenesis. IL-5 has been implicated in esophageal remodeling and esophageal dysmotility in mouse models of EoE.[64,65] However, anti–IL-5 therapy did not lead to clinical improvement or complete histologic remission despite consistent decreases in esophageal eosinophil count. These results suggest that eosinophils are not the only cells driving pathophysiology and mediating clinical symptoms in these patients.

It is possible that using a validated scoring system for methodological tracking of symptoms in future clinical trials may provide more granularity regarding the true clinical effects of mepolizumab. Furthermore, similar to the results of mepolizumab for eosinophilic asthma, mepolizumab may provide benefit in subsets of patients with EoE, and future research efforts focused on defining these subsets may be of benefit.

Anti–Interleukin-13

IL-13 has been implicated in EoE pathogenesis in murine models and human studies. Delivery of IL-13 into the trachea of mice can induce eosinophilia in the esophagus but not the stomach.[66,67] Intraperitoneal injection with anti–human IL-13 antibody abrogated the development of esophageal eosinophilia.[67] In humans, IL-13 expression is increased in the esophagus of patients with EoE, and IL-13 treatment of esophageal epithelial cells induced a previously described distinct, EoE-specific esophageal transcriptome profile.[68,69] IL-13 has also been implicated in the dysregulation of desmosomal cadherin desmoglein-1, which leads to impaired esophageal epithelial barrier function.[70]

Clinical trial

Rothenberg and colleagues, 2015 The first study investigating an anti–IL-13 antibody, *QAX576*, as a potential treatment of adult EoE was published in 2015.[39] Patients (18–50 years of age; n = 25) with greater than or equal to 24 eosinophils per HPF and proton pump inhibitor–resistant esophageal eosinophilia were randomly assigned to QAX576 (6 mg/kg) or placebo every 28 days for 3 doses with 6-month follow-up.

QAX576 was well tolerated and led to a decrease in mean esophageal intraepithelial eosinophil counts. Normalization of EoE-related gene expression in eotaxin-3, periostin, carboxypeptidase A3, and desmoglein-1 was seen after treatment. Transcriptomal changes differed between responders and nonresponders to QAX576. Three genes in particular were associated with response to anti–IL-13: CXCL1, CXCL6, and DHRS9. In addition, there was a trend toward improvement in dysphagia severity as measured by the Mayo Dysphagia Questionnaire, although the change was not statistically significant.

Summary

Isolated IL-13 blockade did not lead to a significant improvement in clinical symptoms despite significantly decreasing esophageal eosinophilia. Similar to results from trials investigating anti–IL-5 therapy, this shows that abrogating eosinophils alone is insufficient for symptom resolution in EoE. Again, note that symptom score tracking varied between each anti–IL-5 trial and this anti–IL-13 trial, as described earlier.

Anti–Immunoglobulin E

Several studies suggest that mast cells play an important role in EoE pathogenesis. Mast cells can affect smooth muscle contractility in the EoE esophagus via production of TGFβ1 and phosphorylation of phospholanban.[71,72] Carboxypeptidase A3 and tryptase, but not chymase, are increased in the esophagi of patients with EoE,[73] and mast cells have been identified as a possible diagnostic marker differentiating EoE from gastroesophageal reflux.[74,75] Mast cells were also implicated in EoE pathogenesis in a post-hoc analysis of patients with EoE treated with mepolizumab. This analysis showed that esophageal intraepithelial mast cell numbers were significantly decreased 12 weeks after mepolizumab treatment, and that esophageal mast cell numbers correlated with EoE symptom severity in patients who had a greater than 70% decrease in esophageal mast cell numbers after mepolizumab treatment.[37] Blocking the binding of IgE to its high-affinity receptor, FcεRI, can inhibit IgE-mediated activation of mast cells.

Clinical trials

Foroughi and colleagues, 2007 One study has been published investigating the use of anti-IgE for eosinophilic gastrointestinal disorder (defined as presence of typical gastrointestinal symptoms, greater than or equal to 25 eosinophils per HPF in stomach or duodenum, and negative work-up for other causes of gut eosinophilia).[40] In this single-center open-label study, 9 patients were treated with omalizumab subcutaneously during week 0 and then every 2 weeks for 8 total doses. Seven of these patients had esophageal eosinophilia at baseline. It is of interest that, although omalizumab led to significant decreases in the levels of serum eosinophils and tissue eosinophils in the duodenum, gastric antrum, and gastric body, esophageal eosinophil counts trended upward. Symptom scores improved significantly after omalizumab treatment.

Clayton and colleagues, 2014 In this prospective, double-blind, randomized, placebo-controlled study, patients greater than or equal to 15 years old were randomized to omalizumab (n = 16) or placebo (n = 14) every 2 to 4 weeks for 16 weeks.[41] Omalizumab did not improve symptoms or decrease esophageal eosinophil counts compared with placebo. However, this study provided interesting new data suggesting a possible role for IgG4 in EoE pathogenesis. Patients with EoE had 45-fold greater levels of IgG4 by immunohistochemistry in their esophagi and had higher serum IgG4 levels that reacted to food allergens, such as milk, wheat, egg, and nuts, compared with controls.

Loizou and colleagues, 2015 In an open-label, single arm, unblended trial, omalizumab was administered to 15 pediatric and adult patients (aged 12–35 years) with EoE every 4 weeks for 12 weeks.[42] Symptoms assessed by Crohn Disease Activity Index improved in 7 of the 15 subjects. Disease remission (defined as histologic improvement to <15 eosinophils per HPF and endoscopic resolution of disease) was seen in 5 patients. There were significant decreases in esophageal eosinophil and mast cell counts. Changes in mast cell numbers but not eosinophil numbers were associated with improvements in endoscopy scores.

Summary

Despite growing evidence supporting the role of mast cells in EoE, inhibiting mast cell activation and degranulation seems to be insufficient for clinical and histologic disease remission in the small numbers of patients studied. Mast cell numbers were associated with endoscopy scores, providing further evidence that mast cells are involved in EoE pathogenesis. Possibly, a combination of therapies inhibiting mast cells and eosinophils could provide sufficient benefit for symptom remission.

Prostaglandin D2 Receptor Antagonists

Prostaglandin D2 (PGD2) is rapidly produced and released by mast cells after cross-linking of FcεRI on mast cell surface. PGD2 exerts downstream inflammatory effects via the CRTH2 receptor, promoting recruitment and activation of CRTH2 receptor–expressing leukocytes such as T_H2 lymphocytes, eosinophils, and basophils.[76] OC000459 is an oral CRTH2 antagonist that holds promise as a therapeutic in T_H2-type inflammatory disorders.

Clinical trial

Straumann and colleagues, 2013 In a double-blind, placebo-controlled trial, 26 patients (aged 18–75 years) with corticosteroid-refractory or corticosteroid-dependent EoE (defined as dysphagia, $\geq$20 intraepithelial eosinophils per HPF in the esophagus, exclusion of other causes of esophageal or systemic eosinophilia) were randomized to either OC000459 100 mg or placebo tablets twice a day for 8 weeks.[43] OC000459 reduced esophageal eosinophil counts, and extracellular eosinophil peroxidase and tenascin C levels. The reduction in esophageal eosinophil counts, although significant, only decreased the posttreatment eosinophil load to 73.26 eosinophils per HPF. Physician's global assessment of disease activity improved significantly for patients on OC000459. However, patient-reported outcome using the visual dysphagia questionnaire was significantly improved in both OC000459 and placebo groups. Endoscopic findings were slightly but not significantly improved in the OC000459 group. Numbers of mast cells, CD3+ T cells, CRTH2 receptor–expressing CD3+ T cells and epithelial cells, and expression of thymic stromal lymphopoietin (TSLP) by epithelial cells were unchanged.

Summary

Taken together, this study suggests that OC000459 is modestly effective for EoE. However, further studies are needed to tailor the administration dose (the dose in this study was based on asthma studies and not dose-ranging studies in EoE) and identify subsets of patients with EoE subtypes for whom therapy with OC000459 would be more effective.

Potential Biologic Therapies for Eosinophilic Esophagitis

Interleukin-4 receptor antagonists (interleukin-4/interleukin-13 blockade)

IL-4 and IL-13 mediate downstream effects via a common heterodimeric receptor, IL-4Rα and IL-13Rα1. It has been proposed that therapies targeting IL-4 and IL-13 separately may be ineffective because IL-4 and IL-13 have overlapping downstream effects.[77] Efforts have been directed toward targeting IL-4Rα to block both IL-4 and IL-13.

Dupilumab, an mAb against IL-4Rα, is arguably the most promising IL-4/IL-13 targeted therapy to date. Dupilumab not only reduced asthma exacerbations in persistent, moderate to severe asthmatics but also improved FEV$_1$, morning PEF, asthma symptoms score, ACQ5 score, and number of short-acting beta-agonist inhalations per day. In addition, levels of biomarkers associated with Th2 inflammation (FeNO, TARC, eotaxin-3, and IgE) all decreased in patients on dupilumab therapy.[78]

Four clinical trials published together in 1 article showed the efficacy of dupilumab in atopic dermatitis. Patients with moderate to severe atopic dermatitis received dupilumab monotherapy (75 mg, 150 mg, or 300 mg every week) for 4 weeks, dupilumab monotherapy (300 mg every week) for 12 weeks, or dupilumab (300 mg every weeks) in combination with topical glucocorticoids for 4 weeks All had symptomatic improvement as assessed by EASI-50 (Eczema Area and Severity Index), pruritus score, and investigator's global assessment score. Dupilumab also led to reduction in Th2 biomarker levels (TARC and serum IgE).[79]

Analysis of skin biopsy specimens from subjects who received 4 weeks of dupilumab as part of these clinical trials showed that genes upregulated/downregulated in atopic dermatitis lesions normalized after dupilumab treatment. Notably, Th2 chemokines were suppressed. Normalization of gene transcription paralleled improvements in clinical scores.[80]

Targeting the IL-4 receptor to completely abrogate downstream signaling of IL-13 may prove to be more effective than isolated IL-13 blockade in EoE.

Anti–thymic stromal lymphopoietin

TSLP is a cytokine expressed by epithelial cells that drives allergic inflammation via activation of dendritic cells,[81,82] mast cells,[83] and CD34+ progenitor cells.[84] Studies suggest that TSLP acts both upstream and downstream of IL-13 to mediate allergic inflammation.[85–87] TSLP levels are increased in IL-13–induced murine allergic inflammation and anti-TSLP inhibits IL-13–induced allergic inflammation in mouse models.[87] TSLP can also induce murine airway inflammation that is reduced in the absence of IL-4 and IL-13.[85,86]

There is evidence that TSLP is involved in EoE pathogenesis. In mice, epithelial TSLP overexpression can induce an EoE-like phenotype via a basophil-dependent and IgE-independent pathway.[88] TSLP expression is upregulated in the esophagi of patients with EoE,[89] and single nucleotide polymorphisms in the TSLP gene have been associated with EoE.[90] It has also been shown that TSLP expression can be induced in esophageal epithelial cells.[90,91] As such, anti-TSLP antibodies could be trialed as a stand-alone therapy or used in combination with other biologics for synergistic effect.

Anti–interleukin-9

T_H2 and mast cells are cellular sources of IL-9. IL-9 promotes mast cell expansion; mast cell expression of TGFβ, IL-5, and IL-13; and enhances B-cell production of IgE.[92] IL-9 contributes to airway mucus production by acting directly and indirectly via IL-13 on airway epithelium.[93] Furthermore, IL-9 is involved in TSLP-mediated allergic inflammation in the lung.[94] IL-9 production by mucosal mast cells was found to be essential for the development of food allergy in murine models.[95]

In murine models of asthma, blocking IL-9 using anti–IL-9 antibody has been shown to attenuate allergic airway inflammation.[96] Anti–IL-9 antibody also reduces eosinophil numbers and IL-4/IL-4/IL-13 levels in bronchoalveolar lavage fluid as well as peribronchial inflammation following OVA challenge.[96,97]

IL-9 may also play a role in EoE pathogenesis. Expression of IL-9 is increased in the EoE esophagus.[68] IL-9 has been implicated in interactions between mast cells and eosinophils in the esophagi of pediatric patients with EoE, and eosinophils have been proposed as one of the cellular sources (but not the only one) of IL-9 in the esophagi of patients with EoE.[37] Other potential sources of IL-9 include Th9 and group 2 innate lymphocyte (ILC2) cells. ILC2 cell numbers are increased in biopsy tissue of patients with active EoE compared with inactive EoE.[98] Similar to anti-TSLP, anti-IL9 antibodies could also be trialed as a stand-alone therapy or used in combination with other biologics for synergistic effect.

SUMMARY

Investigation of biologic therapies in IgE-mediated food allergy and EoE has provided insights into the pathophysiology and treatment of these chronic, allergen-mediated disorders. Much remains to be elucidated. In IgE-mediated food allergy, the use of omalizumab seems to increase tolerability of food allergen and increase safety of desensitization protocols. The results of larger studies evaluating omalizumab with OIT for peanut allergy are anticipated. In EoE, the use of biologics targeting IL-5, IL-13, IgE, and the CRTH2 receptor have had mixed results. Decreases in esophageal eosinophilia are not paralleled by symptomatic remission. Future areas of research include identification of EoE phenotypes that are responsive to biologics and investigating the use of biologics in combination with other therapies.

REFERENCES

1. Sampson HA, Aceves S, Bock SA, et al. Food allergy: a practice parameter update - 2014. J Allergy Clin Immunol 2014;134(5):1016–25.e43.
2. Sicherer SH, Sampson HA. Food allergy: epidemiology, pathogenesis, diagnosis, and treatment. J Allergy Clin Immunol 2014;133(2):291–307.e5.

3. Branum AM, Lukacs SL. Food allergy among children in the united states. Pediatrics 2009;124(6):1549–55.

4. Boyce JA, Assa'ad A, Burks AW, et al. Guidelines for the diagnosis and management of food allergy in the United States: summary of the NIAID-sponsored expert panel report. J Allergy Clin Immunol 2010;126(6):1105–18.

5. Warren CM, Otto AK, Walkner MM, et al. Quality of life among food allergic patients and their caregivers. Curr Allergy Asthma Rep 2016;16(5):38.

6. Wood RA. Food allergen immunotherapy: current status and prospects for the future. J Allergy Clin Immunol 2016;137(4):973–82.

7. Pesek RD, Jones SM. Current and emerging therapies for IgE-mediated food allergy. Curr Allergy Asthma Rep 2016;16(4):28.

8. Bauer RN, Manohar M, Singh AM, et al. The future of biologics: applications for food allergy. J Allergy Clin Immunol 2015;135(2):312–23.

9. Leung DYM, Sampson HA, Yunginger JW, et al. Effect of anti-IgE therapy in patients with peanut allergy. N Engl J Med 2003;348(11):986–93.

10. Rafi A, Do LT, Katz R, et al. Effects of omalizumab in patients with food allergy. Allergy Asthma Proc 2010;31(1):76–83.

11. Sampson HA, Leung DYM, Burks AW, et al. A phase II, randomized, double-blind, parallel-group, placebo-controlled oral food challenge trial of Xolair (omalizumab) in peanut allergy. J Allergy Clin Immunol 2011;127(5):1309–10.

12. Savage JH, Courneya J-PP, Sterba PM, et al. Kinetics of mast cell, basophil, and oral food challenge responses in omalizumab-treated adults with peanut allergy. J Allergy Clin Immunol 2012;130(5):1123–112900.

13. Nadeau KC, Schneider LC, Hoyte L, et al. Rapid oral desensitization in combination with omalizumab therapy in patients with cow's milk allergy. J Allergy Clin Immunol 2011;127(6):1622–4.

14. Bedoret D, Singh AK, Shaw V, et al. Changes in antigen-specific T-cell number and function during oral desensitization in cow's milk allergy enabled with omalizumab. Mucosal Immunol 2012;5(3):267–76.

15. Schneider LC, Rachid R, LeBovidge J, et al. A pilot study of omalizumab to facilitate rapid oral desensitization in high-risk peanut-allergic patients. J Allergy Clin Immunol 2013;132(6):1368–74.

16. Wood RA, Kim JS, Lindblad R, et al. A randomized, double-blind, placebo-controlled study of omalizumab combined with oral immunotherapy for the treatment of cow's milk allergy. J Allergy Clin Immunol 2016;137(4):1103–10.e11.

17. Martorell-Calatayud C, Michavila-Gómez A, Martorell-Aragonés A, et al. Anti-IgE-assisted desensitization to egg and cow's milk in patients refractory to conventional oral immunotherapy. Pediatr Allergy Immunol 2016;27(5):544–6.

18. Barnes PJ. Severe asthma: advances in current management and future therapy. J Allergy Clin Immunol 2012;129(1):48–59.

19. Nadeau KC, Kohli A, Iyengar S, et al. Oral immunotherapy and anti-IgE antibody-adjunctive treatment for food allergy. Immunol Allergy Clin North Am 2012;32(1):111–33.

20. Stokes JR, Casale TB. The use of anti-IgE therapy beyond allergic asthma. J Allergy Clin Immunol Pract 2015;3(2):162–6.

21. Chanez P, Contin-Bordes C, Garcia G, et al. Omalizumab-induced decrease of FceRI expression in patients with severe allergic asthma. Respir Med 2010;104(11):1608–17.

22. Beck LA, Marcotte GV, MacGlashan D, et al. Omalizumab-induced reductions in mast cell FceRI expression and function. J Allergy Clin Immunol 2004;114(3):527–30.

23. Lin H, Boesel KM, Griffith DT, et al. Omalizumab rapidly decreases nasal allergic response and FcepsilonRI on basophils. J Allergy Clin Immunol 2004;113(2): 297–302.

24. Prussin C, Griffith DT, Boesel KM, et al. Omalizumab treatment downregulates dendritic cell FcepsilonRI expression. J Allergy Clin Immunol 2003;112(6): 1147–54.

25. Slavin RG, Ferioli C, Tannenbaum SJ, et al. Asthma symptom re-emergence after omalizumab withdrawal correlates well with increasing IgE and decreasing pharmacokinetic concentrations. J Allergy Clin Immunol 2009;17(2):195–6.

26. Steiss JO, Strohner P, Zimmer KP, et al. Reduction of the total IgE level by omalizumab in children and adolescents. J Asthma 2008;45(3):233–6.

27. Nopp A, Johansson SG, Ankerst J, et al. CD-sens and clinical changes during withdrawal of Xolair after 6 years of treatment. Allergy 2007;62(10):1175–81.

28. Noga O, Hanf G, Kunkel G, et al. Basophil histamine release decreases during omalizumab therapy in allergic asthmatics. Int Arch Allergy Immunol 2008; 146(1):66–70.

29. Noga O, Hanf G, Kunkel G. Immunological and clinical changes in allergic asthmatics following treatment with omalizumab. Int Arch Allergy Immunol 2003; 131(1):46–52.

30. Aceves SS. Eosinophilic esophagitis. Immunol Allergy Clin North Am 2015;35(1): 145–59.

31. Stein ML, Collins MH, Villanueva JM, et al. Anti-IL-5 (mepolizumab) therapy for eosinophilic esophagitis. J Allergy Clin Immunol 2006;118(6):1312–9.

32. Stein ML, Villanueva JM, Buckmeier BK, et al. Anti-IL-5 (mepolizumab) therapy reduces eosinophil activation ex vivo and increases IL-5 and IL-5 receptor levels. J Allergy Clin Immunol 2008;121(6):1473–83.

33. Straumann A, Conus S, Grzonka P, et al. Anti-interleukin-5 antibody treatment (mepolizumab) in active eosinophilic oesophagitis: a randomised, placebo-controlled, double-blind trial. Gut 2010;59(1):21–30.

34. Conus S, Straumann A, Simon HU. Anti-IL-5 (mepolizumab) therapy does not alter IL-5 receptor alpha levels in patients with eosinophilic esophagitis. J Allergy Clin Immunol 2009;123(1):269.

35. Conus S, Straumann A, Bettler E, et al. Mepolizumab does not alter levels of eosinophils, T cells, and mast cells in the duodenal mucosa in eosinophilic esophagitis. J Allergy Clin Immunol 2010;126(1):175–7.

36. Assa'ad AH, Gupta SK, Collins MH, et al. An antibody against IL-5 reduces numbers of esophageal intraepithelial eosinophils in children with eosinophilic esophagitis. Gastroenterology 2011;141(5):1593–604.

37. Otani IM, Anilkumar AA, Newbury RO, et al. Anti-IL-5 therapy reduces mast cell and IL-9 cell numbers in pediatric patients with eosinophilic esophagitis. J Allergy Clin Immunol 2013;131(6):1576–82.e2.

38. Spergel JM, Rothenberg ME, Collins MH, et al. Reslizumab in children and adolescents with eosinophilic esophagitis: results of a double-blind, randomized, placebo-controlled trial. J Allergy Clin Immunol 2012;129(2):456.

39. Rothenberg ME, Wen T, Greenberg A, et al. Intravenous anti-IL-13 mAb QAX576 for the treatment of eosinophilic esophagitis. J Allergy Clin Immunol 2015;135(2): 500–7.

40. Foroughi S, Foster B, Kim N, et al. Anti-IgE treatment of eosinophil-associated gastrointestinal disorders. J Allergy Clin Immunol 2007;120(3):594–601.

41. Clayton F, Fang JC, Gleich GJ, et al. Eosinophilic esophagitis in adults is associated with IgG4 and not mediated by IgE. Gastroenterology 2014;147(3):602–9.

42. Loizou D, Enav B, Komlodi-Pasztor E, et al. A pilot study of omalizumab in eosinophilic esophagitis. PLoS One 2015;10(3):e0113483.

43. Furuta GT, Atkins FD, Lee NA, et al. Changing roles of eosinophils in health and disease. Ann Allergy Asthma Immunol 2014;113(1):3–8.

44. Bel EH, Wenzel SE, Thompson PJ, et al. Oral glucocorticoid-sparing effect of mepolizumab in eosinophilic asthma. N Engl J Med 2014;371(13):1189–97.

45. Ortega HG, Liu MC, Pavord ID, et al. Mepolizumab treatment in patients with severe eosinophilic asthma. N Engl J Med 2014;371(13):1198–207.

46. Rothenberg ME, Klion AD, Roufosse FE, et al. Treatment of patients with the hypereosinophilic syndrome with mepolizumab. N Engl J Med 2008;358(12):1215–28.

47. Moosig F, Gross WL, Herrmann K, et al. Targeting interleukin-5 in refractory and relapsing Churg-Strauss syndrome. Ann Intern Med 2011;155(5):341–3.

48. Kim S, Marigowda G, Oren E, et al. Mepolizumab as a steroid-sparing treatment option in patients with Churg-Strauss syndrome. J Allergy Clin Immunol 2010;125(6):1336–43.

49. Oldhoff JM, Darsow U, Werfel T, et al. Anti-IL-5 recombinant humanized monoclonal antibody (Mepolizumab) for the treatment of atopic dermatitis. Allergy 2005;60(5):693–6.

50. Hulse KE, Stevens WW, Tan BK, et al. Pathogenesis of nasal polyposis. Clin Exp Allergy 2015;45(2):328–46.

51. Gevaert P, Lang-Loidolt D, Lackner A, et al. Nasal IL-5 levels determine the response to anti-IL-5 treatment in patients with nasal polyps. J Allergy Clin Immunol 2006;118(5):1133–41.

52. Gevaert P, Van Bruaene N, Cattaert T, et al. Mepolizumab, a humanized anti-IL-5 mAb, as a treatment option for severe nasal polyposis. J Allergy Clin Immunol 2011;128(5):989.

53. Pavord ID, Korn S, Howarth P, et al. Mepolizumab for severe eosinophilic asthma (DREAM): a multicentre, double-blind, placebo-controlled trial. Lancet 2012;380(9842):651–9.

54. Keating GM. Mepolizumab: first global approval. Drugs 2015;75(18):2163–9.

55. Jenerowicz D, Czarnecka-Operacz M, Silny W. Peripheral blood eosinophilia in atopic dermatitis. Acta Dermatovenerol Alp Pannonica Adriat 2007;16(2):47–52.

56. Kiehl P, Falkenberg K, Vogelbruch M, et al. Tissue eosinophilia in acute and chronic atopic dermatitis: a morphometric approach using quantitative image analysis of immunostaining. Br J Dermatol 2001;145(5):720–9.

57. Tanaka Y, Delaporte E, Dubucquoi S, et al. Interleukin-5 messenger RNA and immunoreactive protein expression by activated eosinophils in lesional atopic dermatitis skin. J Invest Dermatol 1994;103(4):589–92.

58. Islam SA, Chang DS, Colvin RA, et al. Mouse CCL8, a CCR8 agonist, promotes atopic dermatitis by recruiting IL-5+ T(H)2 cells. Nat Immunol 2011;12(2):167–77.

59. Oldhoff JM, Darsow U, Werfel T, et al. No effect of anti-interleukin-5 therapy (mepolizumab) on the atopy patch test in atopic dermatitis patients. Int Arch Allergy Immunol 2005;141(3):290–4.

60. Garrett JK, Jameson SC, Thomson B, et al. Anti-interleukin-5 (mepolizumab) therapy for hypereosinophilic syndromes. J Allergy Clin Immunol 2003;113(1):115–9.

61. Roufosse F, de Lavareille A, Schandené L, et al. Mepolizumab as a corticosteroid-sparing agent in lymphocytic variant hypereosinophilic syndrome. J Allergy Clin Immunol 2010;126(4):828–35.e3.

62. Roufosse FE, Kahn J-EE, Gleich GJ, et al. Long-term safety of mepolizumab for the treatment of hypereosinophilic syndromes. J Allergy Clin Immunol 2013; 131(2):461.

63. Flood EM, Beusterien KM, Amonkar MM, et al. Patient and caregiver perspective on pediatric eosinophilic esophagitis and newly developed symptom questionnaires. Curr Med Res Opin 2008;24(12):3369–81.

64. Mavi P, Rajavelu P, Rayapudi M, et al. Esophageal functional impairments in experimental eosinophilic esophagitis. Am J Physiol Gastrointest Liver Physiol 2012;302(11):G1347–55.

65. Mishra A, Wang M, Pemmaraju VR, et al. Esophageal remodeling develops as a consequence of tissue specific IL-5-induced eosinophilia. Gastroenterology 2008;134(1):204–14.

66. Mishra A, Rothenberg ME. Intratracheal IL-13 induces eosinophilic esophagitis by an IL-5, eotaxin-1, and STAT6-dependent mechanism. Gastroenterology 2003;125(5):1419–27.

67. Blanchard C, Mishra A, Saito-Akei H, et al. Inhibition of human interleukin-13-induced respiratory and oesophageal inflammation by anti-human-interleukin-13 antibody (CAT-354). Clin Exp Allergy 2005;35(8):1096–103.

68. Blanchard C, Stucke EM, Rodriguez-Jimenez B, et al. A striking local esophageal cytokine expression profile in eosinophilic esophagitis. J Allergy Clin Immunol 2011;127(1):208–17.e7.

69. Blanchard C, Mingler MK, Vicario M, et al. IL-13 involvement in eosinophilic esophagitis: transcriptome analysis and reversibility with glucocorticoids. J Allergy Clin Immunol 2007;120(6):1292–300.

70. Sherrill JD, Kc K, Wu D, et al. Desmoglein-1 regulates esophageal epithelial barrier function and immune responses in eosinophilic esophagitis. Mucosal Immunol 2014;7(3):718–29.

71. Aceves SS, Chen D, Newbury RO, et al. Mast cells infiltrate the esophageal smooth muscle in patients with eosinophilic esophagitis, express TGF-β1, and increase esophageal smooth muscle contraction. J Allergy Clin Immunol 2010; 126(6):1198–204.e4.

72. Beppu LY, Anilkumar AA, Newbury RO, et al. TGF-beta-1-induced phospholamban expression alters esophageal smooth muscle cell contraction in patients with eosinophilic esophagitis. J Allergy Clin Immunol 2014;134(5):1100–7.e4.

73. Abonia JP, Blanchard C, Butz BB, et al. Involvement of mast cells in eosinophilic esophagitis. J Allergy Clin Immunol 2010;126(1):140–9.

74. Dellon ES, Chen X, Miller CR, et al. Tryptase staining of mast cells may differentiate eosinophilic esophagitis from gastroesophageal reflux disease. Am J Gastroenterol 2011;106(2):264–71.

75. Kirsch R, Bokhary R, Marcon MA, et al. Activated mucosal mast cells differentiate eosinophilic (allergic) esophagitis from gastroesophageal reflux disease. J Pediatr Gastroenterol Nutr 2007;44(1):20–6.

76. Pettipher R. The roles of the prostaglandin D(2) receptors DP(1) and CRTH2 in promoting allergic responses. Br J Pharmacol 2008;153(Suppl):S191–9.

77. Vatrella A, Fabozzi I, Calabrese C, et al. Dupilumab: a novel treatment for asthma. J Asthma Allergy 2014;7:123–30.

78. Wenzel S, Ford L, Pearlman D, et al. Dupilumab in persistent asthma with elevated eosinophil levels. N Engl J Med 2013;368(26):2455–66.

79. Beck LA, Thaci D, Hamilton JD, et al. Dupilumab treatment in adults with moderate-to-severe atopic dermatitis. N Engl J Med 2014;371(2):130–9.

80. Hamilton JD, Suárez-Fariñas M, Dhingra N, et al. Dupilumab improves the molecular signature in skin of patients with moderate-to-severe atopic dermatitis. J Allergy Clin Immunol 2014;134(6):1293–300.

81. Reche PA, Soumelis V, Gorman DM, et al. Human thymic stromal lymphopoietin preferentially stimulates myeloid cells. J Immunol 2001;167(1):336–43.

82. Soumelis V, Reche PA, Kanzler H, et al. Human epithelial cells trigger dendritic cell mediated allergic inflammation by producing TSLP. Nat Immunol 2002;3(7): 673–80.

83. Allakhverdi Z, Comeau MR, Jessup HK, et al. Thymic stromal lymphopoietin is released by human epithelial cells in response to microbes, trauma, or inflammation and potently activates mast cells. J Exp Med 2007;204(2):253–8.

84. Allakhverdi Z, Comeau MR, Smith DE, et al. CD34+ hemopoietic progenitor cells are potent effectors of allergic inflammation. J Allergy Clin Immunol 2009;123(2): 472–9.

85. Zhou B, Headley MB, Aye T, et al. Reversal of thymic stromal lymphopoietin-induced airway inflammation through inhibition of Th2 responses. J Immunol 2008;181(9):6557–62.

86. Jessup HK, Brewer AW, Omori M, et al. Intradermal administration of thymic stromal lymphopoietin induces a T cell- and eosinophil-dependent systemic Th2 inflammatory response. J Immunol 2008;181(6):4311–9.

87. Miyata M, Nakamura Y, Shimokawa N, et al. Thymic stromal lymphopoietin is a critical mediator of IL-13-driven allergic inflammation. Eur J Immunol 2009; 39(11):3078–83.

88. Noti M, Wojno EDT, Kim BS, et al. Thymic stromal lymphopoietin-elicited basophil responses promote eosinophilic esophagitis. Nat Med 2013;19(8):1005–13.

89. Rothenberg ME, Spergel JM, Sherrill JD, et al. Common variants at 5q22 associate with pediatric eosinophilic esophagitis. Nat Genet 2010;42(4):289–91.

90. Sherrill JD, Gao PS, Stucke EM, et al. Variants of thymic stromal lymphopoietin and its receptor associate with eosinophilic esophagitis. J Allergy Clin Immunol 2010;126(1):160–5.e3.

91. Chandramouleeswaran PM, Shen D, Lee AJ, et al. Preferential secretion of thymic stromal lymphopoietin (TSLP) by terminally differentiated esophageal epithelial cells: relevance to eosinophilic esophagitis (EoE). PLoS One 2016;11(3):e0150968.

92. Noelle RJ, Nowak EC. Cellular sources and immune functions of interleukin-9. Nat Rev Immunol 2010;10(10):683–7.

93. Goswami R, Kaplan MH. A Brief History of IL-9. J Immunol 2011;186(6):3283–8.

94. Yao W, Zhang Y, Jabeen R, et al. Interleukin-9 is required for allergic airway inflammation mediated by the cytokine TSLP. Immunity 2013;38(2):360–72.

95. Chen CY, Lee JB, Liu B, et al. Induction of interleukin-9-producing mucosal mast cells promotes susceptibility to IgE-mediated experimental food allergy. Immunity 2015;43(4):788–802.

96. Cheng G, Arima M, Honda K, et al. Anti-interleukin-9 antibody treatment inhibits airway inflammation and hyperreactivity in mouse asthma model. Am J Respir Crit Care Med 2002;166(3):409–16.

97. Kim MS, Cho K-AA, Cho YJ, et al. Effects of interleukin-9 blockade on chronic airway inflammation in murine asthma models. Allergy Asthma Immunol Res 2013;5(4):197–206.

98. Doherty TA, Baum R, Newbury RO, et al. Group 2 innate lymphocytes (ILC2) are enriched in active eosinophilic esophagitis. J Allergy Clin Immunol 2015;136(3): 792–4.e3.

Adverse Reactions to Biologic Therapy

Sheenal V. Patel, MD*, David A. Khan, MD

KEYWORDS

- Biologic agents • Monoclonal antibodies • Infusion reaction • Delayed reaction
- Drug desensitization • Omalizumab • Rituximab

KEY POINTS

- At the current time, the diagnostic tools, including skin testing and in vitro testing, to evaluate for immediate hypersensitivity reactions for biologic agents are insufficient.
- Desensitization can be considered for reactions suggestive of immunoglobulin E-mediated mechanisms, but allergists/immunologists should be involved in managing these patients.
- Because reactions to desensitizations for biologics occur in approximately one-third of patients, steps to reduce these reactions for subsequent desensitizations are important.

INTRODUCTION

In recent years, there has been a rapid increase in the number of US Food and Drug Administration (FDA) -approved biological agents used to treat a variety of inflammatory conditions and malignancies. As these agents become more widespread in their use, more is likely to be learned about adverse reactions associated with their use, diagnostic approaches, and management strategies. In this review, the authors summarize proposed classification schemes and known adverse reactions to some notable biologic therapies and discuss potential management strategies that are available to physicians with allergist/immunologist involvement.

TYPES OF BIOLOGIC AGENTS

Biologic agents have become a very important therapeutic option for many to help treat inflammatory diseases, autoimmune diseases, and malignancies. Despite their therapeutic potential, the risk of immune-mediated effects by virtue of their mechanism of action is potentially significant.

Disclosures: S.V. Patel has nothing to disclose; D.A. Khan is a speaker for Genentech.
Division of Allergy and Immunology, University of Texas Southwestern Medical Center, 5323 Harry Hines Boulevard, F4.206, Dallas, TX 75390-8859, USA
* Corresponding author.
E-mail address: sheenal.patel@outlook.com

The various biologic agents can be grouped into 3 main categories, including cytokines, antibodies, and fusion proteins. Cytokines are normally secreted proteins with growth, differentiation, and activation functions that regulate and direct the nature of the immune responses.[1] Examples of cytokines used in the form of biologic agents include interferon-α (IFN-α), IFN-β, and interleukin-2 (IL-2). When developed as biologic agents, they are often modified to prolong their half-life in vivo. Biologic agents in the form of monoclonal antibodies have also been developed to soluble proteins like cytokines, to cell surface molecules, to immunoglobulin E (IgE), and to tumor antigens. With advancement in molecular biology techniques, antibody formation has shifted from using monoclonal antibodies derived from mouse origin to chimeric, humanized, or fully humanized monoclonal antibodies. Finally, fusion proteins are essentially soluble forms of natural receptors or ligands that have high affinity for their respective ligands or antibodies. They are designed by fusing proteins with the Fc portion of immunoglobulin (IgG1). Examples of each respective type are shown in **Table 1**.[2]

DIFFERENCES BETWEEN DRUGS AND BIOLOGIC AGENTS

To better understand adverse reactions to biologic agents, it is important to consider some key differences between drugs and biologic agents. Unlike most drugs, which are small compounds with molecular weights less than 1 kDa, biologic agents are larger sized proteins that are designed to be structurally similar to autologous proteins with molecular weights much greater than 1 kDa.[3] Drugs are synthetic compounds, whereas biologic agents are produced with molecular genetic technique and purified from engineered cells.[3] Most biologic agents are administered parenterally as they would otherwise be digested and broken down in the gastrointestinal (GI) tract. Most drugs, however, can be administered either orally or parenterally and are metabolized. The metabolism of drugs is thought to sometimes yield immunogenic intermediates. On the other hand, biologic agents do undergo processing but are not metabolized. Finally, biologic agents have inherent immune-mediated effects as

Table 1	
Types of biologic agents and examples	
Type of Biologic Agents	**Examples**
Cytokines	IFN-α, IFN-β, IL-2
Antibodies directed to:	Soluble proteins like cytokines: anti-TNF-α (infliximab, adalimumab, certolizumab, and golimumab), anti-IL-2 (daclizumab), anti-IL-5 (mepolizumab, reslizumab)
	Cell surface molecules: anti-CD20 (rituximab); anti-IL-2 receptor (basiliximab); anti-LFA-1 (efalizumab)
	IgE (omalizumab) Tumor antigens (eg, EGFR-, cetuximab, anti-HER2- trastuzumab) Receptors (eg, IL-5Rα, benralizumab)
Fusion proteins (soluble receptors for cytokines or soluble cellular ligands)	TNF-αRII (etanercept), CTLA4-Ig (abatacept), IL-1 receptor antagonist (anakinra, which is not a fusion protein but has a similar mechanism of action)

Modified from Pichler WJ. Adverse side-effects to biological agents. Allergy 2006;61(8):913; with permission.

they originate from foreign non-self proteins, which are typically not expected to be seen with drugs because they are smaller synthetic compounds.[2,3]

PROPOSED CLASSIFICATION OF ADVERSE REACTIONS TO BIOLOGIC AGENTS

Adverse reactions to drugs can be classified according to their action. One such classification scheme categorizes adverse reactions to drugs in types A through E. Type A reactions are thought to correspond to the drug's pharmacologic activity, are dose-dependent, and are predictable. Type B reactions are not related to the drug's pharmacologic activity, are unpredictable, and include immune-mediated side effects and hypersensitivity reactions. Type C reactions are due to the chemical structure of the drug itself and its metabolism. Type D reactions are delayed reactions that appear many years after treatment. Finally, type E reactions are those that occur after withdrawal of a specific drug.[4]

Because of the differences highlighted above between drugs and biologic agents, there have been attempts to alternatively classify adverse reactions to biologic agents using classification schemes that focus on their immune target-related adverse reactions. Pichler[2] in 2006 provided such a classification scheme that was further elaborated on by Haussman and colleagues.[5] As shown in **Table 2**, each type of reaction is classified by Greek letters: α, β, γ, δ, and ε.[2,5] Further details about each of the respective types are discussed in the following sections.

Type α: Overstimulation

Type α reactions of biologic agents are similar to type A reactions of drugs in that they are predictable based on the biologic agent's intended pharmacologic activity. It is thought that these types of reactions are due to cytokines administered in high systemic doses in order to achieve a specific therapeutic effect or to the release of high concentrations of cytokines as a result of the specific agent's mechanism of action.[2] This type of reaction was first seen in humans with anti-CD3 monoclonal antibody (muromunab), which was one of the first monoclonal antibodies approved for

Table 2
Proposed classification of adverse reactions to biologic agents

Type	Example Reaction (Causative Medication)
α: Overstimulation	Cytokine release syndrome (cytokine storm) (muromunab, TGN1412)
β: Hypersensitivity	Common acute infusion reactions (rituximab), delayed infusion reactions (etanercept, adalimumab), anaphylaxis (muromunab, cetuximab, omalizumab)
γ: Cytokine or immune imbalance	
Immunodeficiency	Increased risk of tuberculosis (anti-TNF agents) Hypogammaglobulinemia (rituximab)
Autoimmunity	Systemic lupus erythematosus or vasculitis (IFN-γ)
Atopic disorders	Atopic dermatitis (anti-TNF agents)
δ: Cross-reactivity	Acne from anti-EGFR (cetuximab)
ε: Nonimmunologic side effects	Neuropsychiatric side effects including confusion or depression (IFN-α)

Modified from Pichler WJ. Adverse side-effects to biological agents. Allergy 2006;61(8):917; with permission.

use in the setting of acute rejection with organ transplant patients.[6] Symptoms reported attributed to this type of reaction can include fever, arthralgias, nausea, vomiting, diarrhea, capillary leak syndrome with pulmonary edema, headache, altered mental status, and aseptic meningitis. The most severe cases of cytokine release syndrome were seen with the experimental biologic agent TGN1412.[7] TGN1412 was designed as a humanized superagonist anti-CD28 monoclonal antibody. Six healthy men had been administered the study drug as an intravenous bolus all 10 minutes apart. About 1 hour later, they developed severe headaches, low back pain, nausea, vomiting, diarrhea, and fever. They subsequently were transferred to the intensive care unit after developing hypotension, bilateral infiltrates, and respiratory failure requiring intubation, renal failure, and disseminated intravascular coagulation. Laboratory studies showed evidence of cytokine storm with high levels of cytokines such as tumor necrosis factor-alpha (TNF-alpha) and IFN-gamma. Patients were resuscitated and required intensive cardiopulmonary support (including dialysis), high-dose methylprednisolone, and an anti-IL-2 receptor antagonist antibody. Additional clinical features seen later included desquamation of the skin, digital ischemia in one patient, headaches, myalgias, paresthesias, and issues with concentration.[7] Other monoclonal antibodies have been shown to cause cytokine release syndrome with varying degrees of severity, and they include alemtuzumab, rituximab, and tosituzumab.[8]

Type β: Hypersensitivity

Type β reactions of biologic agents are hypersensitivity reactions that are characterized as either immediate or delayed reactions. Factors affecting these types of reactions include the type of immunoglobulin response elicited, possible presence of complement activation, degree of humanization of the monoclonal antibody, and the presence of adjuvants or excipients.[2]

IgE antibodies directed at non-self peptide sequences are possible and may be a cause of immediate reactions. Overall, IgE-mediated immediate hypersensitivity reactions are thought not to be common causes of immediate reactions because many patients will tolerate the same agent infused at a slower rate and possibly with premedications, including antihistamines and steroids.[5] However, IgE-mediated anaphylaxis has been described with multiple biologic agents, including muromunab (anti-CD3 monoclonal antibody), omalizumab (anti-IgE monoclonal antibody), and cetuximab (chimeric mouse and human monoclonal antibody to epidermal growth factor receptor [EGFR]).[9] IgE-mediated anaphylaxis has also been described with cetuximab, which is a chimeric mouse-human IgG1 monoclonal antibody against the EGFR, typically used in cancer therapy. In this case, studies have shown that IgE-mediated anaphylactic reactions to cetuximab were associated with IgE antibodies against galactose-α-1,3-galactose that were present before treatment with cetuximab.[5,10]

Common acute infusion reactions represent a majority of reactions to monoclonal antibodies. These reactions are predictable, common, and usually mild reactions. They may occur with the first dose. Typical symptoms include fevers, rigors, back pain, abdominal pain, nausea, vomiting, diarrhea, dyspnea, flushing, pruritus, or changes in heart rate and blood pressure.[11] The mechanism is not well understood, but the release of proinflammatory cytokines may have some role in some reactions. Complement activation is also thought to play a role in immediate hypersensitivity reactions because complement cleavage products C3a and C5a may directly stimulate mast cells and lead to IgE-independent mast cell activation.[5]

The degree of humanization of monoclonal antibodies has changed significantly over time. As monoclonal antibodies have evolved from murine-derived monoclonal antibodies to humanized and fully human monoclonal antibodies, their immunogenicity has decreased due to the decreasing amount of foreign antigens they contain. Although the risk of forming human antimurine antibodies has decreased, even humanized monoclonal antibodies contain non-self peptide sequences that have the potential to lead to human anti-human antibody formation.[2] The consequence of these antibodies is typically delayed with the production of IgG antibodies and involves inactivation of the drug but typically not many symptoms. Complement is also thought to play a role in delayed reactions by immune complex formation and serum sicknesslike reactions.[2] T-cell–mediated hypersensitivity causing delayed maculopapular exanthema has also been suggested in case reports of abciximab where positive intracutaneous tests were shown after 48 hours.[5]

γ: Cytokine or Immune Imbalance

Type γ reactions are thought to occur as a function of the biologic agent and its effect on altering the balance maintained by a normally functioning immune system. Type γ reactions may therefore lead to impaired function of a normally functioning immune system leading to infections, autoimmunity, or atopic disease.[2] Examples of agents causing an immune system imbalance resulting in increased infections include an increase in tuberculosis infections in those treated with anti-TNF agents and rituximab-induced hypogammaglobulinemia that has been reported to cause an increase in sinopulmonary infections and report of one death from enteroviral meningitis.[12] IFN-gamma has also been described in inducing autoimmune and autoinflammatory diseases, including lupuslike syndrome, systemic sclerosis, Guillain-Barre syndrome, autoimmune thyroid disease, idiopathic thrombocytopenic purpura, vitiligo, and psoriasis.[2] Finally, anti-TNF agents have also been shown to be associated with the appearance of atopic dermatitis.[2,13,14]

δ: Cross-Reactivity

Type δ reactions occur by virtue of a biologic agent targeting an antigen that is expressed on various tissue cells or by targeting an antigen with a similar structure.[2] The clearest example of this is seen with reports of cetuximab causing acneiform eruptions. Cetuximab targets EGFR, which is strongly expressed in carcinomas of different origin and thought to be associated with tumor progression. EGFR is also expressed on normal skin cells. Cetuximab's binding to EGFR on normal skin cells, therefore, is the likely cause of the associated acneiform eruption.[2,15]

ε: Nonimmunologic Side Effects

Type ε reactions are nonimmunologic side effects that are not predictable and unrelated to a biologic agent's mechanism of action. An example of these types of reactions includes the neuropsychiatric adverse effects, such as acute confusional states or depression seen with IFN-alpha treatment.[2]

MANAGEMENT

Although the classification scheme described above is important in understanding the mechanism of adverse reactions of biologic agents, the management of acute reactions is likely facilitated more so by first differentiating an immediate versus delayed reaction and differentiating immediate reactions as common acute infusion reactions versus hypersensitivity reactions.

Common acute infusion reactions are typically characterized by fevers, rigors, back pain, abdominal pain, nausea, vomiting, diarrhea, dyspnea, flushing, pruritus, or changes in heart rate and blood pressure.[11] The mechanism of these reactions is not thought to be IgE mediated. In a study of 14 patients treated with infliximab with infusion reactions, none of the patients were found to have increases in either tryptase levels or IgE levels against infliximab.[16] These types of reactions are typically managed with premedication with corticosteroids, antihistamines, analgesics, and/or slower infusion rates.[17]

Hypersensitivity reactions (eg, IgE-mediated reactions) may have overlapping symptoms and be indistinguishable from common acute infusion reactions. With respect to timing, immediate reactions are thought to occur during or within a few hours from either a first or subsequent infusion, whereas delayed reactions are thought to occur up to 14 days following an infusion.[16,17] The prevalence of anaphylactic reactions is thought to be low, for example, occurring in less than 0.2% of patients treated with omalizumab.[18]

Shared symptoms between common acute infusion reactions and hypersensitivity reactions include GI symptoms, dyspnea, flushing, pruritus, and back pain. Symptoms suggestive of hypersensitivity but not standard infusion reactions may include urticaria, wheezing, frequent coughing, or multiorgan anaphylactic symptoms. Hypersensitivity reactions to biologic agents have been shown to be less common than standard infusion reactions.[19] Hypersensitivity reactions have been reported for rituximab (anti-CD20), infliximab (anti-TNF-α), trastuzumab (anti-HER2), omalizumab (anti-IgE), natalizumab (anti-α4-integrin), basiliximab (anti-IL-2Rα), abciximab (GPIIb/IIIa receptor antagonist), and cetuximab (anti-EGFR).[20]

A REVIEW OF ADVERSE REACTIONS TO SPECIFIC AGENTS

Numerous biological agents have been associated with hypersensitivity reactions, including anaphylaxis. Hypersensitivity reactions to most of these agents share similar characteristic clinical features, and the approach to these reactions in regards to diagnosis and management (eg, desensitization) is quite similar. Therefore, this review focuses on biologics with more robust data on hypersensitivity reactions, those with atypical clinical features and those used more commonly by allergy/immunology specialists.

Biologics for Asthma

Omalizumab

Omalizumab is a humanized monoclonal antibody that binds IgE. In 2007, a joint task force was formed between the American Academy of Allergy, Asthma and Immunology and the American College of Allergy, Asthma and Immunology Executive Committees to examine Genentech's Xolair (omalizumab) clinical trials and postmarketing surveillance data on anaphylactic reactions. In this report, the anaphylaxis reporting rate was found to be 0.09% (35 patients reported to have anaphylaxis out of 39,510 patients receiving omalizumab over an approximate 2.5-year period).[21] With respect to timing of reactions, they found that many reactions, especially reactions occurring after the first to third doses, occurred greater than 1 hour after injection. This report led to recommendations for a 2-hour observation period for the first to third doses of omalizumab and 30-minute observation periods for subsequent doses.[21] A follow-up report published in 2011 showed that most reactions occurred during these recommended waiting times ($\sim$77%).[22] Additional recommendations for patients being treated with omalizumab from this task force report included education regarding signs and symptoms of anaphylaxis and the prescription of epinephrine autoinjectors to all patients.[21,22]

The mechanism for omalizumab anaphylaxis is not well understood. Because omalizumab is composed of 5% mouse polypeptide, it is possible that IgE-mediated reactions may occur against the murine sequences. However, the unusual delayed nature of these reactions and infrequent skin test positivity suggest that this is not the primary mechanism. Excipients have also been proposed to be a cause of anaphylactic reactions to omalizumab. Price and Hamilton[23] reported 2 patients who developed anaphylaxis after more than a year of successful omalizumab administration. Both of these cases were thought to be anaphylactoid in nature and possibly due to an excipient, polysorbate, which has also been found to cause similar allergic reactions since the 1970s.[24] Whether this is the cause of most anaphylactic reactions to omalizumab remains unproven.

Diagnostic testing for IgE-mediated hypersensitivity reactions can involve skin prick and intradermal testing, but it is critical to determine nonirritating concentrations for drug testing. Omalizumab is the only biologic agent in which nonirritating concentrations were determined in a systematic fashion. Different dilutions of omalizumab for both skin prick and intradermal testing were studied in 2010 to establish safety and determine interpretable results for likely IgE-mediated immediate hypersensitivity reactions. Dilutions in sterile water were found to cause irritant reactions, so dilutions with saline were subsequently used. The investigators established a nonirritating concentration of a dilution with saline of 1:100,000 (concentration of 1.25 μg/mL).[25] However, the utility of omalizumab skin testing and further data about the positive and negative predictive values are still unknown.

Desensitization with biologic agents has emerged as an option to manage hypersensitivity reactions; however, results have been mixed with omalizumab. In 2006, a case of a 32-year-old woman was reported who had developed generalized erythema and itching 5 minutes after her first dose of omalizumab 300 mg in the treatment of her asthma and idiopathic chronic urticaria and angioedema.[26] She was treated with epinephrine and additional nonsedating antihistamines. As the patient had seen clinical benefit over the subsequent few weeks in the control of both her asthma and her chronic urticaria, the risks and benefits of further doses were discussed, and she elected to pursue options to receive additional doses. Subsequent doses were given per a desensitization protocol as follows: 7.5 mg, 15 mg, 30 mg, 60 mg, 45 mg (remaining dose) every 30 minutes. During the subsequent doses, she experienced marked generalized erythema and pruritus beginning with the last 3 injections and persisting for several hours. She also was noted to have fever and hypertension suggesting a systemic component to these reactions. With subsequent infusions, she was premedicated with ibuprofen 600 mg and did not develop any further signs of hypersensitivity. However, despite premedication before the seventh dose, she developed a petechial rash 1 to 2 days after the dose that was thought to represent a possible serum sicknesslike reaction, and no further doses were given.[26]

Further cases were published in patients with mild to moderate reactions in 2011. A case series of 3 patients included those with mild to moderate reactions with symptoms of cough/dyspnea, urticaria, and angioedema. Two of the 3 patients were noted to also have vocal cord dysfunction. The investigators utilized a desensitization protocol that started with 0.0625 mg with doubling doses every 30 minutes up to 40 to 55 mg maximum doses with a cumulative dose of 113 to 190 mg. All 3 patients had mild to moderate reactions during the protocol, but 2 of the 3 patients were able to receive weekly omalizumab doses thereafter.[27] This case series contrasts with the experience of an attempt at desensitization in a patient who had an anaphylactic reaction (dyspnea, nausea, hypotension) 1 hour after the second dose of omalizumab

150 mg. Desensitization in this case was then performed after negative skin prick testing, but after the fourth dose (31 mg), the patient was again noted to have an anaphylactic reaction with nausea, chest tightness, and a significant drop in forced expiratory volume in 1 second.[28]

Mepolizumab

Mepolizumab is a humanized monoclonal antibody that binds to and inactivates IL-5, which is a cytokine that is thought to play a role in eosinophil recruitment, persistence, and activation.[29] Mepolizumab has been shown to decrease the frequency of asthma exacerbations in patients with severe persistent eosinophilic asthma and decrease maintenance oral glucocorticoids in severe persistent eosinophilic asthma patients as well.[29] The most common adverse reactions observed with mepolizumab include headache, injection site reactions, back pain, fatigue, nasopharyngitis, rash, and pruritus. Injection site reactions have been reported to occur in as much as 8% of patients treated with mepolizumab. An increased incidence of herpes zoster was also seen compared with placebo in some trials.[30]

Reslizumab

Reslizumab is also a monoclonal antibody against IL-5 that is indicated for add-on maintenance treatment of patients with severe persistent eosinophilic asthma. Anaphylaxis was observed to occur with reslizumab infusion in 0.3% of patients in placebo-controlled trials. Anaphylaxis was seen as soon as the second dose and either during the infusion or within 20 minutes of completion of the infusion. Therefore, patients should be observed for symptoms and signs of anaphylaxis after administration of reslizumab. The most common adverse reaction observed was oropharyngeal pain.[31] In addition, some trial data also showed an increase in the rate of malignancies reported within less than 6 months of exposure to reslizumab (0.6% reported in patients receiving reslizumab vs 0.3% reported in patients receiving placebo). There was no specific type of malignancy that was found to be most common. Increases in creatine phosphokinase, myalgias, and other musculoskeletal complaints were also seen more frequently in patients receiving reslizumab compared with placebo.[31,32]

Benralizumab

Benralizumab is a humanized monoclonal antibody designed to target the IL-5 receptor α chain and block the effects of IL-5 on eosinophils. Unlike mepolizumab and reslizumab, it is not yet FDA approved for the treatment of severe eosinophilic asthma and is continuing in investigational trials. To date, the most common adverse reactions seen with benralizumab include headaches, nasopharyngitis, and nausea. Injection site reactions have also been reported.[33,34]

Other Biologics Notable for Specific Adverse Drug Reactions

Rituximab

Two main categories of adverse reactions to rituximab include immunodeficiency and hypersensitivity. Rituximab is a chimeric monoclonal antibody that binds to CD20. It is used to treat B-cell lymphomas and many autoimmune diseases. It causes rapid depletion of CD20 expressing B-cell precursors and mature B cells, which remain low for 6 to 9 months.[35]

Because of its peripheral B-cell–depleting effects, many studies have sought to determine immune-mediated consequences in those treated with rituximab. In 2013, a large retrospective study was published to determine the long-term safety of rituximab in rheumatoid arthritis patients. They included 3194 patients including

627 patients who were followed for greater than 5 years. They showed that the most common adverse events were common acute infusion-related reactions that mostly occurred with the first dose and were categorized as mild or moderate based on common terminology criteria for adverse events. With respect to immune-related adverse events, they demonstrated hypogammaglobulinemia at the following rates: low IgM, 22.4%; low IgG, 3.5%; and low IgA, 1.1%. Their data showed that hypogammaglobulinemia was not associated with increased infections.[36] However, another study in 2014 reported 19 cases of symptomatic, persistent hypogammaglobulinemia after rituximab with most of these cases seen in hematologic malignancies.[12] The mean interval since last rituximab dose was about 3 years, and 18 of the 19 patients were treated with gammaglobulin replacement because prophylactic antibiotics were not helpful in decreasing risk of infectious illness in this group of patients. Most these patients had sinopulmonary infections, and one died from enteroviral meningoencephalitis.[36] Therefore, it is important to consider that rituximab-induced hypogammaglobulinemia may persist for years after rituximab infusion and is not always associated with symptoms. However, in those patients who have increased infections, consideration for gammaglobulin replacement should be made on a case-by-case basis.

As mentioned above, common acute infusion-related reactions are the most common adverse effect seen with rituximab use. Up to 77% of patients will have infusion-related symptoms with the first dose. Also, up to 80% of fatal reactions occur with the first dose.[37] Premedication with acetaminophen, antihistamines, and corticosteroids is typically recommended. Delayed reactions have also been observed with rituximab with reports of serum sicknesslike reactions occurring in patients with a mean of 7 days following infusion. Most of the patients reported in a systematic review had reactions following their first cycle and most commonly had symptoms of fever (79%), arthralgia (73%), and rash (70%). Most patients were treated with corticosteroids with good response. Attempts at premedication for 4 patients were mixed, because they reported 2 patients tolerated repeat doses, whereas one had recurrent serum sickness and one had angioedema.[38]

Etanercept/adalimumab injection site reactions

Etanercept and adalimumab are both subcutaneously administered TNF blockers used in a variety of inflammatory joint and bowel diseases. One of the most common adverse reactions with their use is an injection site reaction. Zeltser and colleagues[39] retrospectively reviewed etanercept use in patients receiving therapy for various inflammatory arthritic conditions or inflammatory bowel disease and found injection site reactions were reported in 20% of patients. They found that all occurred within the first 2 months of therapy, typically occurred 1 to 2 days after the last injection and resolved within a few days, and were observed to wane with time. They performed skin biopsies in patients who experienced these injection site reactions and showed they had inflammatory infiltrates composed of mostly lymphoid cells and some eosinophils, in a perivascular cuffing pattern, without evidence of leukocytoclastic vasculitis. Further analysis of the lymphoid cells showed that most of them were cytotoxic CD8+ T cells. They suggested the mechanism of these reactions may be a delayed-type hypersensitivity reaction that is T-cell mediated, which wanes over time due to induction of tolerance. Immediate hypersensitivity reactions including anaphylaxis have also been reported with etanercept and adalimumab.[40]

Bavbek and colleagues[41] examined the role for subcutaneous desensitization protocols for both etanercept and adalimumab in the setting of injection site reactions or immediate type hypersensitivity reactions. For etanercept, they included 6 patients who had injection site reactions to etanercept 10 minutes to 24 hours after subsequent injections and one patient who had experienced urticaria, angioedema, wheezing, vomiting, and hypotension 5 hours after the fifth injection. All the patients had negative prick tests, positive intradermal tests at 15 minutes, and negative readings from intradermals at 24, 48, and 72 hours. All 7 patients underwent subcutaneous desensitization protocols and were able to tolerate subsequent etanercept doses with only mild local erythema when premedicated with cetirizine. For adalimumab, they included 4 patients with injection site reactions 1 to 6 hours after subsequent doses and one patient who had urticaria 2 to 3 hours after the third injection. Prick testing was positive in 4 patients; intradermal testing was positive in one patient, and delayed intradermals were negative in all the patients at 24, 48, and 72 hours. All 5 patients underwent successful subcutaneous desensitization; however, they all experienced local erythema that was smaller than the initial reactions. They were all able to tolerate subsequent adalimumab doses with premedication and tolerated spacing of their adalimumab doses to every other week.

DIAGNOSTIC EVALUATION OF BIOLOGICAL HYPERSENSITIVITY REACTIONS, GENERAL PRINCIPLES

Beyond a careful history, various diagnostic testing modalities are used in the evaluation of immediate hypersensitivity reactions and include skin prick testing, intradermal testing, in vitro testing, and drug challenges. The experience with respect to skin prick and intradermal testing for monoclonal antibodies is increasing rapidly. In a study published in 2009, Brennan and colleagues[20] described their center's experience with desensitizations to monoclonal antibodies, including rituximab, infliximab, and trastuzumab. They performed intradermal skin tests using 1:100 and 1:10 dilutions in patients before rapid desensitizations; however, no controls were tested to determine nonirritating concentrations. They had positive intradermal tests in 4/6 patients for infliximab, 6/9 patients for rituximab, and 2/2 patients for trastuzumab and suggested their reactions may be due to immediate hypersensitivity. In cases of positive skin test results, desensitizations were recommended. In the largest desensitization study published to date by Sloane and colleagues,[42] they included 32 patients with hypersensitivity reactions to biologic agents and performed skin prick and intradermal testing. Their skin test results were as follows: rituximab 9/15 positive tests, infliximab 4/9 positive tests, trastuzumab 3/3 positive tests, bevacizumab 2/2 positive tests, tocilizumab 1/1 positive test, and cetuximab 1/1 positive test.

With respect to in vitro testing, the experience is rather limited. Chung and colleagues[10] reported that in patients with cetuximab anaphylaxis, they were able to detect IgE antibodies directed toward cetuximab using the ImmunoCAP assay in 17 of 25 patients who had anaphylaxis.

In addition, elevated tryptase levels may confirm mast cell activation in cases of immediate hypersensitivity, but normal serum tryptase levels in the setting of a reaction should not be interpreted as reassuring. Basophil activation tests have not been evaluated in large studies, and their accuracy in evaluating immediate hypersensitivity with monoclonal antibodies is not known. Finally, drug challenge may be considered in patients with milder reactions with features not suggestive of IgE-mediated reactions, but there are no clear data on the safety of this approach for more moderate-severe allergic reactions.

Overall, the data regarding various testing modalities typically used to evaluate immediate hypersensitivity reactions are limited but expanding. Skin testing has been performed, but nonirritating concentrations for most agents are not well established and predictive values (negative or positive) are not known. For moderate to severe reactions, the lack of sufficient methods to evaluate for immediate hypersensitivity often leads to empiric desensitization, if there is no other feasible alternative.

RAPID DRUG DESENSITIZATIONS TO BIOLOGICAL AGENTS

Rapid drug desensitizations to biologic agents should only be performed when the agent is needed as first-line therapy. Delayed reactions are contraindicated and include Stephens-Johnsons syndrome, toxic epidermal necrolysis, drug rash with eosinophilia with systemic symptoms, acute generalized erythematous pustulosis, erythema multiforme, serum sickness, and so forth. Successful desensitizations have been reported to multiple agents, including rituximab (anti-CD20), trastuzumab (anti-HER2), infliximab (anti-TNFα), cetuximab (anti-EGFR), bevacizumab (anti-VEGF-A), tocilizumab (anti-IL-6R), ofatumumab (anti-CD20), brentuximab (anti-CD30), alemtuzumab (anti-CD52), etanercept (fusion protein against TNF-αRII), and adalimumab (anti-TNFα).[19] Premedications are important for desensitizations and include the use of antihistamines, corticosteroids; and acetominophen may also be considered to reduce fever. Aspirin has been used to prevent flushing and montelukast to prevent bronchospasm in chemotherapy desensitizations. Because of infrequent administrations of most of biologic agents, repeat desensitizations are then typically required as well. Sloane and colleagues[42] showed that when patients are chosen carefully with respect to type of reactions and stratified according to risk, desensitizations are a safe and feasible alternative to allow patients to remain on first-line therapies they have previously had immediate hypersensitivity reactions to. They performed a total of 120 rituximab desensitizations and had no reactions with 86 desensitizations (72%), mild reactions with 23 desensitizations (19%), and moderate or severe reactions in 11 patients (9%). One patient required epinephrine. No deaths were associated with these desensitizations. Overall, most reactions to monoclonal antibodies occurred at the twelfth step and were mostly cutaneous reactions. Based on their overall experience including both chemotherapeutics and monoclonal antibodies, they provided prognostic information and determined patients with an initial grade 1 or 2 hypersensitivity reaction have a 91% to 92% chance of having no (grade 0) or minimal (grade 1) symptoms during their first rapid drug desensitization. They also reported that patients with an initial severe (grade 3) hypersensitivity reaction have an 86% chance of having no or a minimal hypersensitivity reaction during their first desensitization, but continue to have a 9% chance of having a severe hypersensitivity reaction during the first desensitization.

Because reactions to desensitizations for biologics occurs in approximately one-third of patients, steps to reduce these reactions for subsequent desensitizations are important. In addition to adding premedications as discussed above, adding additional steps to the desensitization protocol may also be helpful. Although some investigators suggest adding an additional more dilute bag with an extra 4 steps to the beginning of the protocol, the authors have found that adding additional steps to the last bag (when most reactions occur) is more helpful. An example of this is shown in **Table 3** for a patient who reacted to rituximab during his initial desensitization, but with modifications to the protocol subsequently, tolerated 3 desensitizations without reaction.

Table 3
Modification to rapid desensitization protocol for rituximab

Original rituximab desensitization protocol

Step	Solution	Rate (mL/h)	Time (min)	Volume infused per step (mL)	Dose administered with step (mg)	Cumulative dose (mg)
	Solution (10 mg/250 mL) Conc. = 0.04 mg/mL					
1	1	2	15	0.5	0.02	0.02
2	1	5	15	1.25	0.05	0.07
3	1	10	15	2.5	0.1	0.17
4	1	20	15	5	0.2	0.37
	Solution (100 mg/ 250 mL) Conc. = 0.4 mg/mL					
5	2	5	15	1.25	0.5	0.87
6	2	10	15	2.5	1	1.87
7	2	20	15	5	2	3.87
8	2	40	15	10	4	7.87
	Solution (992 mg/ 250 mL) Conc. = 3.968 mg/mL					
9	3	10	30	5	19.84	27.71
10	3	20	30	10	39.68	67.39
11	3	32.5	30	16.25	64.48	131.87
12	3	45	30	22.5	89.28	221.15
13	3	57.5	30	28.75	114.08	335.23
14	3	70	30	35	138.88	474.11
15	3	82.5	30	41.25	163.68	637.79
16	3	95	30	47.5	188.48	826.27
17	3	100.5	26	43.75	172.8	999.07

Modification to rituximab desensitization protocol

Step	Solution					
Solution (10 mg/250 mL); Conc. = 0.04 mg/mL						
1	1	5	10	0.83	0.033	0.033
2	1	10	10	1.66	0.066	0.099
3	1	20	10	3.33	1.33	1.462
Solution (100 mg/250 mL); Conc. = 0.4 mg/mL						
4	2	5	10	0.83	0.33	1.792
5	2	10	10	1.66	0.66	2.452
6	2	20	15	5	2	4.452
7	2	40	15	10	4	8.452
Solution (492 mg/125 mL); Conc. = 3.936 mg/mL						
8	3	10	15	2.5	9.84	18.292
9	3	20	15	5	19.68	37.972
10	3	25	15	6.25	24.6	62.572
11	3	30	15	7.5	29.52	92.092
12	3	35	15	8.75	34.44	126.532
13	3	40	15	10	39.36	165.892
14	3	45	15	11.25	44.28	210.172
15	3	50	15	12.5	49.2	259.372
16	3	55	15	13.75	54.12	313.492
17	3	60	15	15	59.04	372.532
18	3	65	15	16.25	63.96	436.492
19	3	70	14	16.33	64.27	500.762

SUMMARY

Biologic therapies are emerging as a significant therapeutic option for many with debilitating inflammatory and autoimmune conditions. As expansion in the number of FDA-approved agents continues to be seen, more unanticipated adverse reactions are likely to occur. At the current time, the diagnostic tools including skin testing and in vitro testing to evaluate for immediate hypersensitivity reactions are insufficient. Desensitizations can be considered for reactions suggestive of IgE-mediated mechanisms, but allergists/immunologists should be involved in managing these patients.

REFERENCES

1. Adkinson NF, Bochner BS, et al, editors. Middleton's allergy principles in practice: Chapter 5: cytokines in allergic inflammation. Philadelphia: Elsevier Sanders; 2014.
2. Pichler WJ. Adverse side-effects to biological agents. Allergy 2006;61(8):912–20.
3. Aubin F, Carbonnel F, Wendling D, et al. The complexity of adverse side-effects to biological agents. J Crohns Colitis 2013;7(4):257–62.
4. Naisbitt DJ, Gordon SF, Pirmohamed M, et al. Immunological principles of adverse drug reactions: the initiation and propagation of immune responses elicited by drug treatment. Drug Saf 2000;23:483–507.
5. Hausmann OV, Seitz M, Villiger PM, et al. The complex clinical picture of side effects to biologicals. Med Clin North Am 2010;94(4):791–804.
6. Vasquez EM, Fabrega AJ, Pollak R. OKT3-induced cytokine-release syndrome: occurrence beyond the second dose and association with rejection severity. Transplant Proc 1995;27:873–4.
7. Suntharalingam G, Perry MR, Ward S, et al. Cytokine storm in a phase 1 trial of the anti-CD28 monoclonal antibody TGN1412. N Engl J Med 2006;355:1018–28.
8. Bugelski PJ, Achuthanadam R, Capocasale RJ, et al. Monoclonal antibody-induced cytokine-release syndrome. Expert Rev Clin Immunol 2009;5(5): 499–521.
9. Abramowicz D, Crusiaux A, Goldman M. Anaphylactic shock after retreatment with OKT3 monoclonal antibody. N Engl J Med 1992;327:736.
10. Chung CH, Mirakhur B, Chan E, et al. Cetuximab-induced anaphylaxis and IgE specific for galactose-alpha-1,3-galactose. N Engl J Med 2008;358(11):1109–17.
11. Lenz HJ. Management and preparedness for infusion and hypersensitivity reactions. Oncologist 2007;12(5):601–9.
12. Makatsori M, Kiani-Alikhan S, Manson AL, et al. Hypogammaglobulinaemia after rituximab treatment-incidence and outcomes. QJM 2014;107:821–8.
13. Devos SA, Van Den Bossche N, De Vos M, et al. Adverse skin reactions to anti-TNF-alpha monoclonal antibody therapy. Dermatology 2003;206:388–90.
14. Chan JL, Davis-Reed L, Kimball AB. Counter-regulatory balance: atopic dermatitis in patients undergoing infliximab infusion therapy. J Drugs Dermatol 2004; 3:315–8.
15. Perez-Soler R, Saltz L. Cutaneous adverse effects with HER1/EGFR-targeted agents: is there a silver lining? J Clin Oncol 2005;23(22):5235–46.
16. Cheifetz A, Mayer L. Monoclonal antibodies, immunogenicity, and associated infusion reactions. Mt Sinai J Med 2005;72:250–6.
17. Cheifetz A, Smedley M, Martin S, et al. The incidence and management of infusion reactions to infliximab: a large center experience. Am J Gastroenterol 2003;98:1315–24.
18. Xolair (omalizumab) [Product insert]. South San Francisco: Genentech, Inc; 2007.

19. Galvao VR, Castells MC. Hypersensitivity to biological agents-updated diagnosis, management, and treatment. J Allergy Clin Immunol Pract 2015;3:175–85.
20. Brennan PJ, Rodriguez Bouza T, Hsu FI, et al. Hypersensitivity reactions to mAbs: 105 desensitizations in 23 patients, from evaluation to treatment. J Allergy Clin Immunol 2009;124:1259–66.
21. Cox L, Platts-Mills TA, Finegold I, et al. American Academy of Allergy, Asthma & Immunology/American College of Allergy, Asthma and Immunology Joint task force report on omalizumab-associated anaphylaxis. J Allergy Clin Immunol 2007;120:1373–7.
22. Cox L, Lieberman P, Wallace D, et al. American Academy of Allergy, Asthma & Immunology/American College of Allergy, Asthma & Immunology Omalizumab-Associated Anaphylaxis Joint Task Force follow-up report. J Allergy Clin Immunol 2011;128:210–2.
23. Price KS, Hamilton RG. Anaphylactoid reactions in two patients after omalizumab administration after successful long-term therapy. Allergy Asthma Proc 2007;28: 313–9.
24. Lieberman P. The unusual suspects: a surprise regarding reactions to omalizumab. Allergy Asthma Proc 2007;28:259–61.
25. Lieberman P, Rahmaoui A, Wong DA, et al. The safety and interpretability of skin tests with omalizumab. Ann Allergy Asthma Immunol 2010;105:493–5.
26. Dreyfus DH, Randolph CC. Characterization of an anaphylactoid reaction to omalizumab. Ann Allergy Asthma Immunol 2006;96:624–7.
27. Owens G, Petrov A. Successful desensitization of three patients with hypersensitivity reactions to omalizumab. Curr Drug Saf 2011;6:339–42.
28. Khan DA. Adverse Reactions to Biological Agents: Opportunities for the Allergist American College of Allergy, Asthma, and Immunology National Meeting. San Antonio (TX), November 7, 2015.
29. Bel EH, Wenzel SE, Thompson PJ, et al. Oral glucocorticoid-sparing effect of mepolizumab in eosinophilic asthma. N Engl J Med 2014;371(13):1189–97.
30. Nucala (mepolizumab) [Product insert]. Research Triangle Park (NC): GlaxoSmithKline LLC; 2015.
31. Cinqair (reslizumab) [Product insert]. Frazer (PA): Teva Respiratory, LLC; 2016.
32. Castro M, Zangrilli J, Wechsler ME, et al. Reslizumab for inadequately controlled asthma with elevated blood eosinophil counts: results from two multicentre, parallel, double-blind, randomised, placebo-controlled, phase 3 trials. Lancet 2015; 3:355–66.
33. Laviolette M, Gossage DL, Gauvreau G, et al. Effect of benralizumab on airway eosinophils in asthma with sputum eosinophilia. J Allergy Clin Immunol 2013; 132(5):1086–96.e5.
34. Tan LD, Bratt JM, Godor D, et al. Benralizumab: a unique IL-5 inhibitor for severe asthma. J Asthma Allergy 2016;9:71–81.
35. Gorman C, Leandro M, Isenberg D. B cell depletion in autoimmune disease. Arthritis Res Ther 2003;5(Suppl 4):S17–21.
36. Van Vollenjoven RF, Emery P, Bingham CO 3rd, et al. Extended report: long-term safety of rituximab in rheumatoid arthritis: 9.5-year follow-up of the global clinical trial programme with a focus on adverse events of interest in RA patients. Ann Rheum Dis 2013;72:1496–502.
37. Rituxan (rituximab) [Package insert]. South San Francisco: Genentech Inc; 1997.
38. Karmachayra P, Poudel DR, Pathak R, et al. Rituximab-induced serum sickness: a systematic review. Semin Arthritis Rheum 2015;45(3):334–40.

39. Zeltser R, Valle L, Tanck C, et al. Clinical, histological, and immunophenotypic characteristics of injection site reactions associated with etanercept: a recombinant tumor necrosis factor alpha-receptor: Fc fusion protein. Arch Dermatol 2001; 137:893–9.

40. Quercia Q, Emiliani F, Foschi FG, et al. Adalimumab desensitization after anaphylactic reaction. Ann Allergy Asthma Immunol 2011;106:547.

41. Bavbek S, Ataman S, Akinci A, et al. Rapid subcutaneous desensitization for the management of local and systemic hypersensitivity reactions to etanercept and adalimumab in 12 patients. J Allergy Clin Immunol Pract 2015;3(4):639–40.

42. Sloane D, Govindarajulu U, Harrow-Mortelliti J, et al. Safety, costs, and efficacy of rapid drug desensitizations to chemotherapy and monoclonal antibodies. J Allergy Clin Immunol Pract 2016;4:497–504.

Pharmacoeconomics of Biologic Therapy

 CrossMark

Don A. Bukstein, MD[a,b,*], Allan T. Luskin, MD[c,1]

KEYWORDS

- Severe asthma • Biologic therapy • Pharmacoeconomics • Health care resource use
- Oral corticosteroid • Personalized medicine

KEY POINTS

- Pharmacoeconomics in immune therapy with biologics involves comparing the costs of an intervention with the change in health status to establish value of an intervention.
- Accurate assessments require measuring all disease costs before and after the intervention, including direct disease costs, costs of related comorbidities, and indirect costs.
- Indirect costs include absenteeism, presenteeism, and quality of life of the patient and family/caregivers.
- Proper policy decisions demand that the cost of the intervention be compared with the cost of the lack of the intervention or alternative interventions.
- Costs of lack of the intervention or alternative therapies include both direct and indirect costs, and the direct costs should include the costs of complications of uncontrolled disease and long-term side effects medications such as corticosteroids.

The good physician treats the disease; the great physician treats the patient who has the disease.

—Sir William Osler

INTRODUCTION

Recent years have witnessed tremendous progress in the therapeutic approach to immune-related diseases, such as rheumatoid arthritis, psoriasis, inflammatory bowel disease, and asthma. The introduction of novel biologic agents, including antibodies

Disclosure Statement: D.A. Bukstein has served as a speaker for Merck, Genentech, Novartis Pharmaceuticals, AstraZeneca, Aerocrine, Teva Pharmaceutics, Meda Pharmaceuticals, and Circassia. He has received honoraria from AstraZeneca, Schering-Plough, Merck, Meda Pharmaceuticals, Alcon, and Aerocrine and has commercial interests in Altus Minicampus and the PBL Institute. A.T. Luskin has served as a speaker for Genentech.
[a] Allergy, Asthma & Sinus Center, Madison, WI, USA; [b] Allergy, Asthma & Sinus Center, Milwaukee, WI, USA; [c] Healthy Airways, Madison, WI, USA
[1] Present address: 10 Tower Drive, Sun Prairie, WI 53590.
* Corresponding author. 11 Glen Arbor Way, Fitchburg, WI 53711.
E-mail address: donabukstein@gmail.com

and cytokine inhibitors, has allowed clinicians to achieve improved outcomes for their patients. An important factor that has affected the utilization of novel therapies is their acquisition costs, which far exceed those for older drugs. Nevertheless, these are serious chronic conditions, which can cause substantial morbidity and accelerated mortality for affected individuals. Alternative therapeutic choices often involve the use of agents such as systemic corticosteroids with potentially costly side effects. Both undertreatment with uncontrolled disease and treatment with alternative therapies have severe economic consequences to patients and their families as well as to society. Therefore, appropriate pharmacoeconomic analyses demand we take into account all relevant costs, not only of the treatments but also of the disease itself and that of alternative treatments. In this way, the value of therapies can be correctly estimated.

Previous articles have emphasized the clinical burden of severe asthma. The authors summarize the pharmacoeconomic data obtained for biologic agents in patients with inadequately controlled severe persistent allergic asthma despite high-dose inhaled corticosteroids (ICSs) plus a long-acting β-agonist (LABA) and discuss the cost-effectiveness evidence published for biologic agents in this patient population. Although there is a great deal of evidence highlighting the health, economic, and societal burden of asthma, the evidence is highly skewed toward patients with severe uncontrolled asthma, particularly when asthma is inadequately controlled. In patients who do not respond to traditional therapy but do respond to biologic therapy, the cost-effectiveness of biologics often compares well with other treatments for chronic illness in the long terms of costs.

Costs are a measure of resources consumed. By assessing costs, pharmacoeconomic studies complement studies of efficacy and safety, helping to determine the relationships of treatment and outcome. Costs are divided into 3 categories: direct costs, or costs attributable to the intervention; indirect costs, or costs resulting from reduced productivity; and intangible costs, which are incurred from pain and emotional suffering. Insurance companies, patients, doctors, and society each have different perspectives with respect to costs. The authors review different types of cost analyses and their use in studies of asthma as a model. Cost studies influence clinicians', policy makers', and third-party payers' decisions regarding the implementation of particular therapies or programs. Collection of all relevant cost data needs to be facilitated and evaluated along with clinical trials to facilitate these decisions.

This article attempts to provide a more clinically useful perspective on the pharmacoeconomics of new biologics in the treatment of immune diseases, particularly in the area of asthma. Biologics are a cornerstone of personalized medicine but are inherently costly. Therefore—especially for those with the greatest economic burden—a cost-sensitive approach to improve the health of persons who have or are at the highest risk for uncontrolled asthma and other immune disorders must be developed.

Pharmacoeconomic evaluation encompasses a collection of methods that assesses the costs and consequences of comparative health care interventions. **Table 1** summarizes types of pharmacoeconomic evaluation. Evaluating the health and economic impacts of these interventions has been a topic of long-standing interest among clinicians.[1] Such evaluation involves a variety of issues and methods and additionally has major policy implications. This review discusses the main types of pharmacoeconomic evaluation used to assess the use of biologics in asthma and immune disease and will be achieved by analyzing studies to demonstrate how pharmacoeconomic evaluation has been used for asthma care strategies using biologics. Also discussed are the challenges in the practical application of pharmacoeconomic evaluation and related policy implications. This review is designed for clinicians caring for

Table 1		
Types of pharmacoeconomic analyses		
Type	**Description**	**Comparison (X:Y)**
Cost minimization (CMA)	Compares cost in monetary terms of treatment with identical outcomes	Dollars: Outcome unit varies but equivalent in comparatory groups
Cost-effectiveness (CEA)	Compares cost in monetary terms with outcomes in natural units	Dollars: Natural units such as years, blood glucose, LDL, cholesterol
Cost utility (CUA)	Compares cost in monetary terms and outcomes in terms of years of life	Dollars: QALY quality of life-years
Cost benefit (CBA)	Compares costs and outcomes in monetary terms	Dollars: dollars

Abbreviation: LDL, low-density lipoprotein.

individuals with asthma and other immune diseases to assist with understanding and evaluating published economic analyses, and identifying the key costs and benefits associated with their own clinical practices.[1]

Why Should Caregivers, Insurance Companies, Payers, and Society Be Concerned About the Pharmacoeconomics of Immune Diseases?

Health care costs are increasing, and the focus of both government and private insurance on spending places demands on health care providers to reduce costs yet improve outcomes.[2] Although new medical interventions can substantially improve health outcomes, these often come at considerable cost to both the health care system and patients. In order to efficiently use limited health care resources, beyond the standard evaluations of safety and efficacy, it is necessary to also evaluate the relative cost-effectiveness of new medical technologies. First the inflammatory immune disease asthma is discussed as an example one area of medicine that is grappling with the challenge of applying biologic therapies.

ASTHMA

Asthma is considered a high-burden inflammatory disease of the lungs, affecting an estimated 17.7 million adults and 6.3 million children in the United States.[3] Approximately 1 in 2 asthma sufferers, 10.7 million people, reported having at least one asthma attack, and 3651 casualties were a result of asthma in 2014.[3] In 2010, asthma in the United States resulted in 439,435 hospitalizations, 1.8 million emergency department (ED) visits, and 14.2 million physician office visits.[3,4] Although its health implications are frightening enough, asthma's cost burden is astounding as well. Asthma is associated with an estimated $50 billion (2009 dollars) in total direct incremental costs annually.[4] Furthermore, productivity loss related to the illness accounts for an additional $3.8 billion, and productivity loss from mortality accounts for another $2.1 billion.[5]

Typically, physicians take a three-pronged approach to allergy care: minimize exposure to allergens, reduce symptoms with pharmacologic therapy, and alter the immune response with immunotherapy. For severe asthma, physicians have the option to improve control with either biologics or thermoplasty.[6] Although this 3-pronged method has been adopted by most specialty physicians for asthma treatment, to form an overall management strategy that maximizes positive patient outcomes, asthma treatment needs to be a shared decision-making process (SDM) between the patient, clinician, and payer. Each of the main stakeholders, physician, health care delivery system, employer, patient, and society as a whole, have different areas of emphasis.

Physician perspective
- How can I help these patients control asthma symptoms and prevent comorbidities and exacerbations?
- What type and mix of medical care services will achieve control, balancing benefit and risk?
- For managed-care patients:
  - How can I achieve clinical objectives of Accountable Care Organizations (ACOs), satisfy patient preference, and minimize costs?
  - How can I adhere to mandated guidelines (Pay For Performance [P4P]) and ACOs?

Health care delivery system perspective
- How can direct costs be contained? Managing insurance premiums across groups and maximizing the number of insured patients.
- How will we reduce exacerbation? Exacerbation is associated with mortality and likely higher direct costs than chronic daily symptoms.[7]
- How do we meet guidelines or regulated performance requirements, such as Healthcare Effectiveness Data and Information Set and the Affordable Care Act (ACA)?
- How can I use P4P to reduce costs?
- How do we keep plan members satisfied?
- How do we keep asthma off of our list of concerns?

Employer perspective
- How do I reduce medical costs?
- How do I maintain a productive workforce?
  - Ensure a satisfied workforce
  - Reduce workforce absenteeism
  - Reduce workforce presenteeism
  - Reduce workforce turnover

Patient Perspective
- How do I limit out-of-pocket costs?
- How do I improve my quality of life (QOL)?
- How do I prevent exacerbations and avoid going to the ED?

Societal perspective
- What are the societal costs of asthma?
- How do we control these costs in a non-Orwellian world? (ie, *a mandate such as "Get rid of the cat" or "Quit smoking" is not an option!*)
- What is the impact of the disease on family, friends, work or school, and the community?
- How do we sustain public programs?
- What is the cost-effectiveness and lifetime impact of a preventive intervention?

These various stakeholders weigh various costs differently. Health care systems place more importance on direct costs, whereas patients and employers may value indirect costs. Although all of these parties have high concerns with cost, it is vital to note that value does not equate to cost. It is important then that we define what we mean by quality value in health care and how this may outweigh any dollar costs that many fear. Value in health care is generally defined as quality/cost. More specifically, physicians have refined it to the following:

$$\frac{\text{Change in health status} + \text{Satisfaction}}{\text{Cost}}$$

The cost of a biologic intervention equates to the following:

Cost = Cost of drug − Direct Costs − Positive Change in QOL − Change in Patient Productivity

Accurate evaluation of the equation demands that all costs be measured. These costs are hidden direct costs including the costs of asthma, side effects, medications, and comorbid disease. Furthermore, comorbid disease might be favorably affected either directly by medication, such as in the case of allergic rhinitis, or indirectly by improved control, such as in the case of gastroesophageal reflux disease or obstructive sleep apnea.

Therefore, cheaper is not always less expensive when other elements are measured. As clinicians, we need to learn how to develop an understanding of the true pharmacoeconomic value of biologics, so that we can accurately convey this to health care organizations, the government, and, most importantly, patients. The evaluation depends not solely on drug acquisition costs but also on the costs of the disease itself, from short- and long-term side effects of the drug to alternative treatment costs. The most difficult cost to calculate is the change in productivity. This change in productivity is the cost generated by uncontrolled disease resulting in the loss of personal parental and spousal/family productivity. Also challenging to estimate is the long-term societal cost that is generated from the lack of education because of the effect on school performance as well as underemployment of a patient and their family. The different costs listed in the equation above will vary based on the population receiving the biologic and will depend on identifying the patients who are able to respond and those who are able to do so. The Refractory Asthma Stratification Programme in the United Kingdom (RASP-UK) points out that some patients have poorly controlled asthma simply because they are not taking their medicines correctly.[8] Identifying those patients is important, but there is another group that RASP-UK investigators hope to identify: patients with severe asthma characterized by high eosinophil or periostin levels who are taking their medicines correctly yet fail to respond to medication. Even within this group of asthma sufferers who do have the right biomarker profile, physicians may have difficulty determining which patients should receive which biologic.[8,9] The biomarkers linked to each medicine tend to go up and down together, so a patient might have a high eosinophil count in addition to high periostin levels.[9–12]

WHEN IS BIOLOGIC THERAPY COST-EFFECTIVE?

There are many ways to analyze cost data, and cost-effectiveness is a commonly used method (**Table 1**). A biologic therapy is deemed to be a cost-effective strategy when the outcome is worth the cost relative to competing alternatives. In other words, it is a cost-effective strategy when scarce resources are used to acquire the best value on the market considering all alternatives.[13]

Average cost-effectiveness is calculated as:
Cost of drug

Resulting effect = Cost per unit of effect achieved

What is the incremental cost-effectiveness of a biologic in comparison with all other treatment options?

$$\frac{\text{Cost(Option B)} - \text{Cost(Option A)}}{\text{Effect(Option B)} - \text{Effect(Option A)}} = \text{Cost to achieve one unit of effect}$$

Previous articles have discussed many of the efficacies of data variables, or what product (effect) can be consistently expected from the use of drug or health service, which was determined from clinical trials. They seek a direct relationship to morbidity and mortality such as survival/death or, as per the asthma example, asthma exacerbations avoided. These efficacy outcomes may rely on surrogate measures such as the Asthma Control Test, pulmonary function tests, fractional exhaled nitric oxide, or use of oral steroids. A randomized controlled clinical trial is the gold standard for deriving this efficacy data, but observational studies can also add insight into the real-world costs of a biologic.[14,15]

HOW AND WHAT VARIABLES SHOULD WE MEASURE?

What resources are consumed to produce one unit of the effect? There are drug product acquisition costs, drug preparation and administration costs, drug monitoring costs, treatment costs of adverse effects, and indirect institutional costs (discounting other drugs).

In order to draw the most valid conclusion about costs generated over time to achieve an effect in the future, it is necessary to consider that there is a time preference associated with money. The concept of time-value of money states that the amount of money in your hand at this moment is worth more than the same amount in the future. Therefore, future costs must be adjusted to reflect present value. For example, a $1000 cost 1 year from now requires only $930 in hand today assuming a 7% return on investment.

Sensitivity analysis (SA) is another important tool used to assess the cost-benefit ratio of biologics. Basically, by altering important variables and then recalculating the results, we can test the validity of conclusions.[14] SA becomes increasingly important because assumptions are often made without proper analysis.

For example, SA could be used for questions like:

- Would Agent A still be most cost-effective if the effect of Agent B was greater than measured in a clinical trial?
- Would Agent A still be most cost-effective if the monitoring costs of Agent B were actually lower to a much greater degree?

As an example, although oral steroids are the least costly method in terms of initial dollars for asthma treatment, they may actually be costly in the long run, due to the common health complications they cause for the patient.[16–20] Steroid complications place not only an excessive emotional burden on patients but also a financial one, because they will then be forced to pay for additional hospitalization and also potentially for more drugs for treatment. Therefore, clearly physicians need to look deeper.

THE ADOPTION OF BIOLOGICS

Since biologics were brought into the picture, oral steroid use has decreased by 5%, and clinically significant ulcer complications were reduced by 50%.[20] When questioning whether to adopt biologics, the risk of asthma attacks and exacerbations needs to be looked at. Although biologic treatment has shown to prevent these, it is also important to recognize that not all asthma patients have an equal risk of developing an exacerbation.

This then leads to several questions, including the following:

- Is paying extra for exacerbation protection justified in all patients?
- How much can the risk of asthma exacerbation be altered by using biologics?
- What value is really purchased for the extra cost?

All of these factors must be analyzed for each and every patient to determine the most effective treatment option.

What Are the Real-World Practical Applications of Pharmacoeconomics of Biologics to Shared Decision Making?

One must first collect all the data available, and that includes the true costs of medications, copays, deductibles, and prior authorizations at point of service in order to adequately partake in SDM with patients. Risk reduction for complications seen with oral steroids with biologics is unlikely to offset their increased cost in the management of average-risk patients with asthma with no or little history of exacerbations and without the TH-2 phenotype. Clinical decision making and attempts at risk reduction for other complications seen with biologics are unlikely to offset their increased cost in the management of average-risk patients with asthma-control problems with no history of frequent exacerbations and use of oral steroids.

Decreased monitoring costs of biologics and the attenuated risk of future complications with these agents do result in cost-effective care.[21] Thus, the real issue is who is at risk for steroids' adverse events currently cannot be identified, and there is no consistent method of measurement. The higher acquisition cost may then be justified.

Treating the patient on an outpatient basis creates the best value. Better outcomes are achieved at a lower overall cost: the best possible situation.[21–23] Time and money can only be spent once; choice is inevitable. Whether done unconsciously or with a consistent process, health care professionals are constantly evaluating patient care choices and acting on them.

Pharmacoeconomics and outcomes research can enhance the quality of the practice by strengthening the evaluation process and increasing the probability that better value is delivered in patient care.[22]

Will Establishing General Disease Phenotype Influence the Pharmacoeconomic Choice of a Biologic?

There are many reviews on these topics,[24–27] and in principle, it is generally accepted that therapeutic agents should be used when there is a favorable balance between their benefits and potential risks. Examples from other fields suggest that pharmacogenetic data can help predict both the benefit and the toxicity of particular drugs in individual patients.[23] The general use of disease endotypes for allergies and asthma and correct selection of the responder patient population with defined biomarkers remain essential unmet needs in the clinical settings.[24]

Whether it will be possible to define subtypes of patients with asthma who might benefit from more cost-effective, personalized management plans remains to be determined. In the area of profiling, ideally one would be able to use a limited number of reasonably inexpensive tests to predict responses to various forms of treatment rather than to rely on comprehensive analyses of the subject's response to biologics and other medications (trial of 1), waiting until exacerbation costs skyrocket, or until one can search the entire genome, metabolome, and microbiome. The same point can be made with respect to what type of testing would be needed for effectively monitoring and assessment of treatment responses.[24–27]

What Does a Decision Maker (eg, Patient, Physician, Health Maintenance Organization Pharmacy and Therapeutics Committee, Government Agency) Need to Know in Selecting the Most Cost-Effective Management Approach for a Patient?

Although the potential cost of personalized or precision medicine has been widely discussed, the costs to individual patients and health systems will vary by country, and in countries with private health care options, costs will vary further based on one's type of health insurance.[24–28] No matter who is assessing the cost-effectiveness of an intervention, they should ideally consider all of the costs and benefits of the decision, placing values on such important outcomes as long-term wellness and enhanced QOL, cost of time lost at school or work, and reductions in long-term economic productivity.

Hood[25] has emphasized the importance of involving patients, and in the case of children, their guardians, in making decisions about their health care. This participatory aspect of medicine constitutes the fourth "P" of P4 medicine, where the 4 Ps are predictive, preventive, personalized, and participatory.

It might be possible to devise approaches using biometric and other data, including data about one's genetic profile and personal environment, to identify more accurately if those patients with asthma or other immune diseases will or will not respond favorably to treatment with expensive biologics and to assess the likely effectiveness of diverse interventions. It might also be possible to define constellations of biometric and other individual characteristics that could change the trial-and-failure approach currently often used to move from first- to second- to third-line therapeutic approaches. An approach in which the caregiver, in consultation with the patient (and/or her or his guardians), can more quickly select a treatment, which is in some cases biologic, will likely result in a higher probability of success for that person. Such precision care approaches not only will permit health care resources to be used in a more cost-effective manner, but more importantly, would result in improved satisfaction of patients and their families with their management and treatment, along with producing favorable social and economic effects by improving attendance and performance in school or at work. If we can overcome the significant impediments to establishing such new approaches, then we will be able to offer a much brighter future to those subjects at risk of allergic diseases and to those patients who already have them.[24] This is the basis for the process of initiating patient activation, and possibly improved adherence to biologic therapy.[29–31]

We cannot remain stuck in the past. Even if a study done in 2010 says a biologic is not very cost-effective, the criteria available then do not mean in the near future with improved phenotyping and patient selection, that biologic will not be extremely cost-effective in 2017.[24]

Which of the Potential Biologic Agents Will Be the Most Pharmacoecomonically Realistic and Valuable Choice? In Asthma? What Do We Use?

The past decade has been marked by the introduction and expanding use of biologic therapies for the induction and maintenance of response in patients with asthma and other immune diseases. Traditional cost analyses had shown that biologics and medication costs contributed minimally toward the overall costs associated with the disease; however, these studies were all conducted before the introduction of biologic therapies. At that time, a small minority of patients accounted for a disproportionately large percentage of the overall costs.[17,32,33] This suggested that cost savings could be realized if interventions decreased the utilization of health care resources and associated costs. More recent studies have been heterogeneous in their design and findings. Some have suggested that cost savings realized, due to a decrease in the utilization of health care services, may partially offset the higher costs of biologic agents. Incorporation of data on indirect cost savings and QOL improvements into ongoing and future analyses is required to allow for more accurate analyses of overall costs and cost savings.

Uncontrolled diseases, like asthma, are costlier than controlled diseases, regardless of severity. To appropriately stratify the uncontrolled population, we need not only additional medications but also an improved guide to SDM to make sure the specific biologic is appropriate for the underlying phenotype. Without stratification of uncontrolled asthma for anticipated clinical and economic benefit, the pharmacoeconomics of specific biologics are unclear. Data are conflicting regarding the cost-effectiveness of omalizumab, despite the drug being used on patients for over a decade.[34,35] It has been proposed that omalizumab is a cost-saving option only if given to patients who are predicted to be hospitalized 5 or more times, or 20 days, per year, despite maximal medical management.[35] However, these studies evaluated patients only on severity of disease, not the patients most likely to respond, and thus are fatally flawed.

One commonly used approach in cost-effectiveness analyses is to calculate the incremental cost-effectiveness ratio (ICER), in the form of cost per quality-adjusted life-years (QALY). QALY is an index of survival that is weighted or adjusted by the patient's QOL during the survival period.[36] QALY is particularly useful because it allows for comparisons between interventions and across different conditions. For example, the cost-effectiveness of a therapy for asthma can be compared with one for rheumatoid arthritis.[37,38]

In order to provide estimates of ICER, economic modeling is often necessary. Although general methodological guidelines exist offering helpful modeling principles, evaluating treatments for autoimmune disorders remains challenging.[37,38]

What About Gains in Quality-Adjusted Life-Years with the Use of Biologics?

A recent model suggests that omalizumab may cost as much as $117,000 per QALY, compared with standard therapy with ICS/LABA at a much lower cost of $15,000 per QALY.[39,40] Of course, failure of ICS/LABA therapy administered according to Global Initiative for Asthma guidelines is the criterium used to define the patient who might benefit from biologics used in asthma therapy. There are almost no data at this time on the 2 other biologics mepolizumab and reslizumab, and the price for 1 year of mepolizumab is estimated to be more than $32,500.[41] Although often of minimal importance to the patient, these costs certainly put into question the long-term sustainability of these high costs on the health care system. Omalizumab has recently been reviewed by the National Institute for Health and Care Excellence and is recommended as an option for treating severe persistent allergic asthma as an add-on to optimized standard therapy in patients who need continuous or frequent courses of oral corticosteroids (OCSs).[42]

Points to consider:
- How long must a patient stay on this biologic therapy before they are considered a treatment failure[43]?
- What is the timeframe until we see efficacy and the plateau of that efficacy?

- Before initiating and continuing biologic therapy, SDM needs to take place on these issues, but without studies, this is difficult to quantify.
- Rational use in consideration of the underlying phenotype and with real assessment of costs, risks, and benefits, both long and short term, is the basis for rational decision making on biologic use in asthma rather than experimenting until something appears to work.
- Is there a better way of predicting exacerbations[44]?

The significant progress in asthma therapy with the arrival of omalizumab and use of the new biological drugs has increased the focus on the economic aspects because of the very large price tag related to those treatments. Several more recent economic evaluations suggest that current expensive biologics as compared with pharmacotherapy might be cost-effective for asthma therapy in patients who remain uncontrolled per asthma guidelines. To date, the cost-effectiveness of biologics for comorbid allergic problems has not been investigated.[39–56]

Because of the short amount of time mepolizumab has been on the market, there are limited data on its costs. Early reports estimate a cost per year of treatment from $10,000 to $15,000 per patient.[46] After US Food and Drug Administration approval, the real cost is $32,500 per year per patient and approximately $2700 for a single 4-week injection.[46] To the authors' knowledge, the only real cost-effectiveness analysis was recently conducted and published by the Institute for Clinical and Economic Review Group, which was based on a simulation model of asthma outcomes and costs in a representative population of suitable patients to mepolizumab therapy.[41] The investigators evaluated the incremental cost-effectiveness of mepolizumab, applying drug costs obtained from current prices and estimates of reductions in asthma exacerbations and OCS use from available clinical literature data. In a scenario analysis, it was determined that the price of mepolizumab that would produce cost-effectiveness results at willingness-to-pay thresholds of $50,000 per QALY, $100,000 per QALY, and $150,000 per QALY, respectively. At the moment, based on current purchase prices, the cost-effectiveness estimates are not affordable. To obtain a value correlated with the clinical benefit, a discount of two-thirds to three-quarters from the current acquisition costs of mepolizumab would be necessary. According to the authors of this report, mepolizumab should have a value-based cost between $7800 and $12,000 per year, whereas the full list price per patient in the United States is $32,500 per year. Other doubts arise from the lack of clinical trials evaluating benefits in the long term.

Another group of researchers[47] conducted a study with the aim to evaluate the cost-effectiveness of the newest strategies for the treatment of severe refractory asthma, such as biologic drugs (omalizumab and mepolizumab), as well as bronchial thermoplasty. The investigators used a theoretic model based on the US health care perspective, with a cohort of 10,000 adult patients affected by refractory asthma in an annual cycle and 10-year time horizon. The addition of bronchial thermoplasty to biologic treatment in responder patients was found to not be cost-effective. However, in biologic nonresponders, bronchial thermoplasty remained a cost-effective option as an add-on treatment. Mepolizumab without bronchial thermoplasty was the most cost-effective option for biologic responders, with a 10-year per-patient cost of $116,776 and 5.46 QALYs gained (Institute for Clinical and Economic Review: $21,388). Bronchial thermoplasty is a cost-effective treatment option only in the nonresponders group to biologic treatment ($33,161 per QALY).

A recent draft guidance of the National Institute for Health and Care Excellence does not recommend mepolizumab as an add-on therapy for severe refractory eosinophilic asthma. This is most certainly due to the fact that the costs of mepolizumab compared with usual asthma treatments are above the range usually considered to be a cost-effective use of National Health Service resources.[47]

In the authors' opinion, because it occurred in the past for omalizumab, the increase in the number of eligible patients evaluated in clinical trials may dispel doubts about the real cost-effectiveness ratio of mepolizumab in clinical practice. Cost-effectiveness and pharmacoeconomics of the currently available, extremely expensive biologics approved for use in uncontrolled severe asthma (mepolizumab, reslizumab, and benralizumab) are not well-established figures. Studies in the future should be aimed at defining real-life usefulness of these drugs, and establishing their correct position in treatment guidelines. Pharmacoeconomic studies carried out so far are controversial, but it is likely that they will be necessary to work toward a reduction of purchase costs to extend the availability of these promising therapeutic options.

If Biologics Are Used for Asthma, What Is Their Duration of Benefit?

With respect to clinical benefits, economic evaluations of biologics as compared with pharmacotherapy have indicated that the cost-effectiveness of biologics primarily depends on the duration of the clinical benefit of biologics following treatment cessation.[48] For instance, one study showed that a reduction in the time horizon of the analysis had a negative impact on the cost-effectiveness of the biologic therapy omalizumab.[52] Data on the duration of the clinical benefit of biologics used in economic evaluations were derived from clinical trials, observational studies, expert opinion literature, or authors' assumptions. Although assumptions were informed by clinical trials, the quality of the clinical evidence can be questioned, and uncertainty surrounds the quantitative estimate of the duration of clinical benefit following cessation of biologics.[57–59] Data from the XPORT trial suggest that almost 50% of patients can be successfully withdrawn from omalizamab after 5 years of therapy. Factoring this into the pharmacoeconomic models would make omalizamab appear a much more favorable therapy.[57–59]

What Is the Cost Benefit of Biologics Compared with Pharmacotherapy in Asthma Treatment?

With respect to costs, the cost-effectiveness of biologics as compared with pharmacotherapy depends on the break-even point of cumulative costs between treatment alternatives (ie, the point in time when cumulative costs of biologics equal cumulative costs of pharmacotherapy). Biologics (plus drugs as needed) tend to be more expensive during the first years of treatment, but cumulative costs of pharmacotherapy start to exceed those associated with biologics (if pharmacotherapy is able to be decreased or stopped altogether) at a later stage when biologics has stopped, but its clinical benefit is maintained. Although steps down in therapy after control is maintained is suggested, it is rarely practiced. The break-even point tends to differ between economic evaluations and cannot be transferred given that, for instance, cost estimates reported in economic evaluations are specific to the study setting, and is unlikely to be generalizable.[60]

No economic evaluation has involved a direct comparison of biologics with the combination of biologics with subcutaneous immunotherapy[61–64] except for one study that did not give a conclusive answer because of methodological limitations.[64] Therefore, the question of the cost-effectiveness of biologics versus biologics plus immunotherapy has not been resolved to date. The literature does suggest that any future economic evaluation needs to consider such aspects as safety profile, compliance rate, and administrative costs, which may affect the cost-effectiveness of sublingual versus subcutaneous immunotherapy.[64] Also, where the biologic is given—intravenously or subcutaneously in a medical facility or subcutaneously at home—needs to be considered.

The literature on the cost-effectiveness of biologics consists of studies conducted in Europe and in the United States. The results of these studies should be interpreted with care when assessing their generalizability to another country because the patient population and the specific biologics and administrative costs used are likely to vary between countries, as well as the funding, organization, regulation, and real-life practices governing biologic use in asthma.

Existing economic evaluations have used a variety of outcome measures, such as the peak expiratory flow rate, symptom scores, the number of symptom-free days, the number of patients free from symptoms, and the number of exacerbations. This makes it difficult to compare cost-effectiveness results between studies. Existing economic evaluations of respiratory allergy have shown that improvement in these outcome measures resulting from biologics translate into better QOL.[65] However, there is a need for additional economic evaluations that consider QOL by means of instruments such as the EQ-5D (QOIL scale used in europe Don).[66] This instrument can be used to calculate QALYs and to express the cost-effectiveness of immunotherapy in terms of the additional costs per QALY gained as compared with the alternative. Comparing it with the threshold value set by the health care industry, the payer can then assess the cost-effectiveness of asthma biologics. For instance, the National Institute for Health and Clinical Excellence in England and Wales uses a threshold value of £20,000–£30,000 per QALY[42] that determines which health technologies will be recommended for use by the National Health Service. Economic evaluations of biologics like immunotherapy for asthma should be carried out with real world clinical studies. Thus, cost-effectiveness can be based on randomized controlled trials to provide a degree of internal validity, whereas analyses based on observational studies reflect real-life practice. Alternatively, the use of modeling techniques that critically depend on the study design and the quality of data that are extracted from the literature or other sources are used as input in the cost-effectiveness model.[65]

Some economic evaluations included direct health care costs from the perspective of the third-party payer or the health care system. As a result, these studies focused on the costs of biologics and examined the cost impact of biologics on the use of medicines, physician consultations and hospitalization, ED visits, and exacerbations.[65] The central outcome of exacerbations and use of OCSs most often determines biologic use in asthma. OCS use is the way most physicians determine the number of exacerbations in a patient. This exacerbation history is most often not based on pharmacy data of oral steroid use but on patient history. However, data suggest that relying on patient history could miss as many as 58% of patients who have had 3 or more exacerbations in the past year.[44] Identifying these patients can result in additional interventions that would further reduce their risk for future exacerbations, so a review of pharmacy refill data for OCS bursts, rather than patient history alone, should become a routine component of comprehensive care for asthma patients. Also, although OCS may help control asthma and manage exacerbations, it must be considered that OCS side effects may result in additional health care resource use and costs, highlighting the need for OCS-sparing asthma therapies.[19,20]

A central and extremely important issue is that biologic use is predicated on the number of asthma exacerbations, which for most physicians involves asking the patient how many bursts of OCS they have been on in the past year. The issue is that this is often not a reliable number and may underestimate OCS use.[44] Although OCS are economical from a drug-cost and acquisition perspective, OCS have been associated with dose- and duration-dependent debilitating adverse events, including bone fractures, diabetes mellitus, infections, hypertension, and cataracts. Thus, evidence related to the economic costs attributable to OCS-related side effects has the potential to inform health care insurance company about the tradeoffs of OCS use versus trial of biologic for improved asthma control. Thus, it is high-OCS users with possible OCS-related side effects that are more likely to use health care services than those without such side effects.[65]

EMBRACING QUALITY HEALTH CARE IN THE UNITED STATES

There is pressure on medical providers to embrace payment reform models that give incentives to provide the right care, to the right patient, at the right venue, at the right time, and at the right cost. The United States is at the core of multiple experiments aimed to shift care delivery from a volume-based to a value-based system. On April 16, 2015, President Obama signed into law H.R. 2, the Medicare Access and CHIP Reauthorization Act, a bill that ushers in a new era in physician payment for Medicare. Under either the Merit-based Incentive Payment System (MIPS) or alternative payment models, health care providers will assume some level of financial risk for their clinical decisions. On April 27, Centers for Medicare and Medicaid Services published proposed rules on MIPS implementation and the process and requirements Alternative Payment Models must meet in order to be classified as Advanced Alternative Payment Models. Although fee-for-service is all about volume and reinforces work in silos with little incentive to integrate, the new emphasis for physician reimbursement is on value, with the triple aim of improving quality, enhancing the patient consumer experience, and most importantly, constraining cost growth.

There are huge problems with the current pharmacoeconomic analysis of the costs of biologics in asthma and other immune diseases. Because of fragmented, inefficient, and unorganized delivery of care, extreme variability in treatment practices without apparent benefits, misalignment of incentives, lack of transparency in pricing and costs, and inadequate pharmacoeconomic data to assess value (ie, interaction of quality, cost and patient satisfaction, and experience), biologics and asthma treatment costs are on an unsustainable course. Until some of these issues are addressed and repaired, cost-effective utilization of biologics may remain a mystery.

So What Can Insurance Companies, Society, and Caregivers Do to Move the Study of Pharmacoeconomics of Biologics in the Right Direction? Furthermore, How Can Pharmacoeconomics Enhance the Physicians' and Patients' Outcomes and Reduce Direct Costs, Indirect Costs, and Long-Term Complication Costs?

Improvements in the study of pharmacoeconomics are an aid to decision making with strong potential to:

- Mitigate the influence of marketing
- Help put physicians in the driver's seat
- Enhance the position of allergists from payer's perspective
- Help set practice priorities
- Affect Medicare plans to decrease payout to stem the tide of budget deficits
- Help private payers actively develop quality report cards

POTENTIAL PROBLEMS INTERPRETING PHARMACOECONOMIC DATA

1. The cost of uncontrolled asthma and immune disease is significant and increasing.
2. The cost of an intervention is only partly reflected in drug acquisition costs, and a great deal of the accuracy of pharmacoeconomic evaluations depends on ability to measure change in total disease costs.

3. The pharmacoeconomic equation changes based on the variation in importance of the various costs to user of the data. The individual and family will place more importance on sleep and cough, the employer and perhaps society on productivity, and the ACO on direct costs only without full appreciation for QOL or presenteeism.
4. Drug acquisition data have often been obtained from studies of all comers, completely contrary to personalized medicine, and if personalized therapy is the goal, the pharmacoeconomic data of relevance are the cost-benefits in that population. For example, what are the pharmacoeconomic data for anti–IL-5 biologic therapies in all patients versus patients with blood eosinophil levels of 150, 300, and 400 cells per microliter? The equations will look quite different.
5. Only models that look at responders, with discontinuation of drug in nonresponders, is appropriate. Models looking at 5- or 10-year costs with a drug continued is clinically irrelevant.
6. Models must account for all costs. Hidden direct costs are often overlooked. Indirect costs are difficult to measure and typically ignored but are extremely important to many users of pharmacoeconomic data.
7. Most importantly, pharmcoeconomic data are most appropriately evaluated not using drug versus no drug, but drug versus alternative therapy.
8. That leads to the importance of evaluating all costs of alternative therapy, including the costs of side effects. Because alternative therapy is typically OCSs, it is critical to better understand the costs of side effects of OCSs, both medical and psychiatric.
9. The hidden direct costs and indirect costs, including the ability to put a cost on QOL, are critical for evaluating omalizamab for hives and dupilumab for atopic dermatitis, in which direct costs may not be as great as with respiratory disease.
10. The omilizamab pediatric indication and upcoming dupilumab atopic dermatitis approval make it even more important to understand the costs of disease on parents and caregivers. This is almost invariably overlooked.

SUMMARY

Poorly controlled, therapy-resistant asthma negatively impacts QOL and health care costs. Medication adherence, socioeconomics, and other factors complicate asthma biologic treatments. Cost-effective models of biologic use commonly evaluate the benefit of treatments using QALYs that incorporate both the quantity and the quality of life. Cost-effectiveness information on biologic use can thus assist decision makers in evaluating the overall value of a new treatment or new technology. Long-term savings to the health care system do not always result in short-term patient or payer savings. Pharmacoeconomics and outcomes research can enhance the quality of the practice by strengthening the evaluation process and increasing the probability that better value in patient care is delivered. More of the costs in biologics will be borne by the patients in the future because these patients already have high indirect costs. The international literature suggests that biologics may be cost-effective as compared with pharmacotherapy for certain asthma phenotypes. One economic evaluation has suggested that biologics as compared with pharmacotherapy is unlikely to be cost-effective for asthma. The reader should note that this evidence originated from a limited number of economic evaluations that suffered from several methodological shortcomings. The question of the cost-effectiveness of biologics versus pharmacotherapy has not been resolved to date. No economic evaluation has examined the cost-effectiveness of biologics in asthma taking into account the comorbidities that the biologic also improves. Time and money can only be spent once, so choice is inevitable. Whether done unconsciously or with a consistent process, health care professionals are constantly evaluating care choices and acting on them.

REFERENCES

1. Eisenberg JM. Clinical economics: a guide to the economic analysis of clinical practices. JAMA 1989;262:2879–86.
2. Trueman P, Drummond M, Hutton J. Developing guidance for budget impact analysis. Pharmacoeconomics 2001;19:609–21.
3. Centers for Disease Control and Prevention. Most recent asthma data. In: CDC website. 2016. Available at: http://www.cdc.gov/asthma/most_recent_data.htm. Accessed June 30, 2016.
4. Centers for Disease Control and Prevention. Asthma facts: CDC's National Asthma Control Program Grantees. In: CDC website. 2013. Available at: http://www.cdc.gov/asthma/pdfs/asthma_facts_program_grantees.pdf. Accessed November 18, 2015.
5. Bahadori K, Doyle-Waters MM, Marra C, et al. Economic burden of asthma: a systematic review. BMC Pulm Med 2009;9:24.
6. Reddel HK, Bateman ED, Becker A, et al. A summary of the new GINA strategy: a roadmap to asthma control. Eur Respir J 2015;46:622–39.
7. Healthcare Cost and Utilization Project (HCUP). Chronic Condition Indicator (CCI) for ICD-9-CM. In: HCUP website. 2016. Available at: http://www.hcup-us.ahrq.gov/toolssoftware/chronic/chronic.jsp. Accessed July 8, 2016.
8. Heaney LG, Djukanovic R, Woodcock A, et al. Research in progress: medical research council United Kingdom refractory asthma stratification programme (RASP-UK). Thorax 2016;71(2):187–9.
9. Nair P, Pizzichini MM, Kjarsgaard M, et al. Mepolizumab for prednisone-dependent asthma with sputum eosinophilia. N Engl J Med 2009;360:985–93.
10. Haldar P, Brightling CE, Hargadon BN, et al. Mepolizumab and exacerbations of refractory eosinophilic asthma. N Engl J Med 2009;360:973–84.
11. Ortega HG, Liu MC, Pavord ID, et al. Mepolizumab treatment in patients with severe eosinophilic asthma. N Engl J Med 2014;371:1198–207.
12. Bel EH, Wenzel SE, Thompson PJ, et al. Oral glucocorticoid-sparing effect of mepolizumab in eosinophilic asthma. N Engl J Med 2014;371:1189–97.
13. Cangelosi MJ, Ortendahl JD, Meckley LM, et al. Cost-effectiveness of bronchial thermoplasty in commercially insured patients with poorly controlled, severe, persistent asthma. Expert Rev Pharmacoecon Outcomes Res 2015;15(2):1–8.
14. Einarson TR, Bereza BG, Nielsen TA, et al. Systematic review of models used in economic analyses in moderate-to-severe asthma and COPD. J Med Econ 2016;19(4):319–55.
15. Antonova E, Trzaskoma B, Omachi TA, et al. Poor asthma control is associated with overall daily activity impairment: 3-year data from the EXCELS study of omalizumab. J Allergy Clin Immunol 2016;137(2 Suppl 1):AB14.
16. Morishima T, Ikai H, Imanaka Y. Cost-effectiveness analysis of omalizumab for the treatment of severe asthma in Japan and the value of responder prediction methods based on a multinational trial. Value Health Reg Issues 2013;2:29–36.
17. Barnett SBL, Nurmagambetov TA. Costs of asthma in the United States: 2002–2007. J Allergy Clin Immunol 2011;127(1):145–52.

18. Rowe B, Spooner C, Ducharme F, et al. Corticosteroids for preventing relapse following acute exacerbations in asthma. Cochrane Database Syst Rev 2007;(3):CD000195.

19. Liu D, Ahmet A, Ward L, et al. A practical guide to the monitoring and management of the complications of systemic corticosteroid therapy. Allergy Asthma Clin Immunol 2013;9(1):30.

20. Luskin AT, Antonova E, Broder MS, et al. Healthcare resource use and costs associated with possible side effects of high oral corticosteroid use in asthma: a claims-based analysis. Presented at: Academy of Managed Pharmacy NEXUS 2015. Orlando (FL), October 26–28, 2015.

21. Dominguez-Ortega J, Phillips-Angles E, Barranco P, et al. Cost-effectiveness of asthma therapy: a comprehensive review. J Asthma 2015;52:529–37.

22. Zelger RS, Schatz M, Dalal AA, et al. Utilization and costs of severe uncontrolled asthma in a managed-care setting. J Allergy Clin Immunol Pract 2016;4:120–9.

23. Diaz RA, Charles Z, George E, et al. NICE guidance on omalizumab for severe asthma. Lancet Respir Med 2013;1:189–90.

24. Galli SJ. Toward precision medicine and health: opportunities and challenges in allergic diseases. J Allergy Clin Immunol 2016;137:1289–98.

25. Hood L. Systems biology and P4 medicine: past, present, and future. Rambam Maimonides Med J 2013;4(2):e0012.

26. Ferkol T, Quinton P. Precision medicine: at what price? Am J Respir Crit Care Med 2015;192:658–9.

27. Joyner MJ, Paneth N. Seven questions for personalized medicine. JAMA 2015; 314:999–1000.

28. Akdis CA, Akdis M. Advances in allergen immunotherapy: aiming for complete tolerance to allergens. Sci Transl Med 2015;7:280ps6.

29. Marcum ZA, Sevick MA, Handler SM. Medication nonadherence: a diagnosable and treatable medical condition. JAMA 2013;309(20):2105–6.

30. Goldberg EL, Dekoven M, Schabert VF, et al. Patient medication adherence: the forgotten aspect of biologics. Biotechnol Healthc 2009;6(2):39–42, 44.

31. Bender BG. Overcoming barriers to nonadherence in asthma treatment. J Allergy Clin Immunol 2002;109(6 Suppl):S554–9.

32. Cisternas MA, Blanc PD, Yen IH, et al. A comprehensive study of direct and indirect costs of adult asthma. J Allergy Clin Immunol 2003;111:1212–8.

33. Colice GJ, Wu EQ, Birnbaum H, et al. Healthcare and workloss costs associated with patients with persistent asthma in a privately insured population. Occup Environ Med 2006;48:794–802.

34. Norman G, Faria R, Paton F, et al. Omalizumab for the treatment of severe persistent allergic asthma: a systematic review and economic evaluation. Health Technol Assess 2013;17(52):1–342.

35. Humbert M, Beasley R, Ayres J, et al. Benefits of omalizumab as add-on therapy in patients with severe persistent asthma who are inadequately controlled despite best available therapy (GINA 2002 step 4 treatment): INNOVATE. Allergy 2005; 60(3):309–16.

36. Drummond MF, Jefferson TO. Guidelines for authors and peer reviewers of economic submissions to the BMJ. The BMJ Economic Evaluation Working Party. BMJ 1996;313:275–83.

37. Maetzel A, Tugwell P, Boers M, et al. Economic evaluation of programs or interventions in the management of rheumatoid arthritis: defining a consensus-based reference case. J Rheumatol 2003;30:891–6.

38. Economics Working Group report. a proposal for a reference case for economic evaluation in rheumatoid arthritis. J Rheumatol 2003;30:886–90.

39. Oba Y, Salzman G. Cost-effectiveness analysis of omalizumab in adults and adolescents with moderate-to-severe allergic asthma. J Allergy Clin Immunol 2004; 114:265–9.

40. Zafari Z, Sadatsafavi M, Marra CA, et al. Cost-effectiveness of bronchial thermoplasty, omalizumab, and standard therapy for moderate-to-severe allergic asthma. PLoS One 2016;11(1):e0146003.

41. Tice JA, Ollendorf D, Campbell JD, et al. Mepolizumab (Nucala, GlaxoSmithKline plc.) for the treatment of severe asthma with eosinophilia: effectiveness, value and value-based benchmarks: final report. Boston: Institute for Clinical and Economic Review; 2016.

42. National Institute for Health and Care Excellence (NICE). Omalizumab for treating severe persistent allergic asthma. In: NICE website. 2013. Available at: https://www.nice.org.uk/guidance/ta278. Accessed July 10, 2016.

43. Rodrigo GJ, Neffen H, Castro-Rodriguez JA. Efficacy and safety of subcutaneous omalizumab vs placebo as add-on therapy to corticosteroids for children and adults with asthma: a systemic review. Chest 2011;139:28–35.

44. Bukstein D, Steven G, Luskin A. Pharmacy data more reliable at predicting asthma exacerbations. Presented at: American College of Allergy, Asthma and Immunology (ACAAI) annual meeting. Baltimore (MD), November 7–11, 2015. [abstract: 72].

45. UK Medicines Information. New drugs online report for mepolizumab. In: UK Medicines Information website. Available at: http://www.ukmi.nhs.uk/applications/ndo/record_view_open.asp?newDrugID4675. Accessed March 6, 2016.

46. Institute for Clinical and Economic Review (ICER). ICER draft reports on Nucala® (mepolizumab) for asthma and Tresiba® (insulin degludec) for diabetes posted for public comment edit. In: ICER website. 2015. Available at: http://www.icer-review.org/icer-draft-reports-on-nucala-mepolizumab-for-asthma-and-tresiba-insulin-degludec-for-diabetes-posted-for-public-comment. Accessed March 5, 2016.

47. Bogart M, Roberts A, Wheeler S. Cost-effectiveness of refractory asthma treatment strategies: a decision tree analysis. Value Health 2015;18:A174.

48. Kuprys-Lipinska I, Piotr Kuna P. Loss of asthma control after cessation of omalizumab treatment: real life data. Postepy Dermatol Alergol 2014;31(1):1–5.

49. Molimard M, Mala L, Bourdeix I, et al. Observational study in severe asthmatic patients after discontinuation of omalizumab for good asthma control. Respir Med 2014;108(4):571–6.

50. Nopp A, Johansson SG, Adedoyin J, et al. After 6 years with Xolair: a 3-year withdrawal follow-up. Allergy 2010;65:56–60.

51. Bonifazi F, Jutel M, Bilo BM, et al. EAACI Interest Group on Insect Venom Hypersensitivity. Prevention and treatment of hymenoptera venom allergy: guidelines for clinical practice. Allergy 2005;60:1459–70.

52. Turner SJ, Nazareth T, Raimundo K, et al. Impact of omalizumab on all-cause and asthma-related healthcare resource utilization in patients with moderate or severe persistent asthma. Am J Respir Crit Care Med 2014;189:A6580.

53. Bégin P, Dominguez T, Wilson SP, et al. Phase 1 results of safety and tolerability in a rush oral immunotherapy protocol to multiple foods using Omalizumab. Allergy Asthma Clin Immunol 2014;10(1):7.

54. Schneider LC, Rachid R, LeBovidge J, et al. A pilot study of omalizumab to facilitate rapid oral desensitization in high-risk peanut-allergic patients. J Allergy Clin Immunol 2013;132:1368–74.

55. Pauwels B, Jonstam K, Bachert C. Emerging biologics for the treatment of chronic rhinosinutis. Expert Rev Clin Immunol 2015;11(3):349–61.

56. Umetsu DT. Targeting IgE to facilitate oral immunotherapy for food allergy: a potential new role for anti-IgE therapy? Expert Rev Clin Immunol 2014;10(9):1125–8.

57. Busse WW, Trzaskoma B, Omachi TA, et al. Evaluating omalizumab persistency of response after long-term therapy (XPORT). Presented at the Annual Meeting of the American Thoracic Society (ATS). San Diego (CA), May 16–21, 2014. [abstract: A31].

58. Busse W, Trzaskoma B, Omachi TA, et al. Evaluating omalizumab persistency of response after long-term therapy (XPORT). Presented at the Annual Meeting of the European Respiratory Society (ERS). Munich (Germany), September 6–10, 2014. Eur Respir J 2014;44(Suppl 58):P3485.

59. Antonova J, Trzaskoma B, Raimundo K, et al. Longitudinal change in asthma symptom control in patients who continued vs discontinued omalizumab: results from the XPORT study. Presented at the 71st American College of Allergy, Asthma & Immunology (ACAAI) annual scientific meeting. Atlanta (GA), November 8–11, 2014.

60. Campbell JD, McQueen RB, Briggs A. The "e" in cost-effectiveness analyses: a case study of omalizumab efficacy and effectiveness for cost-effectiveness analysis evidence. Ann Am Thorac Soc 2014;11(Suppl 2):S105–11.

61. Larenas-Linnemann D, Wahn U, Kopp M. Use of omalizumab to improve desensitization safety in allergen immunotherapy. J Allergy Clin Immunol 2014;133(3):937–937.e2.

62. Kamin W, Kopp MV, Erdnuess F, et al. Safety of anti-IgE treatment with omalizumab in children with seasonal allergic rhinitis undergoing specific immunotherapy simultaneously. Pediatr Allergy Immunol 2010;21(1 Pt 2):e160–5.

63. Casale TB, Stokes JR. Future forms of immunotherapy. J Allergy Clin Immunol 2011;127:8–15.

64. Casale TB, Busse WW, Kline JN, et al. Omalizumab pretreatment decreases acute reactions after rush immunotherapy for ragweed-induced seasonal allergic rhinitis. J Allergy Clin Immunol 2006;117:134–40.

65. Sullivan PW, Campbell JD, Ghushchyan VH, et al. Characterizing the severe asthma population in the United States: claims-based analysis of three treatment cohorts in the year prior to treatment escalation. J Allergy Clin Immunol 2014;133(Suppl 2):AB41.

66. Pickard AS, Wilke C, Jung E, et al. Use of a preference-based measure of health (EQ-5D) in COPD and asthma. Respir Med 2008;102(4):519–36.

Future Prospects of Biologic Therapies for Immunologic Diseases

Santhosh Kumar, MD[a],*,[1], Brant R. Ward, MD, PhD[a,b,c,1],
Anne-Marie Irani, MD[a]

KEYWORDS

- Asthma • Atopic dermatitis • Biologic • Churg-Strauss syndrome
- Hemophagocytic lymphohistiocytosis • Immune dysregulation • Immunodeficiency
- Mastocytosis

KEY POINTS

- Currently used or in-development biologic therapies have unexplored potential in treating various allergic and immunologic disorders.
- There is a substantial need for newer biologic therapies targeting specific disease pathways.
- Biologic therapies represent not only an innovative approach but also a substantial advance to disease management in the twenty-first century.

INTRODUCTION

Although biologic therapies like insulin have been used for nearly a century, improvements in recombinant technology and production techniques have led to an explosion of biologic therapies over the past 2 decades. Biologic therapies are currently used for

Funding Sources: Investigator-Initiated Studies Program, McNeil Consumer Healthcare (Dr S. Kumar); Merck Investigator Studies Program, Merck Sharpe & Dohme Corp (Dr B.R. Ward); Novartis research grants (Dr A.-M. Irani).
Conflict of Interest: Advisory Board Consultant for Horizon Pharma (Dr B.R. Ward); Speaker's Bureau: Merck, Advisory Board: Grifols, Merck; Royalties: spouse receives royalties from Thermofisher (Dr A.-M. Irani).
[a] Division of Allergy and Immunology, Children's Hospital of Richmond, Virginia Commonwealth University, CHoR Pavilion, 5th Floor, 1000 East Broad Street, Richmond, VA 23298-0225, USA; [b] Division of Rheumatology, Allergy, and Immunology, Virginia Commonwealth University, McGuire Hall, Room 4-115A, 1112 East Clay Street, Richmond, VA 23298-0263, USA; [c] Department of Microbiology and Immunology, Virginia Commonwealth University, 1101 East Marshall Street, P.O. Box 980678, Richmond, VA 23298, USA
[1] These authors contributed equally to this work.
* Corresponding author.
E-mail address: santhosh.kumar@vcuhealth.org

treating many disease conditions in humans as either an adjunct to conventional therapy or a sole therapeutic intervention. Several of these biologic agents are available on the market in the United States and are approved by the US Food and Drug Administration (FDA) for specific indications.

Outside of approved indications, the use of certain biologics to treat immunologic disease is supported by case series or small studies. In other instances, potential therapeutic benefit may merely be inferred from animal studies or knowledge of the mechanisms of action. The goal of this review is to explore future potential therapeutic use for currently available biologic therapies, based solely on the mechanism of action of the specific agent considered. The pathophysiologic targets and disease states described herein do not represent an exhaustive list. Rather, they represent a selection of potential therapies that may prove useful for the treatment of specific conditions in the near future.

THERAPIES TARGETING CYTOKINES OR CYTOKINE RECEPTORS

Cytokines are soluble low-molecular-weight proteins that mediate communication between immune cells. As such, they are critically linked to the pathophysiology of immunologic disease.[1] Although there is some degree of overlap in the function of certain cytokines, in general, these proteins function in a predefined circuit. That is, release of given cytokine from a specific cell source will trigger a specific effector function by the receiving cell (**Table 1**). This makes cytokines an attractive target for therapeutic intervention, for neutralization of a particular cytokine may, in theory, abate a specific disease process without causing wholesale immunosuppression.[1,2]

Tocilizumab: Anti-Interleukin-6 Receptor Antibody

Interleukin-6 (IL-6) and the IL-6 receptor (IL-6R) were discovered by Tadamitsu Kishimoto in Japan in the 1980s. IL-6 binds to and forms a complex with IL-6R and another cell membrane protein, gp130. Formation of this complex results in the activation of the Jak/STAT pathway through gp130. Two forms of the IL-6R subunit can be found—membrane bound (mIL-6R) and soluble (sIL-6R).[3-5] Membrane anchoring of the IL-6R subunit is not required for signaling, and indeed signaling can occur when IL-6 forms a complex with sIL-6R and gp130. Signaling through soluble receptor is termed trans-signaling and may result in different functional outcomes.[3,5] Understanding of the role of these molecules in various inflammatory pathways has led to numerous clinical trials with therapeutic agents that interfere with their mechanism of action.

Tocilizumab (Actemra) is a recombinant humanized anti-human IL-6R monoclonal antibody of the immunoglobulin G1 (IgG1) subclass. It is currently approved by the FDA for use in moderate to severe rheumatoid arthritis, systemic juvenile idiopathic arthritis, and polyarticular juvenile idiopathic arthritis.

Allergic asthma

IL-6 appears to play a role in allergic asthma. Patients with allergic asthma have high serum levels of sIL-6R at baseline, which is increased approximately 24 hours after an allergen challenge compared with controls.[6] Allergen-induced airway inflammation, specifically with house dust mite and cockroach, has been shown to induce mixed granulocytic inflammation in the airway of mice.[7,8] One may postulate that blockage of IL-6R would result in controlling mixed granulocytic inflammation in allergic asthma, potentially leading to clinical benefit. In a mouse model of allergen-induced asthma, cockroach-induced airway inflammation was shown to be attenuated by intranasal

Table 1
Selected cytokine targets for therapeutic intervention

Cytokine	Principal Sources	Acts on	Function	Therapeutic Agents[a]
IL-6	APCs MCs Th2 cells Multiple somatic cells	Activated T cells B cells MCs Multiple somatic cells	Promotes T cell & neutrophil recruitment Induces Th2 & Th17 differentiation Promotes B-cell survival & differentiation into plasma cells ↑ Histamine & FcεRI expression by MCs Triggers acute phase response	Tocilizumab
IL-12	APCs Neutrophils	Activated T cells NK cells	Induces Th1 differentiation ↑ Cytotoxicity of CD8+ T cells & NK cells	Ustekinumab
IL-18	APCs MCs Multiple somatic cells	Multiple immune cells Multiple somatic cells	Promotes T-cell activation ↑ T-cell cytokine production ↑ Cytotoxicity of CD8+ T cells & NK cells Promotes somatic cell cytokine, chemokine, and adhesion molecule production	*GSK1070806* *Tadekinig alfa*
IL-23	APCs Neutrophils	Activated T cells Memory T cells	↑ IL-17 production by Th17 cells Promotes survival of memory T cells	Ustekinumab
IFNγ	NK cells Th1 cell	Multiple immune cells Multiple somatic cells	↑ MHC class I & II expression ↑ IL-12 production by APCs Triggers antiviral responses in many cells Primes macrophages for activation Induces cell cycle arrest & apoptosis in many cells	*NI-0501*
TNF-α	Multiple immune cells Multiple somatic cells	Multiple immune cells Multiple somatic cells	↑ MHC class I & II expression Promotes activation of multiple immune cells ↑ Vascular permeability ↑ Cytokine, chemokine, and adhesion molecule expression by somatic cells Triggers acute phase response	Adalimumab Certolizumab pegol Etanercept Golimumab Infliximab

a Medications in italic are not yet FDA approved, but currently undergoing clinic trials.

treatment with anti-IL-6R antibody. This effect was also demonstrated in a small sample size human study.[9]

However, the heterogeneity of asthmatic patients presents a special challenge to this strategy. It is important to undestand the concept of asthma endotypes[10]—if a specific group of asthma patients can be identified with high IL-6R levels in the sputum (ie, a "high IL-6" endotype), then it is reasonable to suspect that anti-IL-6R antibody would be a viable therapeutic option. However, endotypes may need to be refined even further given the differential responses noted with anti-IL-6R antibodies. For example, in murine models, activation of sIL-6R induces IL-17A production by γδ T cells and downstream airway neutrophilia. This effect is not seen with classical (membrane-bound) IL-6R stimulation, which activates conventional αβ T cells, leading to downstream airway eosinophilia.[11] The observation in murine studies that roach-induced airway inflammation was attenuated by anti-IL-6R antibody, while house dust mite allergen challenge induced an eosinophilic response in mice treated with anti-IL-6R antibody, has led to speculation regarding differential IL-6R activation (ie, soluble vs membrane bound) by different allergens.

There is already some evidence in murine systems that an anti-IL-6R antibody like tocilizumab is effective in specific models of allergic asthma. Further investigation may uncover a role for this biologic agent in a specific endotype of human asthma.

Atopic dermatitis

The pathogenesis of atopic dermatitis (AD) includes a mixed inflammatory infiltrate, with identification of both T helper 1 (Th1) and Th2 lymphocytes in normal and involved skin, respectively. CD4+ T cells have been shown to release IL-6 when activated, contributing to a proinflammatory state. Other cells like B lymphocytes, fibroblasts, and monocytes also secrete IL-6 and might play a role in the pathogenesis of AD.

Tocilizumab use would be expected to dampen the inflammatory state in AD and may be effective in the treatment of severe, refractory forms of the disease. Navarini and colleagues[12] reported improvement in the Eczema Area and Severity Index in a small number of subjects with AD after treatment with tocilizumab. However, they noted an increased incidence of bacterial skin infections. Further understanding of the heterogeneity of susceptibility to bacterial infections in subjects with AD may improve the prospects for the use of anti-IL-6 therapeutic regimens in these patients.

STAT3 gain-of-function mutations

Next-generation sequencing technologies have fostered an incredible expansion in the understanding of the genetic basis of immunodeficiency and immune dysregulatory disorders. One consequence has been the discovery of activating mutations in the transcription factor STAT3 causing a syndrome very similar to autoimmune lymphoproliferative syndrome (ALPS).[13,14] These patients typically have notable autoimmune cytopenias and lymphoproliferation, with a tendency toward solid organ autoimmunity and recurrent or severe infections. Unlike patients with ALPS, who typically respond to standard immunosuppression with sirolimus, those with gain-of-function mutations in STAT3 may require substantial immunosuppression. In fact, many have failed multiple different immunosuppressive regimens.[15]

Mechanistic studies suggested that the mutations in these patients resulted in decreased dephosphorylation of STAT3, prolonging the activity of the transcription factor after stimulation through cytokine receptors. IL-6 is a major activator of STAT3 in immune cells, and therefore, it was theorized that blockade of IL-6 signaling could help to normalize the cumulative STAT3 activity in these patients.[13] Trials of tocilizumab in several patients have been very encouraging—in all cases, an improvement in their clinical status, especially with regards to solid organ autoimmunity, was observed.[13,15] STAT3 gain-of-function mutations are relatively rare, although as additional patients are identified, tocilizumab may prove to be a cornerstone of treatment.

Ustekinumab: Anti-Interleukin-12/23 p40 Antibody

Ustekinumab (Stelara) is a fully humanized monoclonal IgG1 antibody against the p40 subunit shared by IL-12 and -23. IL-12 is essential to the development of Th1 cells due to its ability to stimulate interferon gamma (IFNγ), and also increases the cytotoxic activity of CD8+ T cells and natural killer (NK) cells. On the other hand, IL-23 is involved in the development and proliferation of Th17 cells.[16,17] Currently, this biologic agent is approved by the FDA for the treatment of plaque psoriasis or psoriatic arthritis in subjects ≥18 years old.

Asthma

A form of chronic asthma that is not responsive to conventional therapy can be conceptualized as a Th17-dominant disease, wherein neutrophils and eosinophils are recruited to the airways via IL-17-dependent pathways. In this subpopulation of neutrophil-predominant asthma, ustekinumab may be useful to control airway inflammation by limiting the proliferation of Th17 cells. Indeed, Amarnani and colleagues[18] have described a patient with both psoriasis and asthma who was treated with ustekinumab. The patient's asthma improved to the extent that he was able to discontinue controller medication while on ustekinumab. Further studies are needed to replicate these results, but ustekinumab is an attractive therapy for the often difficult-to-treat neutrophilic asthma.

Atopic dermatitis

As previously discussed, ustekinumab inhibits Th1 and Th17 inflammatory pathways, and this results in a decrease in IFNγ and tumor necrosis factor-alpha (TNF-α) production. Although AD is typically considered to be a Th2-mediated disease, elevated levels of IL-17 have been demonstrated in the skin during acute eczema flares.[19] Ustekinumab has been shown to be effective in decreasing symptoms of AD based on SCORAD and visual analogue scores in a few case reports.[20,21] Clearly more data are required on the roles of Th1 and Th17 cells in AD, but ustekinumab may find a role as an adjuvant therapy in the disease.

Inflammatory gastrointestinal disorders

Th1 cells are essential to the pathology of multiple inflammatory gastrointestinal diseases. Almost 2 decades ago, researchers discovered increased IL-12 and a predominance of IFNγ-producing T-helper cells in the affected tissue of patients with Crohn disease.[22–24] Research that is more recent has suggested an additional role for Th17 cells in the development of lesions in Crohn disease. With this in mind, several trials were conducted to evaluate the efficacy of ustekinumab in Crohn disease, and the results were positive, particularly in patients who had failed prior therapy with anti-TNF-α therapies.[25] These data have reportedly been submitted to the FDA in hopes of obtaining an indication in the treatment of Crohn disease.

Furthermore, a common theme in immune-mediated disorders of the gastrointestinal tract is the involvement of Th1 and/or Th17 cells. For example, enteropathy in patients with common variable immunodeficiency (CVID) is associated with increased production of IL-12, but not IL-17, by T lymphocytes.[26,27] In contrast, patients with immune dysregulation, polyendocrinopathy, enteropathy X-linked syndrome (IPEX), which is characterized by severe enteropathy, have increased numbers of Th17 cells and a relative reduction in Th1 cytokines.[17] The fact that the IL-12/23 p40 subunit is shared in both pathways makes this an appealing target in these syndromes. To this end, a small study exploring the usefulness of ustekinumab in CVID enteropathy is currently underway.

GSK1070806: Anti-Interleukin-18 Antibody/Tadekinig Alfa: Recombinant Interleukin-18 Binding Protein

GSK1070806 is a humanized monoclonal antibody of the IgG1 isotype that binds to and neutralizes IL-18.[28] It is currently being evaluated as an adjunctive therapy for preventing solid organ graft rejection. Tadekinig alfa is a recombinant form of human IL-18 binding protein and is undergoing evaluation for use in adult-onset Still disease.

IL-18 is a member of the IL-1 family and, like IL-1, is produced as a protein precursor that must be processed by caspases after activation of the inflammasome complex. The full functions of IL-18 are still being elucidated, but it is known to play a role in inflammation and increases the production of other cytokines, such as IFN and IL-17, by immune cells.[29]

Cryopyrin-associated periodic syndromes

The cryopyrin-associated periodic syndromes (CAPS) comprise a spectrum of disorders, including familial cold autoinflammatory syndrome, Muckle-Wells syndrome, and neonatal-onset multisystem inflammatory disease. All are characterized by recurrent fevers and tissue inflammation in the absence of an infectious or autoimmune source. CAPS is caused by activating mutations in NLRP3, also known as cryopyrin, which is a component of the inflammasome complex. Autoactivation of the inflammasome leads to unregulated production of cytokines like IL-1 and IL-18.[30]

The mainstay of therapy for CAPS is blockade of IL-1, and several medications are currently approved for this. In many cases, treatment is very effective.[30,31] However, in certain cases, typically those presenting at a very young age or with very severe features, continual upward titration of the dose is required. One theorized cause for this phenomenon is the effect of excess IL-18, which is not neutralized with current treatments. Data from animal models of CAPS suggest that IL-1 and IL-18 contribute differently to the overall inflammatory phenotype and may be responsible for different stages of the disease process.[31] It is tempting to speculate that when used together with IL-1 blockade, IL-18 antagonists could improve disease control and long-term outcomes in patients with difficult-to-control CAPS.

Hemophagocytic lymphohistiocytosis

Hemophagocytic lymphohistiocytosis (HLH) is a life-threatening disorder characterized by overwhelming inflammation and cytokine release and can be viewed as the most severe incarnation of the cytokine storm.[32] The causes of HLH are diverse and include both inheritable and environmental factors—thus, the syndromes can be classified as familial or reactive. Treatment has centered on removal of the inciting stimulus (in the case of reactive HLH) and potent immunosuppression to control the runaway inflammation.[33,34]

One of the first functions ascribed to IL-18 was its ability to augment dramatically the production of IFNγ by Th1 cells after stimulation with IL-12.[35] Knowing the importance of IFNγ in the pathology of HLH (see later discussion), it is hence easy to expect a role for IL-18 in the disease. Indeed, IL-18 is highly elevated in persons with HLH, and levels correlate better with symptoms in humans than do IL-12 or TNF-α.[36] Furthermore, in murine models of HLH, animals treated with IL-18 binding protein showed significant improvement in multiple disease parameters.[37] Consequently, IL-18 blockade may represent another avenue of therapy for this potentially lethal disease.

NI-0501: Anti-Interferon γ Antibody

IFNγ is the quintessential Th1 cytokine but also has diverse roles in the immune response. It is a type II IFN produced by NK cells, cytotoxic T cells, and Th1 cells. IFNγ functions to prime macrophages, increase major histocompatibility complex (MHC) class I expression on somatic cells, increase MHC class II on antigen-presenting cells (APCs), boost the activity of NK cells and cytotoxic T cells, and promote the differentiation of Th1 cells.[38] NI-0501 is a fully human monoclonal antibody that neutralizes IFNγ. It was granted orphan drug status by the FDA and European Medicines Agency in 2010.

Hemophagocytic lymphohistiocytosis

Animal models of the disease revealed a unique role for IFNγ in the initiation and maintenance of the inflammatory cascade in HLH. In fact, blockade of IFNγ, but not several other cytokines, leads to complete resolution of the syndrome in animal models.[39] Accordingly, IFNγ has been an interesting target to treat the disorder in humans. Early results from phase 1 and 2 studies of NI-0501 in patients with familial HLH have been promising, combining improvements in clinical status with fewer side effects than the typical regimens.[40,41] Because of this, the FDA has designated NI-0501 a Breakthrough Therapy, which may help to shorten the time to the drug's final approval. Based on its mechanism of action, it is reasonable to suspect that the medication will be similarly effective in reactive HLH. If the efficacy is confirmed with additional subjects, NI-0501 could soon become a primary therapy for all forms of HLH.

Adalimumab/Certolizumab/Golimumab/Infliximab: Anti-Tumor Necrosis Factor-α Antibody

TNF-α is generated by multiple cell types early in the inflammatory process, and as such, is part of a first line of defense against tissue injury and foreign antigens.[42] TNF-α has also been shown to cause dysregulation of the immune response in asthmatics. Adalimumab (Humira) is a humanized monoclonal antibody that blocks the binding of TNF-α to its receptors. Its use in rheumatologic conditions and inflammatory bowel disease is well established. Other biologics with similar mechanisms include certolizumab pegol (Cimzia), golimumab (Simponi; Simponi Aria), and infliximab (Remicade).

Asthma

After allergen challenge, lung mast cells (MCs) and macrophages release TNF-α.[43] Further evidence for the role of TNF-α in asthma includes the observations that TNF-α is elevated in the airway of asthmatics,[44] and, when administered to normal mice via inhalation, causes airway hyperresponsiveness (AHR). Hence, blockage of TNF-α by adalimumab has been shown in clinical studies to reduce asthma exacerbations and AHR and to improve asthma quality of life, albeit inconsistently. One reason for the variability in response may be due to polymorphisms in the TNF-α receptor (eg, TNF-308G/A[45]). These and other factors need to be considered when designing future studies to test TNF-α blockade in asthmatics. Regardless, adalimumab may prove to have a role in a subpopulation of asthmatics with refractory symptoms.

THERAPIES TARGETING CELLULAR ACTIVATION OR FUNCTION

Many immunologic diseases arise from a failure to properly regulate potent immune effector functions. As the knowledge of this immune dysregulation has grown, treatment strategies have shifted from nonspecific immunosuppression toward restoring the correct balance between effector and regulatory elements. Current approaches include elimination of the APCs that generate effector cells, inhibiting the activation of effectors, and enhancing the function of natural regulatory cells (**Fig. 1**).

Abatacept and Belatacept: CTLA-4-hIgG1-Fc Fusion Proteins

Costimulation is necessary for optimal T-cell responses, and this is usually provided via the binding of CD28 on T cells to CD80 or CD86 on APCs. Absence or inhibition of costimulation during T-cell activation can lead to anergy or self-tolerance. CTLA-4 is preferentially expressed on activated T cells and regulatory T cells (Tregs) and binds to CD80 and CD86 with much higher affinity than CD28, competing for the costimulatory molecules on the APCs.[46] In addition, CTLA-4 contains an inhibitory signaling motif, in contrast to the activating motif on CD28.[47,48]

Abatacept (Orencia) and belatacept (Nulojix) are fusion proteins containing the extracellular domain of CTLA-4 with the Fc portion of human IgG1. The molecules are designed such that the Fc portion of the molecule is unable to fix complement or mediate antibody-dependent cellular cytotoxicity. These drugs are FDA approved for the treatment of rheumatoid arthritis and juvenile idiopathic arthritis (abatacept) and for the prevention of allograft rejection (belatacept).

Allergen-specific immunotherapy adjuvant

Allergen-specific immunotherapy (SIT) is a very effective therapy aimed at inducing tolerance to an allergen over a period of time. The mechanisms by which this therapy works are only partially understood, but seem to involve the preferential development of allergen-specific Tregs.[49] CTLA-4 signaling has been shown to increase the proliferation and suppressive activity of Tregs as well as to induce anergy in effector T cells.

In an experimental murine model, administration of a CTLA-4-Fc fusion protein concomitantly with allergen-specific SIT was shown to result in an increased number of Tregs, inhibition of activated T cells, and improved induction of tolerance to that allergen. Other effects included decreased airway hyperreactivity and airway eosinophilia in treated mice.[50] One clinical benefit of CTLA-4-Fc fusion proteins as an

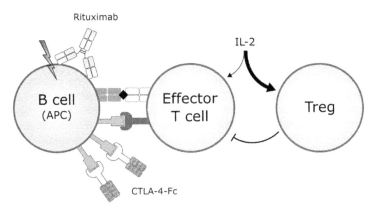

Fig. 1. Mechanisms for inhibiting cellular effector function. The regulation of cellular effectors may be manipulated at several points during the immune response. The use of rituximab may prevent T activation by the elimination of self-reactive B cells that can present self-antigens in germinal centers. CTLA-4-Fc fusion proteins bind to the costimulatory molecules CD80 and CD86, present on APCs. The therapeutic affect is likely due to competitive inhibition of T-cell co-stimulation through CD28. Low-dose IL-2 preferentially stimulates Tregs, which in turn are able to control the activation and proliferation of effector T cells.

adjuvant for SIT would be the ability to use lower doses of the allergen, with the potential for a decrease in systemic hypersensitivity reactions, while maintaining an excellent and possibly improved tolerogenic effect.

Immunodeficiencies with autoimmune features

CVID is a heterologous disease. Although all patients by definition have immune deficiency, some exhibit additional features of autoimmune disease and lymphoproliferation. Next-generation sequencing is slowly identifying individual genetic mutations that make up the group of diseases labeled as CVID. Within the past couple of years, investigators have identified mutations in *CTLA4* and *LRBA* that result in immunodeficiency with striking autoimmune elements.[51–53]

Studies of these patients have revealed decreased CTLA-4 expression on T cells in both disorders. Moreover, in both disorders, the numbers and suppressive function of Tregs are significantly reduced. Based on the pathophysiology, it was theorized that treatment with CTLA-4-Fc fusion protein would help offset the lack of T-cell inhibition. In vitro studies confirmed a beneficial effect of the medication, and its use in a small number of patients was extremely promising.[52,54,55]

Rituximab: Anti-CD20 Antibody

Rituximab (Rituxan) is a chimeric monoclonal anti-CD20 antibody that targets B cells for elimination via antibody-dependent cellular cytotoxicity, complement-dependent toxicity, and apoptosis.[56] CD20 is expressed on pre-B cells and mature B cells but not plasma cells. Hence, rituximab therapy preserves the function of pre-existing plasma cells.[57] This biologic drug is currently approved by the FDA for use in B-cell non-Hodgkin lymphoma, chronic lymphocytic leukemia, rheumatoid arthritis, granulomatosis with polyangiitis, and microscopic polyangiitis.

Atopic dermatitis

There is clear evidence for the role of both B and T cells in the pathogenesis of atopic eczema.[58,59] B-cell involvement is reflected in higher total and allergen-specific IgE in AD patients than controls.[60] Suppression of B cells with rituximab leads to a decrease in T-cell stimulation, total and specific IgE levels, and chemo-attraction of other immune cells. These effects are likely due to a reduction in antigen presentation and other immunomodulatory functions by B cells rather than antibody reduction.[61] Rituximab has been shown to be effective in the treatment of severe AD resistant to conventional therapy in a few case reports and case series.[62] However, immune suppression following the use of rituximab can be prolonged and severe. Thus, as with any other therapeutic modality, the use of this drug should follow a careful analysis of the risk/benefit ratio and should be reserved for the most severe cases, either refractory to treatment or steroid dependent.

Anticytokine autoantibody syndromes

Clinicians are increasingly identifying persons with features that mimic inherited immunodeficiencies but develop relatively late in life. In many cases, these patients lack genetic mutations in recognized pathways, but rather they acquire autoantibodies that interfere with specific inflammatory pathways.[63] For example, persons with neutralizing autoantibodies to IL-12 or IFNγ develop susceptibility to invasive mycobacterial infections, whereas those with autoantibodies to IL-17 may develop recurrent fungal infections and those with autoantibodies to granulocyte-monocyte colony stimulating factor develop pulmonary alveolar proteinosis. In fact, the International Union of Immunological Societies created a new category that includes these disorders in their most recent classification scheme—phenocopies of primary immunodeficiencies.[64]

Despite the fact that rituximab spares plasma cells, it carries an FDA indication for the treatment of rheumatoid arthritis and is an effective therapy for multiple autoimmune conditions characterized by autoantibody production. As mentioned above, this may reflect the pathogenic roles of self-reactive B cells other than antibody production, including interactions with self-reactive T cells, for example, Rituximab's effect in these disorders makes it a logical choice for the treatment of anticytokine autoantibody syndromes. Several groups have reported successes in a small number of patients which has prompted a more rigorous phase 1 trial, currently being conducted by the National Institutes of Health.[65-67]

Aldesleukin: Recombinant Interleukin-2 Protein

Aldesleukin (Proleukin) is a recombinant form of human IL-2. This cytokine signals through a receptor complex consisting of a high-affinity α chain (also called CD25), a β chain, and a common γ chain that is shared with the receptor complexes for IL-4, IL-7, IL-9, IL-15, and IL-21.[68] CD25 is expressed at a modest level on activated T cells and is highly expressed on Tregs. Signaling through this receptor complex promotes cellular survival and activation. Aldesleukin is currently approved by the FDA for the treatment of metastatic renal cell carcinoma and metastatic melanoma.

Immunodeficiencies with autoimmune features

Studies examining the causes of inherited syndromes of immune dysregulation have revealed the importance of Tregs in controlling autoimmunity. Disorders such as autoimmune polyendocrinopathy-candidiasis-ectodermal dystrophy syndrome, CTLA-4 deficiency, IPEX, and LRBA deficiency are all associated with reduced numbers and function of Tregs.[51-53,69,70] In addition, in studies of subjects with CVID for whom a genetic cause was not known, a similar trend was evident,[71-73] although it should be noted that these studies were performed before several genetic causes (ie, LRBA and CTLA-4) had been identified.

Initial trials with recombinant IL-2 focused on activating effector T cells to help fight cancer.[74] Although efficacy was demonstrated, this treatment also famously leads to severe side effects such as capillary leak syndrome. A renewed interest in recombinant IL-2 was generated after it was postulated that Tregs, with their high level of CD25 expression, might be preferentially activated by low doses of IL-2. Small case series and a large volume of mechanistic studies have demonstrated positive responses in treating autoimmunity.[75] Further trials in immunodeficiencies and immune dysregulatory disorders are certainly needed, but recombinant IL-2 may represent an ideal treatment wherein autoimmunity can be controlled without nonspecific immunosuppression—a boon for individuals who are already immunocompromised.

THERAPIES TARGETING IMMUNOGLOBULIN E

Many allergic and immunologic conditions are IgE mediated. Soluble IgE is found in peripheral blood and in the interstitial space, whereas membrane-bound IgE (mIgE) is present on IgE-expressing B lymphoblasts and memory B cells as part of the B-cell antigen receptor complex. IgE also binds to the high-affinity IgE receptor (FcεRI) present on the surface of basophils and MCs. Cross-linking of IgE-bound FcεRI by an antigen causes stimulation and degranulation of these cells. The pharmacologic mediators released are responsible for many allergic and immunologic symptoms. Targeting the IgE pathway can therefore lead to alteration of disease related pathomechanisms.

Quilizumab: Anti-CemX Antibody/Omalizumab: Anti-Immunoglobulin E Antibody

Anti-CemX is a newer biologic undergoing clinical trials for the treatment of IgE-mediated disease. CemX is a 52-amino-acid residue located between the CH4 domain and the C-terminal membrane anchor peptide of the ε chain of mIgE on human B cells. Binding of anti-CemX antibody to this unique domain has been shown to cause apoptosis of IgE class-switched B cells due to a lack of costimulatory signaling. However, it may secondarily cause antibody-dependent cellular cytotoxicity with destruction of the IgE-bearing B cell which ultimately prevents the generation of IgE-secreting plasma cells, resulting in decreased production of IgE.[76,77] As the CemX protein is highly conserved, a high degree of specificity and safety is seen with this drug. This treatment does not target free IgE in the serum, and hence, its effectiveness does not depend on the concentration of IgE in the blood. Quilizumab has been proposed for use in patients with very high serum IgE levels who do not qualify other therapies.

Omalizumab (Xolair) is a humanized monoclonal IgG1 antibody to IgE, which binds to free serum IgE. Binding by this monoclonal antibody occludes the FcεRI binding site, therefore preventing the IgE from binding to receptors on MCs and basophils. In turn, this leads to downregulation of cell-surface FcER1 on these cells.[78] Omalizumab is currently approved by the FDA for treatment of allergic asthma and chronic spontaneous urticaria.

Allergic bronchopulmonary aspergillosis

Allergic bronchopulmonary aspergillosis (ABPA) is a syndrome characterized by an exaggerated Th2 response to fungi of the genus *Aspergillus* (most commonly *Aspergillus fumigatus*) in the lower airways. This Th2 immune response to the fungi can, in turn, lead to an acute or subacute worsening of asthma control. In addition to worsening severity of asthma symptoms, patients display elevated total and aspergillus-specific serum IgE levels as well as positive skin prick tests to aspergillus allergens.[79] The elevated total serum IgE level is thought to play a role in the pathogenesis of this condition.

Various treatment options have been tried, including antifungal therapy, systemic corticosteroids, and others. In recalcitrant cases, treatment with Omalizumab resulted in a reduced number of asthma exacerbations, decreased fractional exhaled nitric oxide levels, and decreased night awakenings.[80] Immunologic studies in omalizumab-treated patients demonstrated a decrease in basophil sensitivity, defined as the amount of allergen required to induce 50% maximal basophil reactivity as measured by CD63 expression on basophils. One can postulate that Omalizumab therapy in patients with ABPA would potentially prevent disease progression and might eventually result in a decreased incidence of progression to bronchiectasis.[81]

Churg-Strauss syndrome

Churg-Strauss syndrome, also known as eosinophilic granulomatosis with polyangiitis (EGPA), is a small-vessel vasculitis associated with blood and tissue eosinophilia.[82] Up to 30% to 40% of patients are positive for serum antineutrophil cytoplasmic antibodies. The pathogenesis of this disorder is still unknown, but marked elevations of IgE and IgG4 are reported in this condition.[83,84] If one postulates that the increased IgE levels play a role in the pathogenesis of this disease, or at least the secondary atopic symptoms associated with it, it would be reasonable to assume that treatment with IgE-targeted therapy may result in clinical benefit in affected patients.

Unfortunately, several cases were reported of Churg-Strauss syndrome developing in asthmatic patients treated with omalizumab.[85,86] A causative relationship between the disorder and drug has largely been disproven, and the association is thought to be due to an unmasking effect after reduction of the steroid dose while on omalizumab therapy.

EGPA remains a therapeutic challenge for most patients, because conventional therapy is not always effective. Omalizumab is a safe biologic therapy that has shown promise in inducing partial or full-treatment response and can also be used as a corticosteroid-sparing agent in EGPA with atopic symptoms such as asthma or sinusitis.[87]

Chronic rhinosinusitis with nasal polyps

Chronic rhinosinusitis with nasal polyps (CRS w/NP) is a complex inflammatory condition. Treatment with conventional therapy such as topical corticosteroids has proven to be frustratingly ineffective, with a lack of improvement in most patients. Nasal polyps show significant eosinophilic infiltration on histologic examination, and Th2-type inflammation with evidence for local IgE production and increased IgE levels has been observed within the polyp tissue.[88] The increase in local IgE production is possibly due to stimulation by superantigens such as staphylococcal enterotoxins and is likely to be polyclonal. Furthermore, because the IgE is produced locally within the polyp tissue, it may not always be evident in the serum.[89] In patients with CRS w/NP and concomitant asthma, there appears to be further increases in local IgE production. This IgE has been demonstrated to play a role in perpetuating the chronic inflammation in these tissues.[90] Thus, inhibiting IgE-induced chronic inflammation is a potential therapeutic target in this condition.

In double-blind placebo-controlled trials conducted in patients with CRS w/NP and comorbid asthma, omalizumab has been shown to improve total polyp score as well as quality of life as measured by the Asthma Quality of Life Questionnaire and Short Form-36 Health Survey validated questionnaires.[91] This beneficial effect did not differ between patients with and without allergic rhinitis. As a consequence, IgE-targeted therapies are attractive as add-on therapy for patients with CRS w/NP and comorbid asthma, not controlled with conventional therapy.

Mastocytosis

Mastocytosis is a disorder characterized by an increased MC burden within the tissues. This increase in MC number can be associated with an increase in the total amount of FcεRI and/or a decrease in the activation threshold of the MCs. One of the more serious symptoms of MC disorders is recurrent anaphylaxis, either idiopathic or due to hypersensitivity to allergens such as foods or insect venoms.[92] No large-scale studies have examined the use of IgE-targeted therapy in mastocytosis, but several case reports have highlighted a reduction in the number of further anaphylactic episodes, the severity of the reactions, baseline serum tryptase levels, and total serum IgE levels.[93,94] Omalizumab has been successfully used as an adjunct therapy in patients with mastocytosis undergoing immunotherapy for venom hypersensitivity reactions; this strategy has been especially beneficial in patients undergoing rush protocols.

Although the exact mechanism of action of omalizumab in the treatment of mastocytosis is not definitively known, it is thought that by preventing free IgE from binding to FcεRI, treatment leads to a reduction in the surface FcεRI expression MCs, leading to an increase in the activation threshold. However, the effect of omalizumab for the treatment of chronic idiopathic urticaria, another disorder of spontaneous MC activation, does not appear to depend on the serum IgE level. Accordingly, omalizumab may affect MC activation through other mechanisms, and it is unclear if other IgE-target therapies will have similar affects in these patients. Further studies are needed.

SUMMARY

The promise of precision or personalized medicine has been evident for nearly a decade.[95] Although the promise has yet to be wholly fulfilled, the field of medicine has made fantastic strides toward this goal. Biologics, due to their inherent specificity, have led the charge in many disciplines and will likely continue to do so in the future. The medicines described above represent a sample of therapies "just in front of us"— ones that physicians may see in their practices in the near future. As the understanding of the pathophysiology of immunologic and allergic diseases expands, and additional therapeutic targets are identified (eg, IL-33 in Th2-predominant disorders), undoubtedly progressively more biologics approved for broader indications will be seen in the decades to come.

REFERENCES

1. Feldmann M. Many cytokines are very useful therapeutic targets in disease. J Clin Invest 2008;118(11):3533–6.
2. Scheinecker C, Redlich K, Smolen JS. Cytokines as therapeutic targets: advances and limitations. Immunity 2008;28(4):440–4.
3. Ataie-Kachoie P, Pourgholami MH, Richardson DR, et al. Gene of the month: interleukin 6 (IL-6). J Clin Pathol 2014;67(11):932–7.
4. Conti P, Kempuraj D, Di Gioacchino M, et al. Interleukin-6 and mast cells. Allergy Asthma Proc 2002;23(5):331–5.
5. Scheller J, Chalaris A, Schmidt-Arras D, et al. The pro- and anti-inflammatory properties of the cytokine interleukin-6. Biochim Biophys Acta 2011;1813(5): 878–88.
6. Doganci A, Eigenbrod T, Krug N, et al. The IL-6R alpha chain controls lung CD4+CD25+ Treg development and function during allergic airway inflammation in vivo. J Clin Invest 2005;115(2):313–25.
7. Page K, Lierl KM, Hughes VS, et al. TLR2-mediated activation of neutrophils in response to German cockroach frass. J Immunol 2008;180(9):6317–24.
8. Phipps S, Lam CE, Kaiko GE, et al. Toll/IL-1 signaling is critical for house dust mite-specific helper T cell type 2 and type 17 [corrected] responses. Am J Respir Crit Care Med 2009;179(10):883–93.
9. Ullah MA, Revez JA, Loh Z, et al. Allergen-induced IL-6 trans-signaling activates γδ T cells to promote type 2 and type 17 airway inflammation. J Allergy Clin Immunol 2015;136(4):1065–73.
10. Muraro A, Lemanske RF Jr, Hellings PW, et al. Precision medicine in patients with allergic diseases: airway diseases and atopic dermatitis—PRACTALL document of the European Academy of Allergy and Clinical Immunology and the American Academy of Allergy, Asthma & Immunology. J Allergy Clin Immunol 2016;137(5): 1347–58.
11. Nish SA, Schenten D, Wunderlich FT, et al. T cell-intrinsic role of IL-6 signaling in primary and memory responses. Elife 2014;3:e01949.
12. Navarini AA, French LE, Hofbauer GF. Interrupting IL-6-receptor signaling improves atopic dermatitis but associates with bacterial superinfection. J Allergy Clin Immunol 2011;128(5):1128–30.
13. Milner JD, Vogel TP, Forbes L, et al. Early-onset lymphoproliferation and autoimmunity caused by germline STAT3 gain-of-function mutations. Blood 2015;125(4): 591–9.

14. Wienke J, Janssen W, Scholman R, et al. A novel human STAT3 mutation presents with autoimmunity involving Th17 hyperactivation. Oncotarget 2015;6(24): 20037–42.

15. Castro-Wagner JB, Kumar AR, Jolley C, et al. Treatment with IL-6 blockade in patients with gain of function STAT3 mutations. In: Final Program of the Clinical Immunology Society 2016 Annual Meeting: Immune Deficiency & Dysregulation North American Conference. Boston (MA), 2016. p. 17.

16. Cingoz O. Ustekinumab. MAbs 2009;1(3):216–21.

17. Marwaha AK, Leung NJ, McMurchy AN, et al. TH17 cells in autoimmunity and immunodeficiency: protective or pathogenic? Front Immunol 2012;3:129.

18. Amarnani A, Rosenthal KS, Mercado JM, et al. Concurrent treatment of chronic psoriasis and asthma with ustekinumab. J Dermatolog Treat 2014;25(1):63–6.

19. Toda M, Leung DY, Molet S, et al. Polarized in vivo expression of IL-11 and IL-17 between acute and chronic skin lesions. J Allergy Clin Immunol 2003;111(4): 875–81.

20. Agusti-Mejias A, Messeguer F, Garcia R, et al. Severe refractory atopic dermatitis in an adolescent patient successfully treated with ustekinumab. Ann Dermatol 2013;25(3):368–70.

21. Fernandez-Anton Martinez MC, Alfageme Roldan F, Ciudad Blanco C, et al. Ustekinumab in the treatment of severe atopic dermatitis: a preliminary report of our experience with 4 patients. Actas Dermosifiliogr 2014;105(3):312–3.

22. Matsuoka K, Inoue N, Sato T, et al. T-bet upregulation and subsequent interleukin 12 stimulation are essential for induction of Th1 mediated immunopathology in Crohn's disease. Gut 2004;53(9):1303–8.

23. Parronchi P, Romagnani P, Annunziato F, et al. Type 1 T-helper cell predominance and interleukin-12 expression in the gut of patients with Crohn's disease. Am J Pathol 1997;150(3):823–32.

24. Peluso I, Pallone F, Monteleone G. Interleukin-12 and Th1 immune response in Crohn's disease: pathogenetic relevance and therapeutic implication. World J Gastroenterol 2006;12(35):5606–10.

25. Simon EG, Ghosh S, Iacucci M, et al. Ustekinumab for the treatment of Crohn's disease: can it find its niche? Therap Adv Gastroenterol 2016;9(1):26–36.

26. Mannon PJ, Fuss IJ, Dill S, et al. Excess IL-12 but not IL-23 accompanies the inflammatory bowel disease associated with common variable immunodeficiency. Gastroenterology 2006;131(3):748–56.

27. Uzzan M, Ko HM, Mehandru S, et al. Gastrointestinal disorders associated with common variable immune deficiency (CVID) and chronic granulomatous disease (CGD). Curr Gastroenterol Rep 2016;18(4):17.

28. McKie EA, Reid JL, Mistry PC, et al. A study to investigate the efficacy and safety of an anti-interleukin-18 monoclonal antibody in the treatment of type 2 diabetes mellitus. PLoS One 2016;11(3):e0150018.

29. Gracie JA, Robertson SE, McInnes IB. Interleukin-18. J Leukoc Biol 2003;73(2): 213–24.

30. Sarrabay G, Grandemange S, Touitou I. Diagnosis of cryopyrin-associated periodic syndrome: challenges, recommendations and emerging concepts. Expert Rev Clin Immunol 2015;11(7):827–35.

31. Brydges SD, Broderick L, McGeough MD, et al. Divergence of IL-1, IL-18, and cell death in NLRP3 inflammasomopathies. J Clin Invest 2013;123(11):4695–705.

32. Brisse E, Matthys P, Wouters CH. Understanding the spectrum of haemophagocytic lymphohistiocytosis: update on diagnostic challenges and therapeutic options. Br J Haematol 2016;174(2):175–87.

33. Jordan MB, Allen CE, Weitzman S, et al. How I treat hemophagocytic lymphohistiocytosis. Blood 2011;118(15):4041–52.
34. Schram AM, Berliner N. How I treat hemophagocytic lymphohistiocytosis in the adult patient. Blood 2015;125(19):2908–14.
35. Bohn E, Sing A, Zumbihl R, et al. IL-18 (IFN-gamma-inducing factor) regulates early cytokine production in, and promotes resolution of, bacterial infection in mice. J Immunol 1998;160(1):299–307.
36. Takada H, Ohga S, Mizuno Y, et al. Oversecretion of IL-18 in haemophagocytic lymphohistiocytosis: a novel marker of disease activity. Br J Haematol 1999; 106(1):182–9.
37. Chiossone L, Audonnet S, Chetaille B, et al. Protection from inflammatory organ damage in a murine model of hemophagocytic lymphohistiocytosis using treatment with IL-18 binding protein. Front Immunol 2012;3:239.
38. Schroder K, Hertzog PJ, Ravasi T, et al. Interferon-gamma: an overview of signals, mechanisms and functions. J Leukoc Biol 2004;75(2):163–89.
39. Jordan MB, Hildeman D, Kappler J, et al. An animal model of hemophagocytic lymphohistiocytosis (HLH): CD8+ T cells and interferon gamma are essential for the disorder. Blood 2004;104(3):735–43.
40. Jordan MB, Locatelli F, Allen C, et al. A novel targeted approach to the treatment of hemophagocytic lymphohistiocytosis (HLH) with an anti-interferon gamma monoclonal antibody (mAb), NI-0501: first results from a pilot phase 2 study in children with primary HLH. In: Final Program of American Society of Hematology 57th Annual Meeting and Exposition. Orlando (FL), 2015.
41. Jordan MB. A novel targeted approach to the treatment of hemophagocytic lymphohistiocytosis (HLH) with NI-0501, an anti-interferon gamma monoclonal antibody. In: Final Program of the Clinical Immunology Society 2016 Annual Meeting: Immune Deficiency & Dysregulation North American Conference. Boston (MA), 2016. p. 17.
42. Bradley JR. TNF-mediated inflammatory disease. J Pathol 2008;214(2):149–60.
43. Catal F, Mete E, Tayman C, et al. A human monoclonal anti-TNF alpha antibody (adalimumab) reduces airway inflammation and ameliorates lung histology in a murine model of acute asthma. Allergol Immunopathol (Madr) 2015;43(1):14–8.
44. Kim J, Remick DG. Tumor necrosis factor inhibitors for the treatment of asthma. Curr Allergy Asthma Rep 2007;7(2):151–6.
45. Aoki T, Hirota T, Tamari M, et al. An association between asthma and TNF-308G/A polymorphism: meta-analysis. J Hum Genet 2006;51(8):677–85.
46. Buchbinder E, Hodi FS. Cytotoxic T lymphocyte antigen-4 and immune checkpoint blockade. J Clin Invest 2015;125(9):3377–83.
47. Alegre ML, Frauwirth KA, Thompson CB. T-cell regulation by CD28 and CTLA-4. Nat Rev Immunol 2001;1(3):220–8.
48. Sakaguchi S. Naturally arising Foxp3-expressing CD25+CD4+ regulatory T cells in immunological tolerance to self and non-self. Nat Immunol 2005;6(4):345–52.
49. Akdis CA, Akdis M. Mechanisms of allergen-specific immunotherapy. J Allergy Clin Immunol 2011;127(1):18–27 [quiz: 28–9].
50. Maazi H, Shirinbak S, den Boef LE, et al. Cytotoxic T lymphocyte antigen 4-immunoglobulin G is a potent adjuvant for experimental allergen immunotherapy. Clin Exp Immunol 2013;172(1):113–20.
51. Kuehn HS, Ouyang W, Lo B, et al. Immune dysregulation in human subjects with heterozygous germline mutations in CTLA4. Science 2014;345(6204):1623–7.

52. Lo B, Zhang K, Lu W, et al. AUTOIMMUNE DISEASE. Patients with LRBA deficiency show CTLA4 loss and immune dysregulation responsive to abatacept therapy. Science 2015;349(6246):436–40.

53. Schubert D, Bode C, Kenefeck R, et al. Autosomal dominant immune dysregulation syndrome in humans with CTLA4 mutations. Nat Med 2014;20(12):1410–6.

54. Lee S, Moon JS, Lee CR, et al. Abatacept alleviates severe autoimmune symptoms in a patient carrying a de novo variant in CTLA-4. J Allergy Clin Immunol 2016;137(1):327–30.

55. Shields CL, Say EA, Mashayekhi A, et al. Assessment of CTLA-4 deficiency-related autoimmune choroidopathy response to abatacept. JAMA Ophthalmol 2016;134(7):844–6.

56. Jazirehi AR, Bonavida B. Cellular and molecular signal transduction pathways modulated by rituximab (rituxan, anti-CD20 mAb) in non-Hodgkin's lymphoma: implications in chemosensitization and therapeutic intervention. Oncogene 2005;24(13):2121–43.

57. Levesque MC, St Clair EW. B cell-directed therapies for autoimmune disease and correlates of disease response and relapse. J Allergy Clin Immunol 2008;121(1): 13–21 [quiz: 22–3].

58. Lugovic L, Lipozenocic J, Jakic-Razumovic J. Atopic dermatitis: immunophenotyping of inflammatory cells in skin lesions. Int J Dermatol 2001;40(8):489–94.

59. Simon D, Vassina E, Yousefi S, et al. Inflammatory cell numbers and cytokine expression in atopic dermatitis after topical pimecrolimus treatment. Allergy 2005;60(7):944–51.

60. Bruynzeel-Koomen C, van Wichen DF, Toonstra J, et al. The presence of IgE molecules on epidermal Langerhans cells in patients with atopic dermatitis. Arch Dermatol Res 1986;278(3):199–205.

61. Silverman GJ, Weisman S. Rituximab therapy and autoimmune disorders: prospects for anti-B cell therapy. Arthritis Rheum 2003;48(6):1484–92.

62. Simon D, Hosli S, Kostylina G, et al. Anti-CD20 (rituximab) treatment improves atopic eczema. J Allergy Clin Immunol 2008;121(1):122–8.

63. Browne SK. Anticytokine autoantibody-associated immunodeficiency. Annu Rev Immunol 2014;32:635–57.

64. Picard C, Al-Herz W, Bousfiha A, et al. Primary immunodeficiency diseases: an update on the classification from the International Union of Immunological Societies Expert Committee for Primary Immunodeficiency 2015. J Clin Immunol 2015;35(8):696–726.

65. Borie R, Debray MP, Laine C, et al. Rituximab therapy in autoimmune pulmonary alveolar proteinosis. Eur Respir J 2009;33(6):1503–6.

66. Browne SK, Zaman R, Sampaio EP, et al. Anti-CD20 (rituximab) therapy for anti-IFN-gamma autoantibody-associated nontuberculous mycobacterial infection. Blood 2012;119(17):3933–9.

67. Czaja CA, Merkel PA, Chan ED, et al. Rituximab as successful adjunct treatment in a patient with disseminated nontuberculous mycobacterial infection due to acquired anti-interferon-gamma autoantibody. Clin Infect Dis 2014;58(6):e115–8.

68. Waickman AT, Park JY, Park JH. The common gamma-chain cytokine receptor: tricks-and-treats for T cells. Cell Mol Life Sci 2016;73(2):253–69.

69. Bacchetta R, Passerini L, Gambineri E, et al. Defective regulatory and effector T cell functions in patients with FOXP3 mutations. J Clin Invest 2006;116(6): 1713–22.

70. Ryan KR, Lawson CA, Lorenzi AR, et al. CD4+CD25+ T-regulatory cells are decreased in patients with autoimmune polyendocrinopathy candidiasis ectodermal dystrophy. J Allergy Clin Immunol 2005;116(5):1158–9.
71. Arandi N, Mirshafiey A, Abolhassani H, et al. Frequency and expression of inhibitory markers of CD4(+) CD25(+) FOXP3(+) regulatory T cells in patients with common variable immunodeficiency. Scand J Immunol 2013;77(5):405–12.
72. Arumugakani G, Wood PM, Carter CR. Frequency of Treg cells is reduced in CVID patients with autoimmunity and splenomegaly and is associated with expanded CD21lo B lymphocytes. J Clin Immunol 2010;30(2):292–300.
73. Genre J, Errante PR, Kokron CM, et al. Reduced frequency of CD4(+) CD25(HIGH)FOXP3(+) cells and diminished FOXP3 expression in patients with common variable immunodeficiency: a link to autoimmunity? Clin Immunol 2009;132(2):215–21.
74. Rosenberg SA. IL-2: the first effective immunotherapy for human cancer. J Immunol 2014;192(12):5451–8.
75. Klatzmann D, Abbas AK. The promise of low-dose interleukin-2 therapy for autoimmune and inflammatory diseases. Nat Rev Immunol 2015;15(5):283–94.
76. Brightbill HD, Jeet S, Lin Z, et al. Antibodies specific for a segment of human membrane IgE deplete IgE-producing B cells in humanized mice. J Clin Invest 2010;120(6):2218–29.
77. Chen JB, Wu PC, Hung AF, et al. Unique epitopes on C epsilon mX in IgE-B cell receptors are potentially applicable for targeting IgE-committed B cells. J Immunol 2010;184(4):1748–56.
78. Chanez P, Contin-Bordes C, Garcia G, et al. Omalizumab-induced decrease of FcxiRI expression in patients with severe allergic asthma. Respir Med 2010; 104(11):1608–17.
79. Greenberger PA. Diagnosis and management of allergic bronchopulmonary aspergillosis. Allergy Proc 1994;15(6):335–9.
80. Voskamp AL, Gillman A, Symons K, et al. Clinical efficacy and immunologic effects of omalizumab in allergic bronchopulmonary aspergillosis. J Allergy Clin Immunol Pract 2015;3(2):192–9.
81. Perez-de-Llano LA, Vennera MC, Parra A, et al. Effects of omalizumab in Aspergillus-associated airway disease. Thorax 2011;66(6):539–40.
82. Jennette JC, Falk RJ, Bacon PA, et al. 2012 revised International Chapel Hill Consensus Conference Nomenclature of Vasculitides. Arthritis Rheum 2013; 65(1):1–11.
83. Vaglio A, Moosig F, Zwerina J. Churg-Strauss syndrome: update on pathophysiology and treatment. Curr Opin Rheumatol 2012;24(1):24–30.
84. Vaglio A, Strehl JD, Manger B, et al. IgG4 immune response in Churg-Strauss syndrome. Ann Rheum Dis 2012;71(3):390–3.
85. Bargagli E, Madioni C, Olivieri C, et al. Churg-Strauss vasculitis in a patient treated with omalizumab. J Asthma 2008;45(2):115–6.
86. Puechal X, Rivereau P, Vinchon F. Churg-Strauss syndrome associated with omalizumab. Eur J Intern Med 2008;19(5):364–6.
87. Jachiet M, Samson M, Cottin V, et al. Anti-IgE monoclonal antibody (omalizumab) in refractory and relapsing eosinophilic granulomatosis with polyangiitis (Churg-Strauss): data from 17 patients. Arthritis Rheumatol 2016;68(9):2274–82.
88. Bachert C, Gevaert P, Holtappels G, et al. Total and specific IgE in nasal polyps is related to local eosinophilic inflammation. J Allergy Clin Immunol 2001;107(4): 607–14.

89. Zhang N, Gevaert P, van Zele T, et al. An update on the impact of Staphylococcus aureus enterotoxins in chronic sinusitis with nasal polyposis. Rhinology 2005; 43(3):162–8.

90. Zhang N, Holtappels G, Gevaert P, et al. Mucosal tissue polyclonal IgE is functional in response to allergen and SEB. Allergy 2011;66(1):141–8.

91. Gevaert P, Calus L, Van Zele T, et al. Omalizumab is effective in allergic and nonallergic patients with nasal polyps and asthma. J Allergy Clin Immunol 2013;131(1):110–6.e1.

92. Rueff F, Dugas-Breit S, Przybilla B. Stinging hymenoptera and mastocytosis. Curr Opin Allergy Clin Immunol 2009;9(4):338–42.

93. Douglass JA, Carroll K, Voskamp A, et al. Omalizumab is effective in treating systemic mastocytosis in a nonatopic patient. Allergy 2010;65(7):926–7.

94. Paraskevopoulos G, Sifnaios E, Christodoulopoulos K, et al. Successful treatment of mastocytic anaphylactic episodes with reduction of skin mast cells after anti-IgE therapy. Eur Ann Allergy Clin Immunol 2013;45(2):52–5.

95. Woodcock J. The prospects for "personalized medicine" in drug development and drug therapy. Clin Pharmacol Ther 2007;81(2):164–9.

Moving?

Make sure your subscription moves with you!

To notify us of your new address, find your **Clinics Account Number** (located on your mailing label above your name), and contact customer service at:

Email: journalscustomerservice-usa@elsevier.com

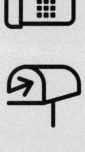

800-654-2452 (subscribers in the U.S. & Canada)
314-447-8871 (subscribers outside of the U.S. & Canada)

Fax number: 314-447-8029

Elsevier Health Sciences Division
Subscription Customer Service
3251 Riverport Lane
Maryland Heights, MO 63043

*To ensure uninterrupted delivery of your subscription, please notify us at least 4 weeks in advance of move.

Printed and bound by CPI Group (UK) Ltd, Croydon, CR0 4YY

03/10/2024

01040392-0007